Medical Assessment Units

The Initial Management of Acute Medical Patients

Edited by

IAN WOOD MA, RN, DipN (Lond)

Lecturer, Department of Nursing & Midwifery
Keele University, Keele

MICHELLE RHODES BSc(Hons), RN, DipN (Lond)

Senior Lecturer, Department of Nursing Studies
St Martin's College, Carlisle

D1117593

W

WHURR PUBLISHERS

LONDON AND PHILADELPHIA

© 2003 Whurr Publishers
First published 2003 by
Whurr Publishers Ltd
19b Compton Terrace, London N1 2UN, England and
325 Chestnut Street, Philadelphia PA 19106, USA

Reprinted 2003

British Library Cataloguing in Publication Data
A catalogue record for this book is available from the British
Library.

ISBN: 1 86156 325 6

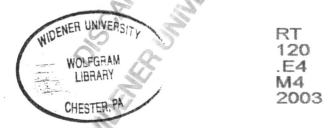
Typeset by HWA Text and Data Management, Tunbridge Wells
Printed and bound in the UK by Athenaeum Press Limited
Gateshead, Tyne & Wear

Contents

Contributors

Brendan Davies *Consultant Neurologist, Department of Neurology, North Staffordshire Hospital NHS Trust*

Michelle Davies *Senior Staff Nurse, MAU, North Staffordshire Hospital NHS Trust*

Carole Donaldson *Night Nurse Practitioner, Medical Division, North Staffordshire Hospital NHS Trust*

Michael Gibbs *Lecturer in Nursing, Department of Nursing & Midwifery, Keele University*

Ruth Harris *Consultant Physician & Gastroenterologist, Countess of Chester NHS Trust*

Susan Hope *Respiratory Nurse Specialist, Department of Respiratory Medicine, North Staffordshire Hospital NHS Trust*

Jane Jervis *Staff Nurse, MAU, North Staffordshire Hospital NHS Trust*

Linda Miller *Lecturer in Nursing, Department of Nursing & Midwifery, Keele University*

Jacqueline Mitchell *Associate Lecturer, Department of Nursing & Midwifery, Keele University and Sister, Intensive Care Unit, Mid Cheshire NHS Trust*

Judith Morgan *Consultant Nurse, A&E Department, Oldchurch Hospital*

Sue Read *Lecturer, Department of Nursing & Midwifery, Keele University*

Michelle Rhodes *Senior Lecturer, Department of Nursing Studies, St Martin's College*

Lorraine Taylor *Staff Nurse, MAU, North Staffordshire Hospital NHS Trust*

Judi Thorley *Team Manager, Combined Healthcare NHS Trust, Stoke on Trent*

Terry Wardle *Consultant Physician, Countess of Chester NHS Trust*

Elizabeth Whelan *Assistant Director of Nursing, Emergency Department, Mater Misercordiae Hospital, Dublin*

Helen Whitehouse *Respiratory Research Nurse, Department of Respiratory Medicine, University Hospital Birmingham*

Ian Wood *Lecturer, Department of Nursing & Midwifery, Keele University*

Acknowledgements

The editors would like to thank the following people for their valuable contributions to the writing of this book.

- The contributors for their hard work in writing and revising their respective chapters

- Stephen Boyce, ICU, Mid Cheshire NHS Trust, for his work on acute respiratory failure

- Janice Bailey, Kathleen Bentley, Sue Pass and Barbara Rickard from the MAU, North Staffordshire Hospital NHS Trust for their contributions to the chapter on initial assessment of acute medical patients (Chapter 2)

- Alison Clarke, Jane Jervis, Michelle Davies, Marsha Holding and Sue Lapper for their ideas and comments when the book was originally conceived

- Debbie Danitsch and Sara Morris for their constructive comments

- Helena Priest and Bernard Beech for their review of the mental health section in Chapter 3

- Sam, Stephanie & Alexander (IW) and Andy (MR) for their support and patience

Normal clinical values

1. Haematology

Haemoglobin	
Male	14.0–17.7 g/dl
Female	12.0–16.0 g/dl
White cell count	$4–11 \times 10^9$/litre
Basophils	$<0.01–0.1 \times 10^9$/litre
Eosinophils	$0.04–0.4 \times 10^9$/litre
Lymphocytes	$1.5–4.0 \times 10^9$/litre
Monocytes	$0.2–0.8 \times 10^9$/litre
Neutrophils	$2.0–7.5 \times 10^9$/litre
Platelet count	$150–400 \times 10^9$/litre
Mean corpuscular haemoglobin (MCH)	27–35 pg
MCH concentration (MCHC)	32–35 g/dl
Mean corpuscular volume (MCV)	80–96 fl
Packed cell volume (PCV)	
Male	0.42–0.53 l/l
Female	0.36–0.45 l/l
Erythrocyte sedimentation rate (ESR)	<20 mm in 1 hour

Coagulation studies

Activated partial thromboplastin time (aPTT)	25–35 s Usually recorded in relation to the laboratory control or reference level
Partial thromboplastin time (PTTK)	24–31 s
Prothrombin time	12–16 s

| International normalised ratio (INR) | 1 |
| Activated clotting time (ACT) | 70–120 s |

2.   Biochemistry

Amylase	<220 U/l
Bicarbonate	22–30 mmol/l
Bilirubin	<17 μmol/l (0.3–1.5 mg/dl)
Calcium	2.2–2.67 mmol/l (8.5–10.5 mg/dl)
Chloride	95–106 mmol/l
Cholesterol	3.5–6.5 mmol/l (ideal <5.2 mmol/l)
Creatinine	0.06–0.12 mmol/l (0.6–1.5 mg/dl)
Creatine kinase (CK)	
Male	24–195 U/l
Female	24–170 U/l
CK-MB fraction	0–5% of total CK
Glucose (fasting)	4.5–6.0 mmol/l (70–110 mg/dl)
Magnesium	0.7–1.1 mmol/l
Phosphate	0.8–1.5 mmol/l
Potassium	3.5–5.0 mmol/l
Sodium	135–146 mmol/l
Urea	2.5–6.7 mmol/l (8–25 mg/dl)

Arterial blood gases (ABGs)

pO_2	10.0–13.3 kPa (75–100 mmHg)
pCO_2	4.8–6.1 kPa (36–46 mmHg)
pH	7.35–7.45
Bicarbonate	24–28 mmol/l
Hydrogen ions (H^+)	35–45 nmol/l
SaO_2	95–98%

Preface

Increasing demands on acute hospital resources, together with a reduction in the number of beds available, have placed greater emphasis on the need for rapid and effective assessment of patients in order to determine their need for hospital admission. These circumstances have led to the widespread emergence of specialist Medical Assessment Units (MAUs) in acute hospitals.

This book provides an up-to-date guide to the initial assessment and management of patients with acute medical conditions. It presents a structured approach based on common presenting features and focuses on the first 24 hours of the patient's hospital stay. The book also provides the reader with sources for further reading in relation to continuing management of the patient.

The requirement for clinically effective practice has increased the need for specific educational preparation for nurses working within these clinical areas. Despite the proliferation of MAUs in the last decade, there is currently little educational provision for MAU nurses and there is a lack of literature relating to the specialism. In 1996, Keele University became the first institution in the United Kingdom to offer an English National Board (ENB) validated course for MAU nurses. Teaching this course has provided the authors with a valuable insight into the educational needs of nurses working in MAUs.

In editing this book, the authors have been able to draw on their own clinical experiences as a charge nurse in Accident & Emergency nursing and a sister in Cardiology nursing, respectively.

Ian Wood
Michelle Rhodes

Introduction

Medical Assessment Units: The Initial Management of Acute Medical Patients aims to meet the need for a nursing text which specifically relates to the assessment and management of patients who present to Medical Assessment Units (MAUs) with acute medical problems. Whilst the book has been written especially for this emerging specialism, the content can be applied equally to any clinical area accommodating medical patients.

Written predominantly *by* nurses *for* nurses, the book has been designed as a quick reference text for use in clinical practice. To act as a source of further reading, the book is extensively referenced throughout, thus increasing its appeal to nurses at all stages of their careers and to those who are undertaking further study.

Each chapter offers clear, concise and down-to-earth information based on a common presenting symptom and provides practical advice, supported by research evidence. The reader is led, step by step, through the initial assessment and management of the patient. Text boxes identify the most common conditions associated with each presenting symptom. A detailed explanation of the causes, pathophysiology, presenting features, investigations and nursing management is given for each condition. The book does not provide information relating to the continuing management of the patient, nor to the less common conditions associated with each presenting symptom. However, sources of further reading are identified.

The book contains a chapter discussing contemporary issues relating to the organisation and delivery of care within MAUs. Other chapters are concerned with principles of initial assessment, management of cardiac arrest, sudden death and vulnerable groups of adults. The latter two chapters are deliberately placed early in the book in recognition of their importance in the provision and organisation of care in MAUs. Normal clinical values are detailed within the prelims.

Specific aims and a reference list are contained within each chapter. Text boxes are used to highlight key points from the text and the book is cross-referenced throughout.

CHAPTER 1

Service organisation in medical assessment units

IAN WOOD

Aims

This chapter will:

- outline the historical development of Medical Assessment Units (MAUs) in the United Kingdom (UK)
- provide a definition of an MAU
- discuss referral patterns, modes of operation and management issues
- discuss resource requirements for the effective assessment and management of MAU patients and their relatives
- discuss nursing roles and skills in delivering optimum care to patients

Historical development

The last 20 years have seen a consistent rise in the number of acute medical admissions to hospitals in the UK. Annual increases of 3% in the 1980s rose to 4% in the early 1990s and climbed even higher in the late 1990s. These increases in medical admissions have had a significant impact on acute hospital services and have led to much debate as to the most appropriate measures for managing demands on the service.

One such measure that has been introduced in many acute hospitals is the establishment of an MAU. The first recorded example of an MAU was at Ninewells Hospital in Dundee where an Acute Admissions Unit was opened when the hospital was built in the mid-1970s. More recently, MAUs have been developed in hospitals across the UK in response to what have been described as 'winter pressures'. Indeed, the Department of Health (DoH) advocated 'the creation of medical assessment and admissions units in all hospitals that do not have them' for relieving the pressure on Accident & Emergency (A&E) department trolley waits (DoH 2000). This has been achieved to some extent by transferring, from the A&E to the MAU, the focus for the acceptance of medical patients referred by their general practitioner (GP).

Whilst many commentators have identified the need to manage more effectively the admissions process for acutely ill medical patients, there has been a distinct lack of consistency in how MAUs have been established and developed. Indeed, at a time when national standards are being set for patient care, no national blueprint exists for the development of MAUs. For this reason, there is wide variation in how MAUs are organised and in their nomenclature (for example: 'Admissions Unit', 'Emergency Medical Unit', 'Assessment Ward' and 'Clinical Decision Unit'). This lack of consistency leads to problems in gathering valid and reliable evidence regarding the effectiveness of these units as it is difficult to compare like with like.

In 1998, the Royal College of Physicians of Edinburgh (RCPE) and the Royal College of Physicians and Surgeons of Glasgow (RCPSG) added to the debate by advocating the 'widespread use of structured receiving areas'. Whilst not favouring one particular approach, the Royal Colleges identified the essential features intended to improve the medical admissions process (Box 1.1).

Box 1.1. Features for improving the medical admissions process

- Short stay with effective discharge planning and support
- Effective involvement of geriatricians
- 'Fast-track' investigations
- Consultant-led service – close consultant guidance

The Royal Colleges saw the establishment of areas for the assessment of acute admissions as having several advantages and disadvantages (Box 1.2).

What is an MAU?

Some attempts to define the purpose of an MAU have been made (Lane 1999, Wood 2000). Lane (1999) coined the term 'Alpha ward' (as many of the titles attributed to these units had an 'A' in their title), which emphasised a concentration of resources, expedited investigations and

Box 1.2. Advantages and disadvantages of receiving areas (RCPE/RCPSG 1998, p 8)

Advantages

- the concentration of medical and nursing expertise in one area and during the critical period
- less disturbance in other wards throughout the hospital
- the reduction or abolition of decanting (except in major crises), provided step-down beds are available
- the introduction of suitable shift systems for junior medical staffing
- overall improvement in morale
- a means of facilitating diagnostic pathways to improve the quality of acute patient care

Disadvantages

- many patients have to move at least once into a step-down area or specialist unit
- the system is highly pressurised with occasional crises
- the possibility of mixed-sex wards
- a major problem of loss of continuity of care for both medical and nursing staff

frequent ward rounds. For the purposes of this book, an MAU has been defined as:

> A dedicated unit or ward in which medical patients undergo rapid and rigorous assessment, investigation and initial treatment with the purpose of establishing their need for admission to or discharge from hospital.

This definition captures the ethos of many MAUs but does not apply to those units that accept non-medical patients (e.g. surgical, orthopaedic, urology) or those units that keep their patients for a number of days. It is open to debate whether these differences are of any consequence to the operation of an individual MAU. This debate raises a number of issues for discussion.

Referral patterns

Little empirical evidence exists regarding referral patterns to MAUs. A study by Hampton and Gray (1998) found that most patients referred to their medical admissions ward were elderly (most commonly 70–79 years) with 58% of all patients being referred from the hospital's A&E following '999' ambulance calls. A further 39% of patients were referred by their GP. Wood's (2000) study also found that many units accepted only medical patients who had been referred by their GP or from the hospital's

A&E. Some units accepted medical patients referred from outpatient clinics and some took patients suffering chest pain brought directly to the unit by ambulance. Paradoxically, other units did not accept any patients with chest pain. In these cases, the individuals were taken either to the local A&E or direct to the Coronary Care Unit (CCU). It is also apparent that some MAUs accept patients with surgical and orthopaedic problems. Rarely, MAUs accept patients who present unannounced as self-referrals.

Given that MAUs were introduced as a measure to manage rising numbers of medical admissions, it could be anticipated that published evidence exists as to their effectiveness in reducing hospital admissions and easing the pressure on acute medical services. This is not the case. Hampton and Gray (1998) found that readmission rates to their admissions ward ranged from 1.9% within one week of direct discharge home down to 0.3% in the third and fourth weeks after discharge. No details as to the reasons for readmission are given but these low rates suggest that appropriate decisions to discharge were made. Many hospitals gather their own data regarding referral patterns, numbers of admissions and discharges from their MAU. Indeed, as in Hampton and Gray's case, some go further and collect data on the number of patients readmitted to the unit or discharged soon after transfer to an inpatient bed. If the effectiveness of MAUs and the acute admissions process is to be evaluated, these data need to be collected to a common standard and on a routine basis to enable analysis of effectiveness.

Modes of operation

MAUs operate in a variety of different ways dependent on a number of factors. Perhaps the most apparent of these is the amount of time a patient is expected to remain in the area. In this respect, MAUs can be divided into two modes of operation.

- Assessment Units, which keep their patients for as short a time as possible and move them to inpatient beds after the decision to admit has been made.
- Admissions Wards, in which patients are rapidly assessed, investigated and treated but then remain on the ward for a longer period (up to 4 days in some cases).

Both modes of operation have their merits and the decision as to which to employ may be best judged by the local facilities available in terms of the number of acute medical beds, other receiving hospitals and numbers of patients referred.

Trolleys or beds

The NHS Plan (DoH 2000) states that by 2004 inappropriate trolley waits for assessment or admission will have been brought to an end in A&E departments. Whilst not explicitly including them in this statement, such waits are an issue for MAUs that use trolleys as opposed to beds. The answer as to why some MAUs use trolleys is not clear but could relate to a number of factors. Firstly, some MAUs evolved as a sub-area of their hospital's A&E in which trolleys were already used. Secondly, space limitations make the use of trolleys more attractive as they occupy a smaller area than beds, hence more trolleys can be used. Finally, and perhaps most importantly, if the ethos of the MAU is that patients are to be rapidly assessed and then moved to another ward, trolleys make this easier in terms of patient transport.

Patients may believe that if they are being cared for in a bed, they have been or are going to be admitted to hospital. Likewise, their relatives may gain this same impression. The use of trolleys, on the other hand, suggests a less permanent arrangement than occupation or ownership of their own bed. Similarly, Wood (2000) suggests that nurses themselves also make distinctions between patients being cared for on trolleys or on beds. He suggests that there is more urgency to assess and move the patient if they are being cared for on a trolley. This notion fits with the NHS Plan philosophy that trolley waits should be kept to a minimum. However, once a patient is in a bed in the MAU, the pressure to find them a permanent inpatient bed is reduced. This situation may be satisfactory in MAUs that are designed to keep patients for a number of days but can cause problems in those units that aim to assess patients and admit or discharge them expeditiously. In these cases, the MAU can become congested with patients who are in beds and, therefore, have little need to be moved out of the unit with any urgency.

Operational policies

Regardless of whether an MAU operates by assessing patients and moving them on to wards or by keeping them in beds for a number of days, the unit needs to have clear operational policies. These policies need to be developed in partnership and collaboration with key stakeholders to ensure that the unit can operate to its fullest potential in helping to manage the acute admissions process. Operational policies need to give clear guidance to clinical and managerial staff on a number of issues regarding patients and their management (Box 1.3).

Box 1.3. Examples of operational issues for consideration

- Specialisms that can accept referrals to the unit (e.g. medicine)
- Specialisms that cannot accept referrals to the unit (e.g. surgery, orthopaedic)
- The types of presenting medical condition that can be referred
- The types of medical condition that cannot be accepted (options for referral should be given)
- Sources of referral (e.g. GP, A&E department, outpatients department)
- Sources of non-referral (e.g. patients self-referring)
- The maximum length of time that a patient can remain in the unit
- Grade of staff who can accept referrals (e.g. Specialist registrar, Sister/Charge nurse)
- Whether referrals can be declined and by whom
- Contingency plans if the unit becomes full
- Contingency plans if a patient is likely to exceed the unit's agreed maximum length of stay
- Which directorate takes operational responsibility for the unit
- Which specialism takes medical responsibility for the unit
- How medical cover for the unit is organised (e.g. physician of the week or on a day-to-day basis)
- What types of audit data are collected

Resource requirements

Two fundamental components of Lane's (1999) definition of an MAU are 'expedited patient investigations' and 'a concentration of resources'. Both aim to ensure that decisions are made rapidly on each patient's need for admission or discharge. The importance of both cannot be over-emphasised. Rapid access to investigation facilities on a 24-hour basis is vital for clinically effective assessment and decision-making (Box 1.4). MAU patients must have access to these services to ensure that they are not delayed by waiting for their results.

Box 1.4. Investigation facilities required on a 24-hour basis

Radiography services (ideally with 'hot' reporting of results)
Haematology
Biochemistry
Blood gas analysis
Electrocardiography
Pharmacy (or other arrangements for out-of-hours supply of discharge medications)

The concentration of resources can also be thought of in terms of medical and nursing expertise. Medical staff need to be on site 24 hours per day and must have sufficient experience to make decisions regarding the patients' best management. This must be supported by rapid and easy access to professional expertise from a range of disciplines (Box 1.5). Portering services must be readily available if patients are moved to and from the unit on a frequent and regular basis.

Box 1.5. Access to professional expertise

District nursing
Physiotherapy
Occupational therapy
Social services
Psychiatric liaison
Learning disabilities liaison
Elderly care liaison

In addition to hospital-based liaison, it is important to remember the value of collaboration with primary and community care providers. Given that many MAUs accept most of their referrals from GPs, bilateral communication links with the local medical liaison committee or Primary Care Trust should be established to ensure that referral patterns can be monitored and action taken as necessary. It is only by taking a multidisciplinary approach with contributions from all the members of the team that the MAU can operate effectively in managing emergency admissions. Hospital management structures must be in place to enable this collaboration.

Facilities

Depending upon its mode of operation, an MAU will need to have the following dedicated facilities for patients.

Resuscitation area

Given the high acuity of many referrals to an MAU, the possibility of patients suffering a cardiac arrest is reasonably high. Similarly, in those MAUs that accept patients directly by ambulance it is possible that some of these individuals will have had an arrest en route to the unit. For this reason, MAUs need an area allocated specifically for the resuscitation of patients who have suffered cardiac arrest. This area must be equipped with a dedicated stretcher-trolley, defibrillator, resuscitation equipment and drugs, and piped oxygen and suction. It must be separated from the main MAU either in a curtained area or, ideally, in a separate room to allow privacy during resuscitation attempts. Having a dedicated resuscitation area means that staffing must be sufficiently high to allow nursing and medical personnel to resuscitate patients without compromising the care of other patients in the unit.

High-dependency area

Units in which the operational policy dictates that patients remain for several days will require an area dedicated to the care of more highly dependent patients. This area must be equipped to allow continuous monitoring and be within easy view of the nurses' station. The unit's nursing and medical establishment needs to take into account the number and acuity of high-dependency patients treated in the unit.

Relatives' room

All MAUs must have a room dedicated for the use of relatives accompanying patients being resuscitated and by the relatives of patients who are extremely ill. The room should have comfortable furnishings, a telephone extension to an outside line (without having to go through the hospital's switchboard) and tea- and coffee-making facilities. Ideally, the room will be in close proximity to the MAU itself and will have toilets nearby. This facility can be used as a quiet area for interviewing relatives and for the breaking of bad news.

Seating area/discharge lounge

Not all patients referred to an MAU will need to be nursed on a trolley or in a bed. To accommodate those who are less seriously ill, a seating area with comfortable chairs should be provided. This serves three purposes. Firstly, it is more comfortable for patients and enhances independence compared with lying on a trolley. Secondly, it allows trolleys/beds to be used for those patients who need them, and finally, from a political perspective, the number of patients waiting for long periods on trolleys is reduced. A seating area can also be used by patients who are waiting to be discharged or for their transport home. The area needs to be supervised by nursing staff at all times.

Nursing roles and skills in MAU

Initial assessment and management

As in most clinical areas, the nursing staff in MAUs provide a 24-hour presence that co-ordinates patient care. Despite the fact that medical colleagues have a high level of commitment to the clinical management of patients, it is often the MAU nursing staff who are the first to meet the patient and initiate appropriate care. The process of initial assessment and management of acutely ill medical patients (see Chapter 2 – Initial assessment) is fundamental to the role of the MAU nurse. It requires a detailed knowledge of presenting medical complaints and their underpinning pathophysiology, relevant investigations and appropriate treatment options. In addition, MAU nurses also need to be skilled in effective communication and co-ordination in respect of patient care.

Undertaking procedures that enable them to initiate first-line treatments and investigations can supplement the MAU nurse's role in initial assessment to ensure that decisions about a patient's need for admission or discharge are made as promptly as possible and that delays in this process are minimised. The patient, their relatives and the MAU itself all benefit if safe and effective decisions are made as promptly as possible. The DoH (2000) outlines key procedures that nurses could undertake. For MAU nurses these might include:

- venepuncture
- cannulation
- defibrillation
- ECG recording
- X-ray requesting
- arterial blood sampling

It is important to remember that the above skills should not replace fundamental nursing skills. By incorporating some or all of these procedures into the initial assessment of patients, MAU nurses could expedite the decision-making process by having the results of investigations available more quickly. Effective communication skills are equally as important as psychomotor skills. MAU nurses need training and education in the care of bereaved relatives and the breaking of bad news (see Chapter 4 – Sudden death).

In addition to the skills outlined above, MAU nurses are in a prime position to develop new roles in their specialism. Many hospitals now have systems that employ nurse-led defibrillation for the first-line management of cardiac arrest (Eastwick-Field 1996, Cooper et al 1998, DoH 2000). Likewise, nurses are leading clinics dedicated to the assessment and treatment of patients with deep vein thrombosis (Pout et al 1999).

Discharge planning

MAU nurses play an important role in discharge planning. They need to be aware of discharge services and recognise that effective discharge planning is based on a multidisciplinary approach with good communication, knowledge and documentation that begins with the initial assessment of patient needs (Chapter 2 – Initial assessment).

The MAU nurse should have a clear understanding of the referral system that operates within their unit. They should have knowledge about how to access help during office hours and from the out-of-hours on-call services. MAUs should have arrangements in place for rapid and easy access to colleagues from district nursing, social work, occupational therapy, pharmacy and physiotherapy. Specialist input from these professional groups can have a positive impact on the smooth transfer of the patient either to their own home or to an appropriate care facility. Social workers may provide counselling and support to patients and/or carers in readiness for discharge. Occupational therapists provide equipment and carry out patient assessments including toilet, bed and chair transfer on the day of admission. They also liaise with medical social workers, home care assessors and physiotherapists and arrange follow-up visits for patients discharged from the unit.

Many hospitals now employ discharge co-ordinators and, although most deal with the early discharge of inpatients, they are a useful source of information and knowledge regarding intermediate or respite beds that are available.

During office hours, patients discharged from an MAU who require medication must be able to access the hospital pharmacy for a supply of the prescribed medication. Similar arrangements must be in place during out-of-hours periods whereby drugs to take home can be dispensed and the patient's discharge not delayed. If a nurse is involved in the issuing of medications out of hours, the indications for, side effects and importance of compliance with the medications must be explained and emphasised to the patient and their carers (UKCC 1992).

Communication about discharge arrangements between patient and MAU staff should be clearly documented to monitor the consistency and standard of advice given (Ferguson 1997). The record of the arrangements made for continuity of patient care on discharge from hospital is an integral and essential part of care and demonstrates that the duty of care has been fulfilled (UKCC 1998). The 1996 Audit Commission report on improving A&E services emphasised the importance of ensuring that patients are sent home with the appropriate advice and are told where to go if symptoms do not resolve. The Audit Commission (1996) also stressed the importance of communication with GPs. Similarly, patients discharged from an MAU must be given a comprehensive letter to take to their GP. This letter should include details of the presenting problem, clinical findings, investigation results, treatment given and follow-up advice. This letter should be written by the discharging doctor and either posted to the GP or given to the patient to deliver. Computer software is available to produce computerised discharge advice sheets and GP letters. Likewise, electronic patient records that can be accessed by all health care professionals provide a speedier and more reliable method of communicating patient information.

The discussion of discharge arrangements offers an opportunity for nurses to provide health advice to patients (McKenna 1993). Time spent giving health education may avoid further visits to the unit or to the patient's GP (Jones 1993). One group for whom this is particularly relevant is homeless people. Planning effective discharge for the homeless can be problematic. Young, single homeless people have difficulty obtaining help from primary care, particularly GPs, and so are often forced to use emergency services instead (North et al 1996). MAU nurses need to have knowledge of local hostels and voluntary services that may be able to help such individuals. Social services have no statutory responsibility for homeless people under pensionable age but may be able to offer advice.

Management of the MAU

The need for MAUs to have clear operational guidelines within which to work has been identified (Box 1.3) and allied to this is the requirement for a unit to have clear lines of managerial responsibility. Wood (2000) found that many units have clearly defined establishments incorporating clinical and managerial leadership from nurses but many respondents commented that the medical management of their MAU could be developed further. Whilst nursing management in MAUs is reasonably well defined, medical management is less clear, with overall responsibility for the unit often resting with a physician whose specialism lies outside acute medicine. In many cases, the management of patients is organised by physicians accepting referrals on a daily basis (physician of the day) or a weekly basis (physician of the week). Whilst these arrangements ensure that effective care is delivered, it is important to remember that if MAUs are to evolve they need medical management from physician(s) who demonstrate a clear commitment to developing the service provided to patients and the hospital. It remains unclear whether this situation is likely to arise given the previous reluctance of the medical Royal Colleges over the introduction of physicians who specialise in acute care (Federation of Medical Royal Colleges 2000). In these circumstances, it may be nurses who become the leading figures in developing practice and managerial responsibility for MAUs.

Summary

This chapter has given a definition of an MAU and has outlined some of the organisational and managerial issues relevant to nurses working in this clinical setting. It is important for both MAU nurses and their medical colleagues that their unit has clear operational guidelines that have been developed in collaboration with key stakeholders. Only by so doing can MAU staff be clear as to their role within the unit and the hospital. It is hoped that this chapter has raised some issues for consideration in your MAU.

References

Audit Commission (1996) By Accident or Design: Improving A&E Services in England & Wales. London: HMSO.

Cooper M, More J, Robb A (1998) A guide to defibrillation. Emergency Nurse 6(3): 16–21.

Department of Health (2000) The NHS Plan. London: HMSO.

Eastwick-Field P (1996) Introducing nurse-initiated management of cardiac arrest. Nursing Standard 10(26): 46–8.

Federation of Medical Royal Colleges (2000) Acute Medicine: The Physician's Role. Proposals for the Future. Edinburgh: Federation of Medical Royal Colleges.

Ferguson A (1997) Discharge planning in A&E. Accident & Emergency Nursing 5: 210–14.

Hampton J, Gray A (1998) The future of general medicine: lessons from an admissions ward. Journal of the Royal College of Physicians of London 32(1): 39–43.

Jones G (1993) Methods of nursing in A&E. Accident & Emergency Nursing 1: 41–8.

Lane D (1999) System Dynamics Modelling of Patient Flows through Acute Hospitals. London: London School of Economics and Political Science.

McKenna G (1993) The scope for health education in the A&E department. Accident & Emergency Nursing 2: 94–9.

North C, Moore H, Owens C (1996) Go Home and Rest – The Use of A&E Departments by Homeless People. London: Shelter.

Pout G, Wimperis J, Dilks G (1999) Nurse-led outpatient treatment of deep vein thrombosis. Nursing Standard 13(19): 39–41.

Royal College of Physicians of Edinburgh and the Royal College of Physicians and Surgeons of Glasgow (1998) Acute medical admissions and the future of general medicine: a review of professional practices in Scotland with recommendations for debate and action. www.rcpe.ac.uk/public/acute.html

UKCC (1992) Standards for the Administration of Medicines. London: UKCC.

UKCC (1998) Guidelines for Records and Record Keeping. London: UKCC.

Wood I (2000) Medical assessment units in the West Midlands region: a nursing perspective. Accident & Emergency Nursing 8(4): 196–200.

CHAPTER 2

Initial assessment of the acute medical patient

MICHELLE DAVIES, JUDITH MORGAN AND IAN WOOD

Aims

This chapter will:

- describe a systematic approach to the initial assessment and management of acute medical patients presenting to the MAU
- discuss the components of physical assessment, history taking and prioritisation
- discuss the principles of documentation and discharge planning as part of the initial assessment process

Introduction

Assessment is the cornerstone of safe and effective practice and goes hand in hand with the process of prioritising patients' needs. It has been compared to the process of house building whereby assessment is the 'foundation on which all care planning and nursing action is built' (Sbaih 1992). If this important first step is inadequate, the whole process is at risk of collapse. The process of assessment starts as soon as the patient arrives in the MAU and incorporates the gathering of information regarding the patient's current physiological status along with a history of the present and any previous episodes. Concurrent to this process, relevant investigations are performed to yield more information about the patient's condition. Early and effective assessment of patients is particularly important in an MAU, where rapid and accurate decisions are made regarding the patient's need for medical attention, hospital admission or transfer to a more appropriate care setting.

14

In this context, patient assessment comprises the following components:

- systematic physical assessment (airway, breathing, circulation, disability, exposure – ABCDE)
- history taking
- prioritisation of needs
- documentation of findings
- discharge planning

Systematic physical assessment (ABCDE)

A rapid and accurate assessment of the patient's airway patency, breathing function, circulatory status and neurological function (disability) are paramount so that immediately or potentially life-threatening abnormalities can be identified and treated promptly. This systematic approach to the initial assessment of all patients is completed by undressing the patient (exposure) and ensures that important clinical indicators are not missed. As a baseline for this assessment, Table 2.1 gives details of normal adult physiological values:

Table 2.1. Baseline physiological values for adults (Woodrow 1999)

Respiratory rate	12–20 per minute
Heart rate:	
Normal	60–100 beats per minute
Bradycardia	Less than 60 beats per minute
Tachycardia	More than 100 beats per minute
Blood pressure:	
Systolic	More than 90 mmHg
Oxygen saturation:	
– normal	95–98%
– hypoxaemia	Less than 85–90%

Airway

Immediately upon their arrival in the unit, assess the patency of the patient's airway. In most cases, this will be a formality as the patient will be alert and talking. However, those patients who are unconscious or semi-conscious on arrival may not be able to maintain a clear airway, particularly if they are positioned supine. Failure to clear the airway will lead to inadequate ventilation of the lungs and reduced oxygenation. Complete airway occlusion will quickly result in respiratory arrest which, without intervention, will proceed to a full cardiac arrest.

Look at the patient's chest for signs of accessory muscle use that may indicate increased respiratory effort caused by airway obstruction. Look at the lips and oral mucosa for cyanosis, pallor (for dark skins this may be difficult to assess), swelling, dryness or cracking. Check whether the patient wears false teeth and if they are well fitting. If false teeth are ill fitting, remove them. Listen for noise in the airway. Inspiratory noise (stridor) can be indicative of upper airway obstruction. Expiratory noise (wheeze) can indicate lower respiratory problems caused by airway collapse on expiration. A swollen, dry or cracked tongue can be indicative of dehydration.

In the unconscious patient, look inside the mouth for saliva, frothy sputum (pulmonary oedema), blood, vomit or foreign bodies. If the patient vomits, use suction to help clear large amounts of material from the mouth and oropharynx and tilt the head of the bed down to reduce the likelihood of pulmonary aspiration. In airway management, nursing interventions include clearing of obstructions (e.g. foreign bodies, vomit and flaccid tongue), administration of suction, insertion of airway adjuncts and moving the patient into the recovery position. If using suction through airway adjuncts, suctioning for more than 15 seconds can deplete the lungs of oxygen, so great care should be taken. If, when checking the airway, there is an inability to open the mouth due to muscle spasm, then trismus is present. Further assessment of the airway includes obtaining any history relating to possible causes of airway problems (e.g. does the patient have any allergies that may have caused an airway problem?).

Breathing

Inadequate breathing may be acute or chronic, continuous or intermittent and can lead to inadequate ventilation of the lungs and subsequent respiratory failure. Initial assessment of breathing focuses on the identification of immediately or potentially life-threatening conditions (Box 2.1; see also Chapter 8 – Shortness of breath and Chapter 9 – Chest pain).

Whilst considering the presence of one or more of these conditions, look at the patient for central or peripheral cyanosis. Observe their posture, count their respiratory rate and assess their depth and effort of breathing. Look at the symmetry of their chest movements. Observe for the use of accessory muscles and for retraction of the skin around the clavicles and ribs indicating increased respiratory effort. Listen for sounds of stridor or wheeze on inspiration (upper respiratory infections), on expiration (bronchospasm) or biphasic (wheeze on inspiration and expiration –

**Box 2.1. Immediately life-threatening and potentially life-threatening
conditions causing breathing problems**

Immediately life-threatening conditions causing breathing problems:
Life-threatening asthma (defined by British Thoracic Society (BTS) guidelines 1997a)
Severe pulmonary oedema
Large pulmonary embolism
Cardiac arrhythmia
Cardiac tamponade
Tension pneumothorax

Potentially life-threatening conditions causing breathing problems:
Acute severe asthma (defined by BTS guidelines 1997a)
Acute exacerbation of COPD/respiratory failure
Chest infection
Myocardial infarction
Pulmonary oedema
Metabolic acidosis
Pulmonary embolism
Simple pneumothorax
Pleural effusion
Anaphylaxis

---

foreign body, laryngospasm or very severe asthma attack). Assess whether
the patient can complete full sentences, short sentences, words only or is
unable to give an oral response. Check the patient's lung expansion by
feeling the chest bilaterally. A more detailed assessment includes
percussion and auscultation of the patient's chest. Percuss anteriorly and
posteriorly in the upper, middle and lower areas bilaterally. Resonance
indicates presence of air whilst dullness indicates fluid underlying the area
percussed. Auscultate the same areas listening for the presence, type and
quality of breath sounds as well as any additional sounds (ALSG 2001).

Ask the patient about any history of asthma, acute/chronic chest
conditions or any deviation from their normal breathing pattern.
Determine if the patient has taken medication (prescribed or not) before or
after their breathing problem started. Make a note of the percentage of
oxygen being given to the patient when they arrive in the unit. This may be
important if the patient has a chronic lung condition.

Nursing interventions at this stage include positioning the patient
upright or in the recovery position as appropriate. Administer 100%
oxygen if required. Patients with chronic pulmonary disorders will require
careful monitoring if given high concentrations of oxygen. Where oxygen
is to be administered for a prolonged period, a humidification device

should be used to prevent drying of the patient's mucous membranes and secretions. Monitor and record oxygen saturation levels using a pulse oximeter probe attached to a finger, toe, nose or earlobe. The blood requires 5 g/dl of haemoglobin to register a value (Chapin and Proehl 1999). Do not use nails coloured with nail polish or henna as they can cause inaccurate readings. Pulse oximetry recordings can also be inaccurate if peripheral vasoconstriction is present or when carbon monoxide has been inhaled (Chapin and Proehl 1999). In patients with chronic obstructive pulmonary disease (COPD), arterial oxygen content can only be measured accurately by arterial blood gas analysis (BTS 1997b). If the oxygen saturation measurement is <85–90% (normal 95–98%) this indicates hypoxaemia (Woodrow 1999). Respiratory exhaustion could be indicative of the need for mechanical ventilation (Collins 2000) (see Chapter 8 – Shortness of breath).

If the patient has an audible wheeze, is a known asthmatic or has an underlying chronic respiratory problem, measure their peak expiratory flow (PEF). To overcome problems with the patient's technique, ask them for three readings and record the highest. Compare this reading with what is normal for the patient. Measurement of PEF is contraindicated for patients with suspected pulmonary embolism or pneumothorax. If the patient is asthmatic, refer to the guidelines for the management of asthma (BTS 1997a) (see Chapter 8 – Shortness of breath).

Circulation

Circulatory problems may be primary or secondary. A primary problem involves the heart not pumping effectively (e.g. following a myocardial infarction (see Chapter 9 – Chest pain)). A secondary problem involves a failure of the circulatory system (i.e. the arterial/venous system) (e.g. severe blood loss). In essence, there is either 'pump' failure or 'pipe' failure. Both primary and secondary problems can lead to tissue hypoxia or 'shock' (Box 2.2; see also Chapter 6 – Shock).

Box 2.2. Potentially life-threatening circulatory problems

Hypovolaemia (see Chapter 6 – Shock)
Severe left ventricular failure (see Chapter 8 – Shortness of breath)
Arrhythmias (see Chapter 5 – Cardiac arrest)
Pulmonary embolism (see Chapter 9 – Chest pain)
Myocardial infarction (see Chapter 9 – Chest pain)
Anaphylactic reaction (see Chapter 6 – Shock)
Sepsis (see Chapter 6 – Shock)
Cardiac tamponade (see Chapter 5 – Cardiac arrest)

Circulatory problems can be assessed through several parameters (Box 2.3).

Box 2.3. Parameters for assessing circulatory problems

Respiratory rate
Pulse site, rate, volume and regularity
Blood pressure
Skin colour, appearance, texture and turgor
Capillary refill
Urine output
Level of consciousness
Peripheral pulses
12-lead ECG

Respiratory rate

The rate and depth of respiration has already been noted when assessing the patient's breathing. However, it is important to remember that an increase in the respiratory rate is often the first physiological response to a reduction in circulating blood volume.

Pulse site, rate, volume and regularity

Check the pulse manually as this enables the patient's pulse rate, volume and regularity to be assessed at the same time as feeling their skin temperature and texture. If the pulse is detectable at the wrist, the systolic blood pressure is at least 80 mmHg (Collins 2000). Absence of a radial pulse on both arms but presence of a brachial indicates a systolic blood pressure of at least 70 mmHg. If this is the case, the patient is profoundly hypotensive and requires immediate treatment.

As other factors (e.g. emotional stress, pain, fitness or drugs) affect the heart rate, it is important that the heart rate alone is not used to assess cardiovascular state. As an example, a patient presenting with a heart rate of 80/min would not normally be associated with cardiovascular compromise. If this patient was a fit athlete with a resting rate of 45/min, a rate of 80/min could be interpreted as a tachycardia. Similarly, patients taking beta-blockers (which slow the heart rate) may not develop a tachycardia. Great care must also be taken when assessing the older person as some have a limited response to catecholamine release (American College of Surgeons (ACS) Committee on Trauma 1988) and do not develop a significant tachycardia even with substantial blood loss.

Blood pressure

Record the blood pressure. A systolic blood pressure of less than 90 mmHg should give immediate cause for alarm as it could indicate significant hypotension that warrants emergency intervention. Remember that patients taking beta-blocker medication may normally have a low systolic pressure. Pay attention to the pulse pressure (difference between the diastolic and systolic). This narrows as the diastolic pressure increases (peripheral vasoconstriction causes an increase in peripheral vascular resistance) in order to increase the circulating volume by moving blood from the venous reservoir (Herbert and Alison 1996). The calculation of a mean arterial pressure (MAP) (one-third pulse pressure added to the diastolic pressure) indicates the pressure that is driving the blood through the circulation (Herbert and Alison 1996). A MAP less than 60 mmHg is an indicator of poor organ perfusion (Hudak and Gallo 1994). The blood pressure may need to be recorded in both arms, as a difference of 10–15 mmHg could be indicative of a dissecting thoracic aortic aneurysm (ACS 1988). Another indicator of blood volume is to assess for distension of the neck veins when the patient is laid flat. If no neck veins can be seen or they do not fill when the patient is positioned upright, dehydration may be present. Conversely, distended neck veins could be a sign of fluid overload, heart failure or an increase in thoracic pressure (e.g. tension pneumo-thorax). Care should be taken when handing over responsibility from one nurse to another, as one may record the diastolic as a muffling of heart sounds (4th Korotkov sound) and the other may record it when the sound disappears (5th Korotkov sound). An electronic sphygmomanometer records the average between the two sounds.

Skin colour, appearance, texture and turgor

Observe the patient for pallor (vasoconstriction, anaemia), flushing (pyrexia, carbon monoxide poisoning), cyanosis or a waxy appearance.

The skin may feel cool and clammy due to vasoconstriction with no heat to evaporate insensible perspiration (Clarke 1996) or hot due to vasodilation or pyrexia. Check skin turgor for signs of dehydration. Pinch some skin over the back of the hand or inner forearm; if the skin stays pinched this indicates severe dehydration (Hinchliff 1996). Care should be taken in testing turgor in the older person, as there is often an insidious loss of elasticity of the skin (Iggulden 1999).

Capillary refill

Record a capillary refill test. Press a fingernail firmly for 5 seconds and when the pressure is released, colour should return within 2 seconds. If the colour takes greater than 2 seconds to restore, then this is indicative of peripheral vasoconstriction and/or marked hypotension. This test can be inaccurate if the patient is cold.

Urine output

In critically ill patients, the placement of a urinary catheter may be necessary to assess their hourly urine output as this is an accurate indicator of tissue perfusion. Trends indicating a urine output less than 0.5 ml/kg body weight per hour indicate inadequate renal perfusion. Exercise greater caution in using this as a measure in the older person as their kidneys have a reduced ability to concentrate urine (Iggulden 1999).

ECG recording

Any patient who is critically ill, has a cardiovascular deficit or a history suggestive of a cardiac cause should have a 12-lead electrocardiogram (ECG) recorded. This will establish the underlying heart rhythm and identify signs of an acute coronary syndrome (e.g. myocardial infarction or unstable angina (see Chapter 9 – Chest pain)). Continuously monitor the cardiac rhythm of critically ill patients and repeat 12-lead ECGs at any rhythm change and during chest pain.

Peripheral pulses

Check for presence of pedal pulses in patients referred with potential arterial or venous problems. Check for a history of sudden onset of pain and numbness in the affected limb. Observe the limbs for pallor and cyanosis and feel for coldness to touch.

Nursing interventions to manage circulatory problems include the insertion of intravenous (IV) cannulae and the collection of blood samples for urea, electrolytes, haemoglobin, white cell count (possibly with differential) and blood glucose levels. If hypovolaemia is suspected, request a group & cross-match or group & save, and administer IV fluids as prescribed via two large bore cannulae (see Chapter 6 – Shock).

Disability (neurological status)

Patients are referred to the MAU with an altered neurological status (conscious level) for a variety of reasons (Box 2.4).

Box 2.4. Potential causes of altered consciousness (see Chapter 7 – Altered Consciousness)

Hypoxia (see Chapter 8 – Shortness of breath)
Cerebrovascular accident (CVA) (see Chapter 7 – Altered consciousness)
Subarachnoid haemorrhage (see Chapter 7 – Altered consciousness)
Hypo- or hyperglycaemia (see Chapter 7 – Altered consciousness)
Transient ischaemic attack (TIA) (see Chapter 7 – Altered consciousness)
Drug overdose (see Chapter 7 – Altered consciousness)
Sepsis (see Chapter 6 - Shock)
Epileptic seizures (see Chapter 7 – Altered consciousness)
Meningitis (see Chapter 7 – Altered consciousness)
Head injury
Acidosis (respiratory and metabolic)
Alkalosis (respiratory and metabolic)
An unidentified reason

A neurological assessment comprises three parts:

1. Use of a neurological assessment tool
2. Assessment of pupil reaction
3. Assessment of limb function

Neurological assessment tool

Two tools can be used: the mnemonic 'AVPU' and the Glasgow Coma Score (GCS). These give a clear indication of how obtunded the patient is and allow a quick assessment of the critically ill patient. AVPU is quick and easy to use and is ideal for initial assessments. The GCS (Table 2.2) is internationally accepted as the measurement of choice. It does not always meet the needs of some patients who have a reduced conscious level solely through drugs, alcohol or a metabolic cause.

AVPU. The AVPU (**A**lert, responds to **V**oice, responds to **P**ain or **U**nresponsive) (ACS 1988) as a scale is self-explanatory. If the patient is conscious and able to talk regardless of whether they are confused or giving inappropriate answers to questions, they are considered to be 'Alert'. If they are not talking but respond to 'Voice' by opening their eyes or obeying commands, their conscious level is obtunded. If they do not respond to voice but respond to a 'Pain' stimulus (trapezium squeeze: by using the thumb and two fingers, 5 cm of the trapezius muscle where the head meets the shoulders are held and then twisted (Shah 1999)), their conscious level is even further reduced. If they do not respond to pain, the patient is completely 'Unresponsive'.

GCS. The GCS (Table 2.2) was developed to facilitate a common language between doctors in tertiary hospitals and neurosurgeons in specialist centres (Teasdale and Jennett 1974). The scale is designed to identify early deterioration in conscious level to facilitate prompt intervention that reduces morbidity and mortality. The tool centres on the determination of three variables: best eye opening response, best verbal response and best motor response. Each area is assessed in turn and scored out of 15. A score of 15/15 considers the patient to be fully conscious. A score of less than 8/15 designates the patient as being in a coma (see also Table 2.3).

Consider the following when using the using the GCS:

- When transferring accountability for care from one nurse to another, the nurses should undertake one set of neurological observations together to ensure continuity of measurements.
- Best eye opening: If the patient has their eyes closed – for whatever reason, including sleep – and opens them at the commencement of the recording, they score 3.
- Best verbal response: To be assessed as orientated, the patient must know their name, that they are in hospital and either the month or the year. If they only answer two correctly, they are considered to be confused.
- Best motor response: To test for obeying commands, the patient should be asked to touch their nose, wriggle their toes and stick their tongue out. Two instructions must be successful to be assessed as obeying commands. Asking the patient just to squeeze fingers should be avoided, as it cannot be ascertained if this was a reflex action. If this method is used, the command should be to squeeze and then let go.

Table 2.2. Glasgow Coma Score

Score	Description	Interpretation
Best eye response		
4	Spontaneously	Eyes open without the need of a stimulus
3	To speech	Eyes open to verbal stimulation (normal, raised or repeated)
2	To pain	Eyes open to pain only
1	None	No eye opening to verbal or painful stimulus
Best verbal response		
5	Orientated	Knows: who they are, where they are and the month or year
4	Confused	Incorrectly answers the above questions
3	Inappropriate words	Responses given do not answer questions posed
2	Incomprehensible sounds	Not able to formulate recognisable words
1	None	No verbal response
Best motor response		
6	Obeys commands	Follows and acts out commands and must undertake 2 out of 3
5	Localises to pain	Purposeful movement to remove a painful stimulus – here supra-orbital pressure should be used as then one can see the patient localising to the pain as they lift their hand to push away the stimulus
4	Withdrawing from pain or normal flexion	Flexes the arm at the elbow without wrist rotation in response to a painful stimulus
3	Abnormal flexion to pain	Flexes arm at elbow with rotation of the wrist with resulting spastic posture in a response to a painful stimulus
2	Extends to pain	Extends arm at elbow with inward rotation of the arm in response to a painful stimulus
1	None	No motor response

Table 2.3. Comparison between neurological scores

AVPU	Glasgow Coma Score
Alert	GCS 14/15
Responding to voice	GCS 8–13
Responding to pain	GCS 4–8
Unresponsive	GCS 3

Pupil reaction

Check pupil reactions using a bright light (not an ophthalmoscope) shone into each eye and record the size and reaction. Whilst shining the light in one eye, check the other to confirm the presence of consensual reflexes. Altered pupil sizes (measured in millimetres) and reaction to light give some indication of underlying pathology. Pinpoint pupils may indicate the presence of opiates or a metabolic disorder, whilst dilated pupils may be present following seizures or the ingestion of some drugs (e.g. cocaine, amphetamines or tricyclic antidepressants). The size and reaction of the pupil may also indicate the site of damage in the brain (Hudak and Gallo 1994). Consider the shape of the pupil, as one that is not round may indicate an underlying brain lesion (Shah 1999). Having unequal pupils without a reduced conscious level is insignificant.

Pupil reaction is an essential component when undertaking a neurological assessment where there is potential for raised intracranial pressure. The pupil becomes fixed and dilated when significant pressure is placed on the third cranial (oculomotor) nerve, which lies just above the tentorium. This is often unilateral. If this pressure continues, the brain will subsequently 'cone' whereby the uncal portion of the temporal lobe herniates through the foramen magnum in the base of the skull (Copstead and Banasik 2000).

Limb assessment

Assessment of the patient's best limb response will determine where specific brain injury has occurred. Limb response is assessed against normal power, mild weakness, severe weakness, flexion, extension and no response (Table 2.4).

Table 2.4. Limb assessment of motor power (based on Shah 1999)

Normal power	Patient is able to match resistance applied by the observer to any joint movement
Mild weakness	Patient is able to move against resistance but is easily overcome
Severe weakness	Patient is able to move his or her limb but not against resistance
Flexion	Flexes the limb to painful peripheral stimulation
Extension	Extends the limb to painful peripheral stimulation
No response	No response

In a co-operative patient, normal power, mild or severe weakness can be confirmed by asking the patient to undertake some actions (e.g. touching their nose, lifting their arm or leg in the air). Take care when assessing the patient's arm weakness because if the patient is asked to squeeze the nurse's fingers, one hand is usually dominant and has greater power. Assess patients with a reduced conscious level by using a peripheral pain stimulus (i.e. by applying pressure to a pen that is held to the proximal side of one of the patient's fingernail beds (Allan et al 1996)). Record subsequent limb movement. To confirm the presence of a mild arm weakness, lay the patient flat, ask them to close their eyes and hold their arms out in front of them. If one arm drifts, there is a mild weakness.

Further assessment of neurological status includes taking a history from the patient or relative regarding disorientation, confusion, fitting and loss of consciousness or head injury.

Exposure

It is not possible to complete a thorough assessment without undressing the patient. Inspect the patient's skin for integrity, colour, rashes, oedema and signs of possible abuse or self-harm. Make a note of any existing pressure sores. Take the opportunity to measure their temperature and blood glucose using a glucometer. Having exposed the patient, remember to keep them warm and to preserve their dignity.

History taking

History is of paramount importance when assessing patients as approximately 90% of diagnoses are derived from the history alone (ACS 1988). When assessing a patient who is critically ill, the MAU nurse must make a clinical decision as to when and how the history will be taken. The aim is to complete an accurate history as soon as possible after the patient's arrival. It is important to identify in chronological order the history of how each of the symptoms has developed and what, if any, events were related to them. Likewise, it is also important to determine how the patient feels about their illness and what aspect of their condition has led them to seek medical advice. The obvious presenting problem should not stop the MAU nurse from questioning the patient further to satisfy themselves that this is indeed the most important complaint. On occasions, the presenting condition is not seen by the patient to be their main problem as other aspects of their physical state may cause them more concern. The 'news reporter's tool' may be a useful mnemonic to use when taking a patient's history (Box 2.5).

Details of the patient's family history of illness can be important as it may highlight the possibility of the patient developing the same condition.

Box 2.5. The news reporter's tool (Who? What? Where? When? Why? How?)

1. Who is the patient?
   - Are they male or female?
   - What is their age?
   - What is their ethnicity and culture?
   - Do they have any particular religious beliefs?
   - How do they appear? Pale, cyanosed or do they have a mobility deficit?
   - Are they appropriately dressed for the time of the year? Does their clothing depict a lack of care or poverty or are they unkempt? Is this related to their social circumstances (e.g. homeless)?

2. What happened to cause them to seek assistance today?
   - Has their condition changed?
   - Is their condition acute or chronic?
   - What is their presenting complaint?

3. Where did the problem start?
   - Was it at home or work?
   - What were they doing at the time?
   - Where exactly is the problem?
   - Does it affect their activities of daily living? If so, what is affected?

4. When did it start?
   - How long have they had it?
   - Was the onset sudden or slow?
   - Was the onset insidious or overt?
   - Has it happened before?

5. Why did this occur?
   - Have they done anything different today that may have caused the problem?
   - Are there any other symptoms in addition to the main problem?

6 How did this happen?
   - Was the problem precipitated by anything?

It may also allow the patient to express fears and anxieties regarding conditions suffered by their family, which they fear may also affect them. Similarly, gathering information about the patient's personal and social history helps to identify their employment status. This may be relevant if their work is associated with particular physical or mental health risks. Consider also the patient's weekly alcohol intake, smoking habits and recreational drug use. Drug use is sometimes a difficult and sensitive subject to discuss and it is often much easier to approach the subject when asking about alcohol and smoking habits.

An insight into a patient's social circumstance is important. Gather details of the patient's next of kin, who they live with, whether they are cared for or whether they themselves act as a carer to someone else. This information helps if the patient needs admission as provision can then be made for dependants. If the patient so wishes, relatives, friends and carers can be kept informed of their hospital admission. This information is also an important aspect of the discharge planning process. Social workers and other members of the health care team benefit from this information in planning the provision of services for the patient if they are discharged. In the context of contemporary issues relating to patient consent and in relevant cases, discussion with the patient about their wishes regarding resuscitation, and if they wish their family to be present, should be considered.

An important component of any history relates to the type of any pain experienced by the patient in relation to their presenting problem. There are many pain assessment tools in use in general nursing; a quick and easy one to remember is the 'PQRST' mnemonic developed by Rogers et al (1989). This assesses what provokes the pain, its quality, whether it radiates, its site and severity and how long it has been present (Box 2.6).

Another mnemonic that may act as an aide mémoire is 'AMPLE' (ACS 1997), relating to allergies, medications, previous medical history, the patient's nutritional/dietary status and the events surrounding the presenting problem (Box 2.7).

The use of the above mnemonics is not compulsory but they act as a guide to the history taking process during which questions should be asked in a tactful and caring way. An MAU nurse requires experience and expertise to obtain this information during the assessment process. Any assessment guide or tool should be designed specifically to help the nurse collect the information necessary to make an accurate and effective assessment. An acute problem has to be clearly differentiated from a chronic condition. This will aid the implementation of the correct plan of care for the patient's needs (Seidel et al 1998, Cagan and Marfell 1998).

Prioritisation of patients' needs

As stated at the beginning of this chapter, patients are referred to the MAU to have their medical needs assessed. Given the variety of presenting medical conditions, it is apparent that some patients will require more urgent attention than others. Jervis (2000) identified the similarities between MAUs and A&E departments as both give emergency care. In

---

Box 2.6. The PQRST mnemonic

Provokes
- What provokes the pain?
- Does anything make it better or worse (e.g. positioning, heat or cold)?
- Is it present only on movement?

Quality
- Ask the patient to describe the pain.
- Is it stabbing, crushing, spasmodic or continuous?

Radiation
- Does the pain radiate anywhere?
- If so, where to? Remember not to ask leading questions.

Site/severity
- Where exactly is the pain?
- Is it localised?
- Can it be pinpointed?
- What is the severity? A pain scoring system may be used
- Is the pain the same now as it was last time?
- Does it impair any bodily functions? If so, which ones?

Time/treatment
- How long has the pain been present?
- Has the patient taken any analgesia? If so what and when?
- If they have taken analgesia, are they presenting a true picture of the severity and quality of their pain?

---

particular, there are similarities in the role of the nurse in assessing and prioritising patients' needs for medical and nursing interventions. In A&E, patients have their presenting complaint assessed and their need for treatment prioritised in a process known as triage. This process has been adopted in some MAUs as a means of assigning priority for medical attention to those patients who have the most urgent physiological needs.

Many patients referred to MAUs have already been assessed, had a provisional diagnosis made and been given treatment by their GP, in the local A&E or outpatients departments or by paramedics. It is good practice, however, for all patients referred to MAU to be reassessed and have their needs prioritised on their arrival in the unit. In most cases, MAU nurses will undertake this assessment and prioritisation process because they are the only professional group with a constant presence in the unit. Best practice suggests that one nurse is nominated to triage patients when they arrive and to allocate them according to their clinical priority and the demands on the unit at that time. In some units, another

---

Box 2.7. The AMPLE mnemonic

Allergies
- Does the patient have any? If so, what are they?
- Are they relevant to your plan of care?

Medications
- Does the patient currently take any medications?
- What medications have they previously taken?
- Are they prescribed, over the counter, herbal, illicit drugs or smoking?
- With what frequency and for how long have they been taking them?

Past medical history
- Is the present problem an exacerbation of a previously experienced condition (e.g. asthma)?
- Are there any underlying conditions that could complicate this presentation (e.g. diabetes mellitus, alcohol dependence, hypertension)?
- Is the patient at risk of pressure sore development?

Last ate
- Is the patient well nourished?
- What type of diet do they eat?
- Do they have any special dietary needs?
- Should they receive food or fluid by mouth?
- Are they likely to have vitamin or mineral deficiencies (e.g. alcoholism)?

Events/environment
- What events led the patient to come to you today?
- What is their home environment like?
- Are they able to return home safely?
- What social support do they receive?
- Does this require cancelling or rearranging?
- Do they care for anyone else?
- Who has come to hospital with them today?

---

nurse conducts a more detailed secondary triage. The emergency triage method (Mackway-Jones 1997) may be beneficial as a framework for this process but, if adopted, would require modification for use in an MAU setting.

Documentation

Having assessed the patient and started initial investigations and treatments, findings and actions should be documented. In an MAU, this serves the purpose of communicating details of nursing care to all members of the team and providing a written record of all activity relating to the patient. When documenting patient care it is important to follow a structured approach to ensure that vital information is not omitted. This also ensures that all relevant information is available to be shared and utilised by the multidisciplinary team. The MAU nurse should also undertake a final evaluation and document the findings before the patient is discharged from their care, irrespective of whether discharge is back into the community or to a ward. There are many approaches to documentation within an MAU depending upon how the unit is organised. The best approach for each unit is adopted after discussion and collaboration between all members of the MAU team. Box 2.8 outlines components of the documentation that should be included

.

Box 2.8. Components of documentation

- Demographic data (name, address, date of birth, next of kin, religion)
- Details of the presenting problem/complaint
- Findings of airway, breathing, circulation, disability assessment, including vital signs:
    respiratory rate and depth
    blood pressure
    heart rate, regularity & pulse volume
    temperature
    oxygen saturation
    PEF
    AVPU/GCS
- Previous medical history
- Current medication
- Any known allergies
- Skin integrity
- The patient's psychological state
- Details of investigations carried out:
    blood glucose
    ECG
    laboratory tests (haemoglobin (Hb), white cell count (WCC), urea and electrolytes (U&E))
    X-rays
    blood gas analysis
- Triage priority – including the time (and scale/flow chart if used)
- Medical and nursing interventions and their effects
- Patient's current condition
- Any changes in the patient's condition
- Date and time of entry
- Name and signature of the nurse completing the documentation

---

It is of the utmost importance that all information is documented accurately. Record the time using the 24-hour format to avoid confusion in using a.m. or p.m. To be effective, documentation must be complete so that all information relating to the patient can be communicated without confusion to the members of the nursing and medical team.

The UKCC (1998) identifies a number of important factors that affect accurate record keeping. These state that the entry should be made as soon as possible after the event to maintain accuracy and to reflect the current condition of the patient. The records should be legible and written in a way that they cannot be erased. Mistakes can occur as a result of illegible handwriting. Jargon, abbreviations (except where there is an explanatory list available to patients and staff) and irrelevant speculation should not be included.

Historically, nursing and medical records have been maintained separately. A collaborative and integrated approach for doctors, nurses and other health care professionals in recording patient care and treatment has many benefits for the patient and MAU staff. Integrated Care Pathways ensure that information is not duplicated needlessly. Each member of the team has access to all the information concerning the patient. This stops the patient being subjected to repetitive questioning and reduces the risk of relevant facts being omitted. Similarly, facts can be presented in a straightforward and comprehensive manner. Integrated Care Pathways can also be provided in the form of computerised records.

Discharge planning

One of the fundamental principles underpinning the development of MAUs is that patients have their medical conditions assessed and investigated thoroughly and that decisions on their need for admission or discharge are made promptly and effectively. On this basis, it is essential that discharge planning is commenced during or as soon as possible after the initial assessment to avoid problems arising when the decision is finally made to discharge the patient home. Vulnerable patients (e.g. the elderly) may require multidisciplinary collaboration and consultation with the family and GP.

During or soon after the initial assessment, the nurse should spend time with the patient's relatives or carers to discuss any concerns about how the patient and family will manage if the patient is discharged. Where appropriate, those involved in the patient's care before admission should be involved in planning their discharge.

Summary

This chapter has focused on the guiding principles involved in a systematic approach to the initial assessment of patients referred to the MAU. It is imperative that all patients are assessed using the same approach, thereby ensuring that all life-threatening or potentially life-threatening conditions are identified and treated as promptly and effectively as possible. As MAU nurses are the only 24-hour professional presence in some units, it is vital that they are all familiar with this approach and use their knowledge and skills to ensure that patient care is optimised. It is also important to remember that the discharge process for many patients starts soon after their arrival in the unit. By using a team approach to the assessment of their patients, MAU nurses can have a significant impact on an effective admissions process.

References

Advanced Life Support Group (ALSG) (2001) Acute Medical Emergencies: The Practical Approach. London: BMJ Books.

Allan D, Nie V, Hunter M (1996) The central nervous system. In Hinchliff S, Montague S, Watson R (eds) Physiology for Nursing Practice, 2nd edn. London: Baillière Tindall.

American College of Surgeons (ACS) Committee on Trauma (1988) Advanced Trauma Life Support for Doctors, 5th edn. Chicago: ACS.

American College of Surgeons (ACS) Committee on Trauma (1997) Advanced Trauma Life Support for Doctors, 6th edn. Chicago: ACS.

British Thoracic Society (1997a) The British Guidelines on Asthma Management: 1995 review and position statement. Supplement to February issue of Thorax 52(1).

British Thoracic Society (1997b) Guidelines on the Management of COPD. Thorax 52 (Supplement 5): S1–S28.

Cagan J, Marfell J (1998) Health Assessment. Chicago: Rush University College of Nursing.

Chapin J, Proehl J (1999) Pulse oximetry. In Proehl J (ed) Emergency Nursing Procedures, 2nd edn. Philadelphia: WB Saunders.

Clarke M (1996) The autonomic nervous system. In Hinchliff S, Montague S, Watson R (eds) Physiology for Nursing Practice, 2nd edn. London: Baillière Tindall.

Collins T (2000) Understanding shock. Nursing Standard 14(49): 35–41.

Copstead L-E, Banasik J (2000) Pathophysiology: Biological and Behavioral Perspectives. Philadelphia: WB Saunders.

Herbert R, Alison J (1996). Cardiovascular function. In Hinchliff S, Montague S, Watson R (eds) Physiology for Nursing Practice, 2nd edn. London: Baillière Tindall.

Hinchliff S (1996) Innate defences. In Hinchliff S, Montague S, Watson R (eds) Physiology for Nursing Practice, 2nd edn. London: Baillière Tindall.

Hudak C, Gallo B (1994) Critical Care Nursing: A Holistic Approach, 6th edn. Philadelphia: JB Lippincott.

Iggulden H (1999) Dehydration and electrolyte disturbance. Nursing Standard 13(19): 48–56.

Jervis J (2000) Brief but to the point. Nursing Times 96(3): 42–4

Mackway-Jones K (ed) (1997) Emergency Triage. London: BMJ Publishing.

Rogers J, Osborn H, Pousada L (1989) Emergency Nursing: A Practice Guide. Baltimore: Williams & Wilkins.

Sbaih L (1992) Accident & Emergency Nursing – A Nursing Model. London: Chapman & Hall.

Seidel H, Ball J, Dains J, Benedict G (1998) Mosby's Guide to Physical Examination, 4th edn. St Louis, MO: Mosby Year Book.

Shah S (1999) Neurological assessment. Nursing Standard 13(22): 49–56.

Teasdale G, Jennett B (1974) Assessment of coma and impaired consciousness. Lancet ii: 81–4.

UKCC (1998) Guidelines for Records and Record Keeping. London: UKCC.

Woodrow P (1999) Pulse oximetry. Nursing Standard 13(42): 42–6.

CHAPTER 3

Vulnerable groups

LINDA MILLER, MICHAEL GIBBS, JUDI THORLEY
AND ELIZABETH WHELAN

Aim

This chapter will:

- discuss the principles involved in assessing and managing the needs of the following groups of vulnerable adults who may be referred to the MAU:
  - older adults
  - individuals with learning disabilities
  - individuals with mental health needs

Introduction

Early assessment and identification of abuse and neglect of vulnerable adults is vital for the protection of the individual and prevention of further abuse. This chapter highlights issues relating to three vulnerable groups of individuals in society: older adults, individuals with mental health problems and those with learning disabilities. The chapter is organised into three sections, each devoted to one vulnerable group. The aim of each section is to offer a framework whereby the needs of these individuals can be assessed and treatment options developed. It is important to remember that individuals from vulnerable groups are as susceptible to 'medical' problems as other members of society. It should also be remembered that individuals with learning disabilities can have co-existing mental health problems. For the purposes of this book, a vulnerable adult is defined as a person:

who is or may be in need of community care services by reason of mental or other disability, age or illness; and who is or may be unable to take care of him or herself, or unable to protect him or herself against significant harm or exploitation. (Department of Health (DoH) 2000a, p 8)

A. ABUSE, NEGLECT AND INADEQUATE CARE OF OLDER ADULTS
(Linda Miller)

Aims

This section will:

- provide nurses working in MAUs with a framework for identifying and assessing abuse and neglect of older adults
- describe the recognition of abuse, neglect or self-neglect in the presenting condition
- discuss the circumstances within which abuse may take place
- discuss how to create a sensitive environment and approach for assessment of potential abuse
- describe the actions to be taken in the event of alleged abuse

Introduction

Since the 1980s, there has been a gradual recognition of abuse and neglect of older people. Similarly, society has come to recognise domestic violence and the abuse and neglect of children as a 'social problem in need of attention' (Kingston and Penhale 1995). In the case of children with certain types of injury, there may be no question as to whether or not the individual has been a victim of violence or abuse. There are, however, times when the picture is not so clear and this is particularly true in the case of vulnerable adults. In this context, Kingston and Penhale (1995) refer to the unique position of A&E nurses in identifying cases of abuse and neglect of older people. MAU nurses will find themselves in a similar position, particularly given that the multiple pathology of older people often means that they are referred directly to the MAU rather than the A&E department.

Concerns have been expressed, however, that health and social care providers have not had the necessary knowledge, skills or experience to enable them to address the issues involved (DoH 2002a, Social Services Inspectorate (SSI) 1993, Kingston and Penhale 1995, 1997). *The Service*

Standards for the National Health Service (NHS) *Care of Older People* (Centre for Policy on Ageing/NHS 1999) and the DoH (2000a) stress the need for health and social care provider groups to work in partnership. This partnership must ensure that there are 'robust procedures' in place to give guidance in respect of the identification and management of abuse of vulnerable adults.

Forms of abuse

Categorisation of abuse has formed the basis of much discussion over a number of years. There now appears to be a general consensus that abuse may 'consist of a single act or repeated acts' (DoH 2000a) and may be 'physical, sexual, psychological, financial/material, neglect/acts of omission or discrimination' (UKCC 1999, DoH 2000a). Definitions of abuse and neglect have occupied the thoughts and time of many commentators but those outlined in Box 3.1 appear to reflect today's thinking.

Box 3.1. Forms of abuse (DoH 2000a)

- Physical: including hitting, slapping, punching, kicking, misuse of medication, restraint or inappropriate sanctions
- Sexual: including rape and sexual assault or sexual acts to which the vulnerable adult has not consented, or could not consent or was pressured into consenting
- Psychological: including emotional abuse, threats of harm and abandonment, deprivation of contact, humiliation, blaming, controlling, intimidation, coercion, harassment, verbal abuse, isolation or withdrawal from services or supportive networks
- Financial/material: including theft, exploitation, pressure in connection with wills, property or inheritance or financial transactions, or the misuse or misappropriation of property, possessions or benefits
- Neglect/acts of omission: including ignoring medical or physical care needs, failure to provide access to appropriate health, social care or educational services, the withholding of the necessities of life (e.g. medication, adequate nutrition, heating)
- Discriminatory: including racist, sexist, that based on a person's disability, and other forms of harassment, slurs or similar treatment

---

An older person may experience more than one form of abuse and there may be more than one perpetrator. In some cases, there may be no identifiable perpetrator. Abuse may occur in the domestic setting or in an institution. Abusers may be relatives, friends, neighbours, formal or informal caregivers or strangers. Neglect or inadequate care may be a result of poor care resources, the inadequate coping strategies of informal carers or the inferior resourcing of health or social care settings. The individual may self-harm or self-neglect; indeed, Brogden and Nijhar (2000) suggest that half the referrals to welfare agencies relate to self-neglect. They further suggest that self-neglect may be a result of wilful or non-wilful behaviour (Box 3.2). Wilful neglect is identified as any behaviour that is a threat to the health, well-being or safety of self. Self-neglect 'occurs frequently in relation to the other forms of abuse and neglect but the mechanisms, motivations and underlying self-neglecting and self-abusive behaviour may be different than that caused by another' (Brogden and Nijhar 2000, p 41).

Box 3.2. Examples of self-neglect

Examples of wilful self-neglect:
    Abuse of illegal drugs
    Abuse of alcohol

Examples of non-wilful self-neglect:
    Forgetting to take one's medication
    Not eating properly

Assessment of possible abuse of older people

When an older person is referred to the MAU, it is imperative that the staff have the knowledge and understanding to recognise whether abuse, neglect or self-neglect is a factor in the presenting condition. There is a need to be aware of the indicators of abuse (CPA 1999) (Box 3.3) and to recognise circumstances in which abuse may have taken place. MAU nurses must have the confidence to take the appropriate action.

Box 3.3. Indicators of abuse (CPA 1999, p 52)

- The patient displays excessive drowsiness, general unhappiness, flinches or withdraws when approached
- Bruising/burns to inner arms and thighs, round wrists or ankles
- Injuries, inconsistent with history given
- Frequent minor injuries
- Sexual interference
- Poor nutrition
- Prescribed medication not being administered by carer
- Use of inappropriate medication in order to control behaviour

---

Where there may be suspicion of abuse or neglect, the assessment process must reflect and be linked to guidance outlined in the unit's/ Trust's policy on vulnerable adults. The assessment will involve the need to ask difficult questions. In order to do this sensitively it is important to create a physical environment where it is possible to talk to the patient in private. Questions need to be asked in such a way that patients are able to talk about their experiences of abuse or neglect.

Assessment of mental status

Bennett and Kingston (1993) state that an individual's mental status should always be ascertained before detailed questioning begins. Bennett and Kingston (1993) and Eastman (1994) suggest that a useful starting point for assessment of mental state is the abbreviated mental test. This consists of ten questions that test short-term and long-term memory, orientation and numeracy. A low score from this test does not necessarily indicate permanent mental impairment but may point to an obvious problem. A more detailed evaluation of memory may be achieved by performing a 'mini-mental state' test that consists of 20 questions (see Section C, Patients with mental health needs). The MAU nurse should note that a poor score does not mean that the patient lacks the capacity to give informed consent. Likewise, it does not mean that a person is totally lacking in judgement or understanding concerning their situation (Bennett 1994).

It is essential that patients are given a full explanation of the assessment process. Having their memory assessed may irritate those who are mentally competent and those who are not mentally competent may become fearful, anxious or agitated by the process. Box 3.4 indicates the information that the MAU nurse should collect in addition to demographic data collected on all patients.

It is important that the MAU has clear guidelines that govern the process of assessing and caring for patients suspected of being abused or neglected. In particular, consideration must be given to the principles governing the sharing of confidential information between members of the multidisciplinary team (SSI 1993, Kingston and Penhale 1995, DoH 2000a). Box 3.5 outlines guidelines for good practice when assessing abuse and neglect of older people.

If the assessment reveals the possibility of abuse, it should then be expanded to evaluate the degree of abuse. A number of factors should be considered when assessing the seriousness of an abusive situation (Box 3.6).

Box 3.4. Components of the assessment

- Assessment of the patient's physical status (ABDCE)
- Assessment of the patient's mental status
- General assessment of:
     hygiene
     skin integrity
     nutritional state
     dehydration
- Visual inspection for and assessment of:
     bruises, lacerations
     pressure sores
     bruising/bleeding of the rectum and genitalia
- Social network:
     relationships with family, friends, significant others
     social support systems
- Usual routines:
     ability to participate in day-to-day activities
     mobility
     medication

Box 3.5. Good practice guidelines for the assessment of abuse and neglect of older people

Assessment should:
- be provided in an environment in which it is possible to talk to the older person in private
- take account of the relationship between the older person and their carer(s)
- involve the older person in decision making where they are competent to do so
- recognise when there is a need for an independent advocate
- consider the needs of the carer(s), their coping resources, stress factors
- respect the need for confidentiality
- be carried out in accordance with the unit/Trust's policy

Box 3.6. Assessing the degree of abuse (DoH 2000a)

- The vulnerability of the individual
- The nature and extent of the abuse
- The length of time it has been occurring
- The impact on the individual
- The risk of repeated or increasingly serious acts involving this or any other vulnerable adult

The DoH (2000a) identifies the implications of the vulnerable adult's capacity to make choices and take risks when decisions need to be made in terms of investigating or managing abusive situations. As an example, older people may refuse offers of help or assistance and have the right to do so. There are circumstances in which the right to self-determination and autonomy may not be upheld, for example 'in situations where the individual is severely cognitively incapacitated and not legally competent to make such decisions' (Penhale and Kingston 1997).

In the case of older people, MAU nurses must have some understanding of the ageing process. They should be able to distinguish between what may be the result of frailty or illness and what may be the result of abuse or neglect. Bennett (1990), Bennett and Kingston (1993) and Eastman (1994) all make the point that the establishment of abuse in older people can be complicated. The physical or behavioural pointers that may indicate the presence of abuse in children are not so easily identified in older people. Bennett (1990) and Bennett and Kingston (1993) suggest that the comparative norms available in childhood are absent in ageing and that 'the physiological changes that occur with ageing are not well known even by most health care professionals dealing with the elderly' (Bennett and Kingston 1993, p 34).

Researchers in the field of abuse and neglect of older people stress that assessment of abuse and neglect must be as holistic as possible and should not be based purely on physical signs. For example, many writers have identified that some older people develop what is known as transparent skin syndrome in which the thinning of the skin is so severe it is easily damaged even in normal handling. Severe bruising, therefore, should not be used as a definitive sign of abuse or neglect but it should be noted (Bennett and Kingston 1993, Eastman 1994). It is essential, therefore, that the assessment should not be rushed. The CPA/NHS (1999) state that all NHS providers must have a policy on elder abuse. Similarly, the 'No Secrets' document (DoH 2000a), which in part was driven by what is now the 1998 Human Rights Act (DoH 2001a), demonstrates the commitment expected of those delivering health and social care services in protecting vulnerable adults.

Nursing actions in the event of suspected abuse

If the assessment process indicates evidence or suspicion of abuse/neglect, options for referral need to be considered. Penhale and Kingston (1997) suggest that assessment frameworks should adequately address risk factors and risky situations and that any decisions should be based on the 'degree of risk and priority of the situation'. A multidisciplinary approach with the agreement of the patient should be taken in any decision making unless the individual is suffering severe cognitive impairment. Once identified, an abusive situation should be monitored following the guidance stated in the unit/Trust policy. This policy should include details of options for referral to appropriate care agencies, how such referrals can be made and by whom. Options for referral need to be available 24 hours per day, 365 days per year.

While the first priority in the case of suspected abuse is the safety and protection of the vulnerable adult, it is also important to deal sensitively with the suspected perpetrator. Consideration should be given to the needs of all those involved. Information should be given in respect of the complaint against the suspected perpetrator and they should be made aware of their rights. It is unlikely that an individual MAU nurse would be directly responsible for reporting serious cases to the police but they do need to be aware of legal concepts that may be relevant (Box 3.7).

Box 3.7. Legislation and legal concepts relevant to the care of the vulnerable adult (Bennett and Kingston 1993)

- The Mental Health Act (1983)
- The National Assistance Act (1948) (Section 47)
- The Chronically Sick and Disabled Persons Act (1970)
- Guardianship
- Power of Attorney
- Enduring Power of Attorney
- Agency

Summary

Responding to the sensitive issues in respect of abuse and neglect can be a daunting and difficult task for MAU nurses. It is essential that they develop the skills and knowledge to enable them t readilyo identify potential victims of abuse and neglect. The nurse's role becomes paramount in identifying, monitoring and supporting older people who are at risk. Assessment frameworks need to be implemented, or adapted, to include full consideration of indicators of risk of abuse and neglect. Appropriate assessment is crucial to the subsequent organisation of care or intervention. If abuse and neglect of vulnerable adults is to be given the commitment it deserves it is not sufficient simply to raise staff awareness. There is a need for all practitioners who work with older people to be trained to detect and manage suspected abuse or neglect.

B. INDIVIDUALS WITH LEARNING DISABILITIES
(Michael Gibbs and Judi Thorley)

Aims

This section will:

- discuss the concept of learning disability, its policy development and theoretical perspectives
- equip the MAU nurse with the knowledge and understanding to effectively meet the needs of people with learning disabilities
- discuss principles of assessment, communication and education
- discuss the role of the liaison nurse in supporting the MAU staff to meet the needs of people with a learning disability by effectively utilising their existing skills

Fundamental principles

People with learning disabilities share the same risk factors relating to cardiovascular and respiratory disease, cancers, mental illness, sexual health and accidents as other individuals in society (Turner and Moss 1996). Indeed, they may even be more susceptible to some health problems (Bailey and Cooper 1997). Similarly, a person with a learning disability has the same feelings and needs as anyone in society and has the capacity to interact and gain from their environment at all levels of functioning. These fundamental principles underpin the assertion that people with learning disabilities have the same right to services including health provision. It is unacceptable to refuse or to offer inferior treatment to anyone because he or she has a learning disability (Lindsey 1998). *The NHS Plan* (Department of Health (DoH) 2000b) takes this philosophy further by suggesting that the NHS must be responsive to the needs of different groups and individuals within society. It states that discrimination on the grounds of age, gender, ethnicity, religion, disability and sexuality must be challenged. The Department of Health's publication *Valuing People* (DoH 2001b) has made a significant contribution to the potential service provision for people with learning disabilities, particularly with the concept of the health care facilitator.

Definitions of learning disability

The concept of learning disability is complex and many definitions have been used over the years. The 1913 Mental Deficiency Act (Malin et al 1980) included 'idiots, imbeciles, feeble-minded and moral defectives'. The 1959 Mental Health Act (Ministry of Health 1959) defined 'subnormality' and 'severe subnormality'. More recently, the 1983 Mental Health Act (Department of Health and Social Security (DHSS) 1983) identified mental impairment as 'a state of arrested or incomplete development of mind ... which includes significant impairment of intellectual functioning and is associated with abnormal aggressive or seriously irresponsible conduct on the part of the person concerned'. These legal definitions emphasise the negative aspects of learning disability and were used to legitimise the use of a range of treatments.

There are other, more humanistic approaches to the definition of learning disability. Classifying an individual's disability by means of various tests to determine their intellectual ability in the form of IQ scales (and hence their ability to perform intellectual tasks and solve problems) is one approach. Another perspective is to assess social competence and the way an individual adapts to the changing demands made by society. On this basis, any individual performing significantly below what might be considered as 'normal' may be assessed as having a learning disability (Gates 1997). Many people without learning disabilities could be so described given that familial and environmental factors impinge on an individual's level of social competence. Another perspective on learning disability is that of the individual's reduced cognitive ability. These people may have reduced ability to understand complex information and situations, may have difficulty in learning and developing new skills and may be unable to live an independent lifestyle.

In 1992, the Department of Health adopted the more socially acceptable term 'learning disability'. In this context, learning disability is categorised as being mild, moderate, severe or profound. Most individuals so defined possess verbal communication skills, whilst those without these skills employ different methods to communicate their thoughts, wishes and values. Most people with learning disability struggle with abstract concepts and complex ideas but have many talents, qualities, strengths and support needs (Lindsey and Russell 1999).

Assessment skills

The skills required when assessing a person with learning disabilities are identical to those employed for any other person referred to the MAU, in that their immediate physiological needs are identified and treated as a priority. The often diverse and complex health needs of the person with learning disabilities (Callan et al 1995) mean that this assessment process is dynamic and a different approach to communication is therefore required. During the assessment, it is essential that the MAU nurse includes the patient's carers, as a source both of effective communication with the patient and of information regarding the patient's previous medical and social history.

MAU nurses already possess the key skills required to assess patients with learning disabilities. The challenge lies in realising that their existing skills as carer, communicator, observer, therapist, advocate and counsellor (Baldwin and Birchenall 1993, Jones 1999) apply to these patients. Many nurses feel that they do not possess the necessary skills and knowledge of learning disabilities to deliver care to a high standard. It is evident that nurses and other health care professionals need to feel confident in caring for people with learning disabilities in order to utilise effectively their skills in delivering appropriate care. This confidence can be gained through an in-depth understanding of communication and through education and training.

Communication

Communication takes many forms ranging from the spoken word to non-verbal facial expressions, gestures, postures and emotional states (Callan et al 1995). For the person with a learning disability, the nurse's interpretation of the individual's non-verbal communication may be of paramount importance. Given that some people with learning disabilities make fewer non-verbal cues, it is often difficult for the nurse to recognise that they are trying to convey a message. If these non-verbal cues are not recognised by the nurse, the patient may reduce the number of cues even further, making communication even more difficult (Ferris-Taylor 1997). This interactive model of communication, in which the interaction may not be verbal, has been described by Bradley and Edinberg (1990). Case example 1 illustrates how effective communication can be developed.

Case example 1

Mary, a 46-year-old woman, is referred to the MAU by her GP. She has been complaining of chest pain for two days. On arrival, she looks well but is constantly hitting herself. When the nurse attempts to ask her questions, Mary starts to shout and scream loudly and uses increasing amounts of force to hit herself. This makes it impossible for the MAU nurse to make an assessment at this time.

The response described in this case may not be a sign of self-injurious behaviour or a physical threat to others, but may be this particular individual's way of communicating her fears of being in a strange and potentially threatening environment. The MAU nurse could attempt to reduce this woman's anxieties and fears by moving her to a smaller and quieter area to be assessed. Another approach may be the use of simple conversation supplemented by the use of pictures, images or signs. Similarly, the nurse may try demonstrating a blood pressure being taken on herself before this procedure is carried out on the patient. Such an approach may help the nurse to gain the patient's confidence and co-operation.

The approach to communication in this case example is time-consuming, but it is important that the person with a learning disability has complete trust in the nurse. Consequently, the nurse may have to delay the completion of a physical assessment and any investigations until the individual is less anxious. Demonstration of procedures can assist with the development of trust. Despite the fact that MAUs operate on the principle of patients being rapidly assessed and treated, it is important for the MAU nurse to recognise that their priorities might need to be directed by the individual's needs rather than by nursing or medical procedures. This can be difficult in MAUs where patient throughput is high and nurses have multiple demands upon their time. To ensure effective communication and assist in patient assessment, a degree of lateral thinking may be required. In order to facilitate social interaction, the principles outlined in Box 3.8 can be applied.

By using these principles, the nurse can facilitate effective interaction and communication. Repeated and continual giving of information and explanations can help to support this process. Using the example of taking a blood pressure, 'ice-breaking' statements that may be used include:

- 'Can I sit here whilst I take your blood pressure?'
- 'I would like to take your blood pressure with this machine, do you want to hold it? This is what is does.'
- 'Let me show you on me first.'

Box 3.8. Principles of communication with learning disabled patients

- Always introduce yourself and all appropriate others
- Use language that the person is likely to understand
- Avoid the use of jargon or abbreviations – these may cause confusion and increase the person's anxiety
- Always re-direct the focus of the conversation to the individual concerned – 'ice-breaking' statements can assist with this process
- Be aware of the importance of body language
- Note the positioning of the patient, relatives and staff – if necessary change positions so that the MAU nurse can observe the non-verbal cues clearly
- Sitting at the same level and trying not to stand over the person creates a better therapeutic relationship
- Assist the person to answer questions by giving them extra time to think
- Be careful not to rush in with predetermined answers

These are simple ways of breaking down barriers and overcoming patients' fears. Be prepared to leave the patient for a short time. This enables the person to familiarise themselves with the situation and seek clarification from their carer. When the nurse returns, ask the patient if they have any questions. Continuing the blood pressure example, this could involve leaving the machine with the patient and their carer to allow them to inspect the equipment. The nurse may return a short time later and ask, 'Are you okay now, shall we take your blood pressure?'

Remember that the patient should be the focus of the nurse's attention. With this in mind, always ask the patient what they want rather than asking their carer. You should be aware, though, of verbal and non-verbal cues from the carer. It is important to realise that the behaviour of the nurse gives cues to the patient. Consequently, if the nurse behaves respectfully the patient is more likely to do likewise.

Education and training

Cullen (1988) stated that in order to improve communication with the client, it is essential first to change the behaviour of the staff. McConkey and Truesdale (2000) support this assertion when they discuss the differing attitudes and reactions of nurses and therapists when they meet people with learning disabilities. In 1998, Mencap produced the results of a national survey that examined health care provision for people with learning disabilities. The results highlighted the continuing need for improvement not only in access and communication but also in the attitudes of health care professionals. This need for improvement is well documented (McConkey and Truesdale 2000, Slevin and Sines 1996, Biley 1994). Since the publication of *Signposts for Success* (Lindsey 1998), the need and specification for improved services for people with learning disabilities in accessing acute and general health care has been widely accepted and implemented across the UK (Cumella and Martin 2000). When developing services, several fundamental questions should be asked in relation to how the MAU staff care for people with learning disabilities (Box 3.9).

Box 3.9. Questions to be asked of the current system

- What are the actual and potential needs of this patient group?
- Are these needs being met by the current system? Whom do we ask to find out?
- Could the system be improved?
- Is there a unit-wide desire to improve the service?
- What are the attitudes of the unit's staff to patients with learning disability?
- Do the staff have educational needs?
- What resources do we have to address issues raised by this exercise?
- What links do we have with learning disability nurses?

In 1998, Lindsey made clear recommendations for staff working throughout the NHS. One recommendation was for learning disability nurses to be available to offer education, advice and support to health care professionals as required, 24 hours a day. In some hospitals (the author's [JT] included), this has been achieved by the establishment of a Liaison Nurse Specialist service. An important aspect of this role is the establishment of aims and objectives not only to meet the learning needs of the professionals but also to ensure a measurable improvement in services offered to people with learning disabilities. If sufficient needs were identified in other hospitals, MAUs could employ liaison nurses more widely. More commonly, arrangements could be made to access expert advice and support through the hospital's existing learning disability manager on-call system. This system could be supplemented by weekly visits to the MAU to facilitate both a support system for staff and a mechanism for the referral of patients requesting or identified as requiring follow-up.

To improve communication with patients with learning disability, nurses need to supplement their verbal communication skills with non-verbal tools such as sign language and pictures. In order to address specific issues regarding staff education, a programme of teaching should therefore concentrate on effective communication techniques. This programme should also recognise the importance of co-morbidity in respect of people with mental health needs and learning disability, general health needs and learning disability, consent and challenging behaviour.

In the authors' own work settings, a communication leaflet using Makaton pictures (Walker 1996) has been devised and implemented along with guidelines for staff. In addition, posters and leaflets have been used to highlight the service available. The service, comprising a liaison nurse, programme of teaching, posters and leaflets, has been running for three years and is currently being evaluated to measure its effectiveness and to identify areas for development. Initially based in the local A&E department, the service has since been extended to provide support to the MAU, surgical assessment unit, central treatment suite, outpatient's department, radiology, pathology and some ward areas. This service needs to continue in order to facilitate the improvement of health care professionals' attitudes and to ensure the provision of a 'complete service' that is able to meet all the health needs of people with learning disabilities.

Case examples 2 and 3, both of which are from clinical practice, demonstrate the value of a liaison service to the person with learning disability, their carers and health care professionals. (To ensure anonymity, pseudonyms have been used.)

Case example 2

David is a 34-year-old man with a mild learning disability and mental health problems in the form of anxiety and depression. He lives alone and manages his day-to-day life very well. David's mother died 3 years previously and he has struggled to come to terms with his loss. David has a community nurse, social worker and consultant psychiatrist with whom he maintains contact when he is feeling well. When his depression is acute, David isolates himself and refuses to attend appointments and declines input from professionals. As David had previously expressed suicidal thoughts, the liaison nurse discussed the situation with David, other professionals involved and A&E colleagues. Arrangements were made that if David attended A&E, the learning disability on-call manager would be contacted as soon as possible. When David did attend the department saying that he had suicidal thoughts, the medical and nursing staff were able to contact the learning disability on-call manager, who arranged for a consultant psychiatrist to speak with David. Subsequently, arrangements were made for David to be admitted for respite care with staff that he knew.

Case example 2 illustrates how a well-planned system enabled early intervention that prevented David having to wait in what to him may have been a threatening and strange environment (the A&E department). It also shows how an admission to an acute psychiatric ward was prevented, thereby removing the need for David to deal with what may have been a potentially difficult situation for him.

Case example 3

Adam is a 40-year-old man with mild to moderate learning disabilities. He lives in a private community home for people with learning disabilities. Adam was admitted to the MAU with a suspected gastrointestinal bleed and, from the MAU, was admitted to a medical ward. When no source of bleeding was found, Adam was discharged home the following day. During his initial assessment on the MAU, nursing staff became concerned about Adam's other health needs. He had previously been diagnosed as asthmatic but seemed to be poorly controlled. He was also obese and smoked at least 25 cigarettes per day. Consequently, the MAU nurses referred Adam to the learning disability liaison nurse to follow up these health issues with him at home.

Having discussed the situation with Adam's community nurse both she and the liaison nurse arranged to meet with Adam to assess his health needs. In this relaxed setting, the liaison nurse was able to assess Adam's understanding of his asthma and his technique when using his inhalers. It was evident that there were learning needs in both of these areas not only for Adam but also for the care staff involved. After some short teaching sessions for both parties, their understanding of asthma was improved and Adam's care more effectively managed. Adam was also encouraged to reduce his smoking by the use of a reward system. He has since reduced to 18 cigarettes per day.

By improving his asthma management, Adam now has more energy and confidence and has taken up walking and gardening. Both these activities have had a positive impact on his weight.

Both of these case examples illustrate how the development of a learning disability liaison service can positively influence the care delivered to this potentially vulnerable group of patients. All nurses have a role in health promotion but nurses working in MAUs are in an enviable position, in that they have the opportunity to assess the overall health and well-being of the patients in their care.

Summary

MAU nurses must maintain the involvement and autonomy of the person with a learning disability and their carers. Their rights to dignity and privacy in the hospital setting must be respected irrespective of their communication ability and the nurse's own limitations and skills. This chapter has highlighted how MAU nurses can positively influence the care of this vulnerable group of patients. They already possess many of the skills required to do so. The knowledge and skills they do not possess can be developed by effective education and training facilitated by a liaison nurse. The challenge lies in recognising the need for education, acquiring new skills and putting those skills into practice.

C. PATIENTS WITH MENTAL HEALTH NEEDS
(Elizabeth Whelan)

Aims

This section will:

- provide a structured approach to the assessment of patients with mental health needs
- describe the components of a combined physical and mental health assessment
- promote understanding of specific assessment tools, including when and how to apply them in the MAU setting

Introduction

Most patients with mental health disorders first present to their general practitioners (GP) with physical complaints such as inability to sleep, lack of energy, or vague aches and pains (Harrison et al 1998, Craig and Boardman 1998). Patients may have co-existing physical and mental health problems (for example, poorly controlled diabetes may lead to depression). Alternatively, the patient's physical illness such as cancer, heart disease or chronic pain may have precipitated mental health problems. Since 12% of patients referred to medical outpatients have psychologically based physical problems (somatisation) (Ramirez and House 1998) and 20% of medical inpatients have a co-existing depressive or anxiety disorder (Harrison et al 1998), it is likely that many patients referred to MAUs will have some kind of mental health need. Health care professionals are not immune to feeling negatively disposed towards patients with mental health disorders, resulting in segregation and avoidance of these patients in the general ward setting (Brinn 2000). It is important, therefore, that nurses have a sound knowledge of mental health issues and their recognition, as effective management has been shown to improve outcome for this vulnerable group of patients (Harrison et al 1998).

Most common mental health disorders

The International Statistical Classification of Diseases (ICD) (WHO 1992) has defined one hundred categories relating to mental health disorders. For ease of use, these are condensed into 10 divisions. The seven relating solely to adults are outlined in Table 3.1. The mental health charity MIND has compiled a frequency of mental health disorders that coincide with several of these classifications (MIND 2001); these are included within the table.

Within the MAU setting, mental health disorders are usually described in one of the following ways:

1. Psychosis is defined as 'gross impairment of reality testing'. Psychoses are disturbances characterised by delusions and hallucinations (Townsend 1999, Davies 1997). Psychotic disorders include schizophrenia, psychotic depression, mania, toxic drug reaction, dementia and delirium. This definition can be further expanded by defining 'delusions' as 'false beliefs which are fixed and are not amenable to logic or explanation' and 'hallucinations' as 'false sensory perceptions that involve any of the five senses such as auditory hallucinations in schizophrenia' (Isaacs 2001).
2. Neurosis refers to disorders in which anxiety or emotional symptoms predominate. Neurotic disorders include anxiety, panic disorders and somatoform disorders. Neurosis is now little used except in literature as it is difficult to define (Townsend 1999, Davies 1997).

Table 3.1. ICD codes for mental health disorders (WHO 1992)

ICD-10 code	Division	Categories include	Frequency
F00–F09	Organic – including symptomatic mental disorder	Dementia in Alzheimer's disease Vascular dementia Delirium not induced by alcohol/substances Brain disease/damage	Dementia – 6% of people over 65 and 20% of people over 80 in the UK (Social Services Inspectorate 1996)
F10–F19	Mental and behavioural disorders due to psychoactive substance abuse	Acute intoxication Dependence syndrome Withdrawal state Psychotic disorder	Alcohol dependence in 4.7% of UK adults Drug dependence in 2.2% of adults living at home (Davies 1997)
F20–F29	Schizophrenia, schizotypal and delusional disorders	Schizophrenia Persistent delusional disorders Acute and transient psychotic disorders Schizoaffective disorders	Schizophrenia – under 1% of UK population with 2–4 cases per 1000 at any one time (Birchwood et al 1989)
F30–F39	Mood (affective) disorders	Manic episodes Bipolar affective disorder Depressive episode Recurrent depressive disorder	Depression – 10% of the population at any one time Lifetime prevalence between 18–25% (Hale 1997)
F40–F49	Neurotic, stress-related and somatoform disorders	Phobic anxiety disorders Obsessive–compulsive disorder Reaction to severe stress Hypochondriacal disorder	Anxiety – 3.1% of adult population A further 7.7% have mixed anxiety and depression 1.2% with obsessive–compulsive disorder (Meltzer 1995)
F50–F59	Behavioural syndromes associated with physiological disturbances and physical factors	Eating disorders Non organic sleep disorders Sexual dysfunction Abuse of non dependence producing substances	For UK women between ages of 15 and 30 years, 1% suffer from anorexia nervosa and 1–2% from bulimia nervosa (Mental Health Foundation 1997)
F60–F69	Disorders of adult personality and behaviour	Personality disorders (borderline) Enduring personality change after catastrophic experience or psychiatric illness Habit and impulse disorders (e.g. gambling) Gender identity disorders	Personality disorder between 2 and 13% (MIND 2001)

The complex presentation of mental health problems with their myriad of potential physical and psychological components increases the vulnerability of this patient group. For this reason, it is important that MAU nurses assess these patients effectively and accurately. Ward (1995) suggests that referral to a hospital involves many stressors for patients with mental health problems. These include:

- admission to hospital
- medication being changed

- being cared for in an unfamiliar environment
- possible exacerbation of mental health problems by acute physical problems including infections or constipation
- discharge from hospital

Repeated visits to their GP and return visits to A&E departments by a patient with a mental health problem would suggest that there has been a failure to address the patient's psychological needs adequately. This can lead to increased difficulty in coping and, eventually, to a crisis. The key to addressing these issues in MAU is a combined physical and mental health assessment, which can provide vital information to measure the patient's level of distress and define the treatment acuity that is essential for effective management. Assessment in this context aims to answer the questions in Box 3.10.

Box 3.10. Initial assessment of the patient with a possible mental health problem

- Does the patient have any life-threatening or potentially life-threatening physical problems?
- Is the patient in distress?
- Are they able to co-operate with the assessment process?
- Is their behaviour likely to be unpredictable (e.g. noisy, aggressive, rude, walking naked, wandering, abusive (Mavundla 2000))?
- Are they at risk because of mental distress or self-harm or are they likely to place others at risk (Atakan and Davies 1997)?
- Are they likely to abscond?
- Is there a supportive person with them?
- What level of supervision do they require?
- Are they likely to be a risk to others?

The assessment of patients with a mental health problem has two components, the physical assessment and the psychological assessment.

Physical assessment

Before physical symptoms can be attributed to a mental health problem, an initial assessment of the patient's airway, breathing and circulation must be carried out to exclude an organic cause. In this way, any acute physical problems can be identified and treated. In addition to the assessment procedures discussed in Chapter 2 – Initial assessment, if a mental health problem is suspected consider adding the components outlined in Box 3.11.

Box 3.11. Additional components of the initial assessment

Observations
- Head to toe observation for injury (signs of self-harm, needle/track marks)
- Neurological: Is the patient lethargic or alert? What is their pupil size and reactivity?
- Psychomotor activity: Do they have any tics or tremors, altered gait or agitated movements?
- Musculoskeletal: Is their co-ordination and movement altered?

Investigations
- Altered blood glucose level may be associated with a change in mental status (e.g. hypoglycaemia can cause anxiety and personality changes or schizophrenia-like features (Good and Nelson 1986)

Patient records
- Past medical and psychiatric history
- Current medication (polypharmacy may cause interactions between medications)

Many physical conditions may cause an alteration in normal behaviour patterns. The MAU nurse should be aware that a number of chronic illnesses could affect neurological or mental status. Table 3.2 outlines some of these conditions.

Table 3.2. Physical conditions that may exhibit psychological symptoms (Good and Nelson 1986, Molitor 1996)

Condition	Presenting features
Addison's disease	Withdrawal, apathy and depression
Hyperthyroidism	Hyperactivity (can mimic 'mania'), irritability
Hypoglycaemia	Personality changes
Lung cancer	Progressive dementia, anxiety or panic attacks
Phaeochromocytomas	Progressive dementia, anxiety or panic attacks
Vitamin B12 deficiency	Visual hallucinations, personality changes, dementia
Hypocalcaemia	Any psychiatric symptom
Alcohol withdrawal	Delirium, hallucinations, acute anxiety
Epilepsy	Repetitive behaviours, manic-like psychosis
Head injury/hypoxia	Altered conscious level
Infection/constipation	Mental confusion

In addition to the conditions outlined in Table 3.2 patients prescribed anti-hypertensives and anti-ulcer medications may display psychological symptoms. Examples of these medications include methyldopa (causes depression) and cimetidine (causes toxic psychosis) (Good and Nelson 1986).

Psychological assessment

All patients should have a mental health assessment completed even when there are no apparent cognitive, emotional or behavioural problems. As a basis for the initial assessment of a patient's mental health status, consider factors relating to their presenting problem and insight, previous psychiatric history, environment, associated risk factors and the potential for violence and/or aggression.

Presenting problem and insight

The patient's answers to the following questions may help to give an indication of their current situation and their level of insight.

- What does the patient think is their main problem?
- What do they think caused it?
- What other problems does the patient have?
- Did the problems start recently or are they part of a chronic illness?
- Does the patient have a current physical illness that may be contributing to the problem?
- Has there been a recent trauma or head injury that could have contributed to the onset of symptoms?
- Is there anything that makes the problem worse or better? How is it affecting their daily lives?
- Does the patient think anything is wrong with them?
- What is their understanding of their present difficulty?

The patient should be encouraged to answer the question in his or her own words, and may need encouragement to remain focused on the current problem. When necessary and appropriate, information may be obtained from friends or relatives. If this is the case, the source of the information must be noted in the patient's notes.

Previous psychiatric history

The patient's previous psychiatric history can provide a valuable insight into their current situation. Details need to be confirmed for accuracy against previous medical records. Information to be collected should include:

- Previous psychiatric episodes/admissions?
- What were the patient's main problems?
- What therapy was given?
- Did they comply with therapy?
- Was the therapy effective?
- What was the mental state between episodes? (i.e. What was their level of recovery? Did any recovery take place with or without therapy?)

Environment

Essential details of the patient's background and social circumstances provide an invaluable context for their problems. Information already available through a patient's GP or hospital notes needs to be confirmed for accuracy. The information collected should include details regarding cohabitation, housing, employment, financial situation and any family history of mental health problems.

Risk factors

According to Harrison et al (1998), a detailed risk assessment is required for those patients who have expressed suicidal intentions, have a history of mood disorder, psychosis or substance abuse or a history of self-harm or violence. The assessment of risk associated with mental health problems is most often related to the danger that the patient presents to others. More commonly, and of equal importance, is the risk of harm to themselves and the risk of absconding prior to treatment. The history, assessment and the context of the present situation may reveal other features that are associated with risk of harm (Box 3.12). (For further information on risk assessment, see Atakan and Davies 1997 and Wyatt et al 1999.)

Box 3.12. Factors associated with risk of harm

- Personal history of self-harm or violent behaviour
- Planning of a suicide attempt
- Recent stress or loss
- Considerable mood disturbances
- Substance misuse
- Chronic painful physical conditions

Violence and aggression

In difficult situations (e.g. the unexpected admission to hospital), almost any patient (or their relatives) may make threats, behave aggressively or violently. Not all will have an underlying mental health problem. No single assessment tool accurately predicts likelihood of violence. However, Atakan and Davies (1997) have identified a number of risk factors which may enable the MAU nurse to predict a potentially violent situation. The risk factors include:

• history of violent behaviour
• threats of violence
• psychotic or neurotic disorders
• misuse of alcohol/illicit drugs (e.g. intoxication or withdrawal)
• behaviour associated with violence (e.g. clenched fists, pacing, shouting)
• metabolic disorders (e.g. hypoxia or hypoglycaemia)

Mental health assessment in more detail

The above information can be collected as the basis of an initial assessment of a patient's mental health status. From this assessment, if a mental health problem is suspected, the MAU nurse can use the following assessment framework to provide a more detailed mental health assessment (Seidel et al 1998, Townsend 1999).

• Appearance
• Behaviour
• Cognitive ability and communication
• Disposition and emotional responses

1. Appearance

The patient's appearance can give an indication of their mental status. However, it is impossible to make generalisations in this respect. The following issues may be useful indicators:

• Clothing – is the patient's clothing appropriate for the time of day, the weather and/or the time of year?
• Neglect – are there obvious signs of self-neglect such as poor hygiene and body odour?

- Nutrition – is the patient unusually thin or emaciated? Is there evidence of weight loss or gain? Recent weight loss may be indicative of physical illness or chronic anxiety.
- Body language – assess the patient's posture. Is it tense? Is the patient slumped?
- Facial expression – is the patient's expression suggestive of irritability or anxiety?
- Substance misuse – is there any suggestion of drug, alcohol or substance misuse? Assess the patient's pupils. Are they dilated or pinpoint? Pupils become pinpoint with the use of opioids, dilated by alcohol.

2. Behaviour

This refers to the patient's observable activities and can include the following:

- Movements – are there any unusual movements such as tremors, tics or ataxia?
- Psychomotor activity – is the patient agitated? Are they pacing about the area? Patients with an elevated mood may be overactive and restless. Patients with a depressive illness may be slow in initiating movement and slow in performing that movement.
- Reaction – how does the patient respond to being assessed? Is the patient angry? Are they over-familiar, fearful, tearful or guarded?

3. Cognitive ability and communication

Cognitive ability

The following aspects can give an indication of a patient's cognitive ability:

- Level of response – is the patient alert, drowsy, responding to stimuli? Stupor (total immobility, no response to stimuli) can be a catatonic feature of schizophrenia or a feature of an organic disorder.
- Orientation – is the patient orientated? Can they remember their name, where they are, what year it is?
- Memory and attention span – can the patient remember three everyday items after 3 minutes?
- Judgement – is the patient able to make accurate judgements about the situation? Are they able to give informed consent to treatment?

- Thought processes – are they well ordered, coherent and relevant? Is the patient preoccupied?
- Content – is there flight of ideas? Is there poverty of thought? A patient with severe depression may complain of an inability to gather or express thoughts.
- Paranoia/delusions – is the patient expressing hypochondriacal delusions of bodily disease, which are rigidly maintained despite medical evidence to the contrary?
- Perceptual distortions – has the patient any auditory hallucinations (described as voices that issue orders or make suggestions)? These are most common in psychotic disorders such as schizophrenia.

Communication

Aspects of verbal and non-verbal communication should be assessed along with the content of the conversation. Remember to consider language barriers and cultural influences when assessing communication.

- Speech – is the verbal rate uninterruptible or is it slow? Is the volume loud or quiet? Is the quality of speech hesitant or slurred? Articulation difficulty can suggest a neurological disorder or the side effect of antipsychotic drugs.
- Content – is the patient confused? Is the patient expressing unusual ideas, using inappropriate word substitutions? Are they expressing ideas of self-harm or harm to others? Do they feel in danger?
- Non-verbal – is eye contact intense, staring or poor (if culturally appropriate)?

4. Disposition and emotional responses

This refers to the patient's mood, emotions and the atmosphere of the interview and includes the following:

- Mood – subjectively, how does the patient perceive his or her own mood? Objectively, note the predominant mood during the assessment. Is it fluctuating? Is it appropriate to the situation? Do the patient's perceptions and your own observations on mood correspond?
- Is the patient angry or agitated? Is the patient sad and despondent (depression) or euphoric and elated (bipolar disorder)? How does the patient feel about himself or herself? Is the patient feeling worthless or unreal (depersonalisation)? Is there an exaggerated sense of ability?

Using the above framework can help to build up a more detailed assessment of a patient's mental status. It is unlikely that any single patient will exhibit all of the above indicators.

Specific assessment tools

Assessment tools are a useful aid to identify a potential problem. Common tools include those for cognitive impairment, alcohol misuse and suicide. These should be used as indicated during the initial assessment.

Cognitive impairment

The mini-mental state examination may be used to provide a numeric rating of cognitive ability. A score of 20 or less is indicative of confusion and/or impaired communication (Table 3.3).

Table 3.3. The mini-mental state examination (Wyatt et al 1999, Seidel et al 1998)

Assess	Method	Score
Orientation for time	Day, date, month, season, year	1 point each
Orientation for place	Country, county, city/town, hospital, name of the ward/unit	1 point each
Learning of new information	Name three unrelated objects (clock, umbrella, carrot) Patient must remember all three objects	1 point each – at first attempt only
Attention and concentration	Spell 'world' backwards	1 point each letter in the correct order
Short-term memory	'Tell me the three items that we named a few minutes ago'	1 point each
Language	Point to a pen and wristwatch and ask the patient to name them.	2 points
	Repeat the phrase 'No ifs, ands or buts'.	1 point
	Tell the patient to follow these instructions 'Take this piece of paper in your right hand, fold it in half and put it on the floor'.	1 point for each part
	Read and obey: show the patient a piece of paper with the phrase 'Close your eyes' written on it and ask them to follow the instructions	1 point
	Ask the patient to write a short sentence	1 point – if it makes sense
	Ask the patient to copy a diagram (e.g. two five-sided shapes that are intersecting)	1 point

Alcohol or drug use

When assessing for potentially problematic alcohol or drug use, the CAGE mnemonic (Mayfield et al 1974) may be used as an aide-mémoire. Using this approach, if the patient admits to drinking alcohol, the following questions could be asked.

- Have you ever thought you should **C**ut down on your drinking?
- Have people ever **A**nnoyed you by criticising your drinking?
- Have you ever felt **G**uilty about your drinking?
- Have you ever had an **E**ye-opener (drink) first thing in the morning?

If the patient answers 'yes' to two or more questions, Mayfield et al (1974) state that the likelihood of alcohol misuse is very high. To make an accurate assessment, this tool relies on the patient answering truthfully.

Suicide

There are many assessment tools for assessing suicide risk. One that may be useful is the 'SAD PERSONS' scale (Patterson et al 1983). Using this approach, objective and subjective information is collected and scores allocated according to the responses. The information and associated scores are as follows:

S sex	female = 0	male = 1
A age	<19 or >45 = 1	other ages = 0
D depression/hopelessness		= 1
P previous attempts		= 1
E excessive alcohol/drug use		= 1
R rational thinking loss (psychotic or organic illness)		= 1
S separated, widowed, divorced		= 1
O organised or serious suicide attempt		= 1
N no social support		= 1
S stated future suicide intent		= 1

When the scores are added together, an indication of the patient's suicide risk is obtained as outlined below:

Total score <3 = low risk
Total score 3–6 = medium risk
Total score >6 = high risk

Management of the patient with a mental health need

The medical and/or mental health diagnosis and stage of the illness will determine the selection of psychological, pharmacological or social options of management. Following the nursing assessment of both medical and mental health needs, an analysis is required to determine the priorities in the plan of care. The analysis may determine needs common to many disorders. The priorities for a plan of care are as follows (after Polli and Lazear 2000):

- identify and treat life-threatening emergencies
- maintain airway, breathing and circulation
- prevent complications
- maintain safety of the patient, other patients, relatives and staff
- administer medications as prescribed and monitor effects
- provide suitable ward environment

A nursing care plan for patients with specific mental health disorders can be seen in Table 3.4, page 64.

Any attendance at hospital is filled with anxiety-provoking stimuli and nurses can help reduce this by providing order and keeping the patient informed so that they can prepare themselves. Allowing the patient choices and including the patient in decisions when possible can increase their sense of being in control of the situation. The provision of information and explanations can also reduce anxiety (Hudak and Gallo 1994).

Nurses also need to manage risk, which encompasses the need for psychiatric referral, risk of self-harm or suicide, and/or risk of aggression/violence (Heslop et al 2000). If a patient has been assessed as being at risk (an ongoing process) of harming themselves or others, then appropriate measures must be employed to prevent them causing harm (Table 3.5). Common law allows reasonable restraint of such patients until appropriate medical/psychiatric personnel arrive. The emergency admission to hospital of a mentally ill patient is covered by the Mental Health Act in England and Wales (Department of Health and Social Security 1983). If the Act is invoked, the correct documentation must be used and completed accurately. It is useful for MAU staff to familiarise themselves with the requirements of the Act and the relevant documentation before they are needed. Methods for managing the patient at risk are identified in Table 3.5.

Table 3.4. A nursing care plan based on the patient's mental health disorder (Selfridge-Thomas 1995, Polli and Lazear 2000, Isaacs 2001)

Disorder	Clinical features	Nursing care
Anxiety	Not always sure what they are anxious about History of panic attacks Precipitating incident Tachycardia, headache, hyperventilation, nausea, diarrhoea, chest tightness, hypertension Tremors, irritability, anger, pacing, restless, crying, Expect the worst outcome Lack of concentration Difficulty sleeping	Acknowledge stress and anxiety Provide support by being available Discuss coping strategy for any physical tests to be performed Provide information on tests and keep patient up to date with the plan of care Encourage calm breathing and relaxation Nurse in quiet area of unit/ward if medical condition allows
Dementia (including Alzheimer's disease)	Loss of memory in union with lack of concentration Confusion about time and place Signs of self-neglect Wanders aimlessly Reasoning slow and muddled Depressed, agitated and restless	Orientate patient to time, place and person at level of ability Reduce environmental stimuli Maintain safety Work with family in setting realistic goals Encourage to follow set routine of rest and activity
Suicidal behaviour	Past medical history – chronic illness and/or mental health disorder Signs of depression Suicidal ideas Respiratory/cardiovascular status may be altered from drug ingestion Self-inflicted injuries Presence of risk factors	Encourage to talk about feelings Listen objectively Provide safe environment in an observable area Specific treatment for any drugs ingested Ensure patient is aware of care plan Orientate to unit/ward Avoid actions that could be viewed as criticism
Depression	History of depression A precipitating incident Quiet, withdrawn, tired Crying Insomnia, hypersomnia Loss of interest Feelings of worthlessness Possible bradycardia Slowed gait and movements	Provide emotional support Discuss with patient possible cause(s) of depression Assess suicide risk Facilitate adequate nutrition Avoid actions that could be viewed as criticism
Bipolar disease	Alternating mania and depression History of bipolar disease Hallucinations Agitation or withdrawal Flight of ideas or flat affect (mood) Delusions or thoughts of grandeur Not sleeping Over-activity or slowed movement	Orientate patient to ward and plan of care Minimise environmental stimulation Administer lithium carbonate if required Monitor nutritional intake – high calorie Promote rest periods if manic Advise patient on importance of taking prescribed medications
Schizophrenia	Delusions Hallucinations Paranoia Bizarre behaviour (e.g. inability to care for self) Pressure of thought Thought blocking Thoughts are being broadcast, being inserted or removed	Observe for early cues of agitation Orientate patient to time, place and person Reduce environmental stimuli Speak softly to induce calm if verbally aggressive Reinforce absence of auditory hallucinations

Table 3.5. Management of the patient at risk

Indications of risk	Nursing action	Monitoring
Extreme agitation, excited behaviour, pacing, shouting, violent gestures, slamming doors, threats, abusive language indicate a high risk of violence May be the result of the effects of excessive use of drugs/alcohol	Always keep an exit clear Always have an escape route Inform security personnel of potential for violence Ask them to attend unit/ward prior to attempting to deal with situation Move other patients quietly Remove potential weapons (e.g. furniture, equipment) Ensure assistance is available from unit/ward staff trained for such situations Talk calmly, be clear and non-threatening. Allow space between self and patient If possible, try to find cause of outburst but avoid confrontation Use a sideways posture (less of target) and keep hands open Contact medical staff and psychiatric liaison team	Security personnel to stay until situation under control Consider physical restraint only if absolutely necessary Monitor continually according to mental health assessment Offer drinks and food Respect space and dignity Ensure other staff are continually aware of situation
Expressing desire to harm self High suicide risk Tries to leave	Seek immediate assistance from available unit/ward staff trained in such situations Contact medical staff and psychiatric liaison team Inform security and ask them to attend the unit Administer medications as prescribed (depending on cause of symptoms) Nurse to be relieved regularly (at least every hour) Review level of observation regularly	One or two nurses to wait with the patient Consider physical restraint only if absolutely necessary Monitor at all times Restrict movement so that there is minimum opportunity to abscond by routes such as windows, fire exits
Frightened, impulsive, may not wait	Seek urgent medical/psychiatric assessment Keep patient informed of plan of care	Sit with patient Offer support and reassurance Monitor closely
Appears to be under the influence of drugs/alcohol but no physical compromise	Monitor clinical signs as indicated by substance Nurse in high observation area	Discreet observation Check regularly for deterioration in physical/mental state
Wandering (Coping mechanism – boredom, hunger)	Check at regular intervals the whereabouts of the patient Keep patient informed of the unit/ward routine (e.g. meals, when they will be reviewed by doctor) At handover, the patient's whereabouts must be confirmed	Discreet observation Check regularly for deterioration in mental status Do not forget nutritional needs
Patient absconds	Inform security personnel, medical staff and manager Contact GP and next of kin Contact the police if patient is at high risk of harm to self or others	

Documentation

As a guide to future patient management, an accurate and concise history of the current problem must be recorded. This should include:

- details of the presenting complaint, duration and intensity, psychiatric and physical assessments, include both positive and negative findings (Brown 1996)
- an estimate of the degree of urgency of treatment in terms of risk to patient and others
- source of information and relationship to patient
- full details of any behavioural problems encountered and any action taken
- risk assessment
- plan of care with treatment goals, medication prescribed and/or reason for referral to any other agency
- evaluation of care given
- date and time of assessment and name of assessor

Referral options

An important minority of these vulnerable patients will require referral to a psychiatric liaison team for an expert assessment of their mental health status, suicide risk or substance dependency. Based on this referral, a decision whether to admit or discharge will be made.

If the patient is discharged with a serious (e.g. chronic illness) but low-risk (of harm to self or others) mental health need, follow-up must include an outpatient's clinic appointment or GP referral. When any patient with a mental health disorder is discharged, their GP, community psychiatric nurse (CPN) and key worker (if they have them) must be informed of their attendance and subsequent discharge. The role of the CPN is to monitor the patient's coping mechanisms in their home environment whilst the key worker (if already allocated) liaises with primary care services, specialist mental health services and local authority housing and social services. A psychiatric social worker may be involved in the assessment of social needs including such issues as housing or social support.

This team approach to caring for vulnerable people with mental health needs can be supported by the development of a psychiatric liaison service between the MAU, local A&E department(s) and stakeholders from local mental health care providers.

Discharge planning

Failure to ensure follow-up for a mental health disorder denies the patient an opportunity for effective treatment and can adversely affect the quality of life for both them and their family. This makes discharge planning vital for effective transfer of information and management of care. Before discharge, ensure that patients (and their carers) are aware of their diagnosis and plan of care. Give instructions regarding prescribed medications, their side effects and where and when to get a follow-up prescription. Details of any support that has been arranged should be given in written form along with details of where to attend in case of a crisis. The date, time and location of outpatient appointments should also be written down. Finally, the patient should know who has been informed of their discharge (e.g. their GP and any community services that are involved in their care).

Summary

Amongst vulnerable groups attending the MAU, one of the most complex are those patients who present with a co-existing mental health need. This vulnerability can be compounded by the patient's own reluctance to acknowledge a mental health disorder. Such patients may be feared by the public, may be vulnerable to assault and may be the victims rather than perpetrators of violence (Atakan and Davies 1997). Their health can be vulnerable as a result of their own behaviour; from the physical injuries of attempted suicide or self-neglect in cases of severe depression. These individuals can be vulnerable to a decline in their social circumstances, to social violence (e.g. assault and battery, sexual abuse, domestic violence) and to the use and abuse of alcohol and drugs (Mavundla 2000). This situation is often compounded on general hospital wards by the insecurity of nursing staff in their skills and knowledge of mental health issues. This leads to apprehension amongst nurses, which is often generated by patients' invasive behaviours and aggression (Brinn 2000, Heslop et al 2000). In these circumstances, care plans often focus on the physical elements of care, as these are perceived as being more familiar and easier to achieve.

This section has aimed to provide a structure for the assessment of patients with mental health needs. By so doing, it is hoped that these patients will receive the individualised care that they require and that nurses will overcome their apprehensions in respect of this vulnerable group of people.

References

Atakan Z, Davies T (1997) ABC of mental health: mental health emergencies. British Medical Journal 314(7096): 1740–2.

Bailey N, Cooper S-A (1997) The current provision of specialist health services to people with learning disabilities in England and Wales. Journal of Intellectual Disability Research 41(1): 52–9

Baldwin S, Birchenall M (1993) The nurse's role in caring for people with learning disabilities. British Journal of Nursing 2(17): 850–5.

Bennett G (1990) Assessing abuse in the elderly. Geriatric Medicine 20(7): 49–51.

Bennett G (1994) Clinical diagnosis and treatment. In Eastman M (ed) Old Age Abuse – A New Perspective. London: Chapman & Hall.

Bennett G, Kingston P (1993) Elder Abuse: Concepts, Theories and Interviews. London: Chapman & Hall.

Biley A (1994) A handicap of negative attitudes and lack of choice: caring for inpatients with disabilities. Professional Nurse 9(12): 786–8.

Birchwood M, Smith J, MacMillan J, Hogg B, Prasad R, Harvey C, Bering S (1989) Predicting relapse in schizophrenia: the development and implementation of an early signs monitoring system using patients and families as observers: A preliminary investigation. Psychological Medicine 19: 649–56.

Bradley J, Edinberg M (1990) Communication in the Nursing Context, 3rd edn. Connecticut: Appleton and Lange.

Brinn F (2000) Patients with mental illness: general nurses' attitudes and expectations. Nursing Standard 14(27): 32–6.

Brogden M, Nijhar P (2000) Crime, Abuse and the Elderly. Devon, USA: Willan Publishing.

Brown A (1996) Emergency Medicine Diagnosis and Management, 3rd edn. Melbourne: Butterworth Heinemann.

Callan L, Gilbert T, Golding K, Lockyer T, Rafter K (1995) Assessing health needs in people with severe learning disabilities: a qualitative approach. Journal of Clinical Nursing 4: 295–303.

Centre for Policy on Ageing/NHS (1999) Service Standards for the NHS Care of Older People. London: Central Books.

Craig T, Boardman A (1998) Common mental health problems in primary care. In Davies T, Craig T (eds) ABC of Mental Health. London: BMJ Books.

Cullen C (1988) A review of staff training: the emperor's new clothes. Irish Psychology 9: 309–23.

Cumella S, Martin D (2000) Secondary Healthcare for People with Learning Disability. London: Department of Health.

Davies T (1997) ABC of mental health: mental health assessment. British Medical Journal 314(7093): 1536–9.

Department of Health (2000a) No Secrets. Guidance on Developing and Implementing Multi-agency Policies and Procedures to Protect Vulnerable Adults from Abuse. London: HMSO.

Department of Health (2000b) The NHS Plan. A Plan for Investment, a Plan for Reform. London: DoH.

Department of Health (2001a) Human Rights Act 1998. London: HMSO.

Department of Health (2001b) Valuing People: A New Strategy for Learning Disability for the 21st Century. London: DoH.

Department of Health and Social Security (1983) The Mental Health Act. London: DHSS.

Eastman M (ed) (1994) Old Age Abuse – A New Perspective. London: Chapman & Hall.

Ferris-Taylor R (1997) Communication. In Gates B (ed) Learning Disabilities, 3rd edn. Edinburgh: Churchill Livingstone.

Gates B (ed) (1997) Learning Disabilities, 3rd edn. Edinburgh: Churchill Livingstone.

Good W, Nelson J (1986) Psychiatry Made Ridiculously Simple, 3rd edn. Miami: MedMaster.

Hale A (1997) ABC of mental health – anxiety. British Medical Journal 315: 43–6.

Harrison P, Geddes J, Sharpe M (1998) Lecture Notes on Psychiatry, 8th edn. Oxford: Blackwell Science.

Heslop L, Eslom S, Parker N (2000) Improving continuity of care across psychiatric and emergency services: combining patient data within a participatory action research framework. Journal of Advanced Nursing 31(1): 135–43.

Hudak C, Gallo B (eds) (1994) Critical Care Nursing: A Holistic Approach, 6th edn. Philadelphia: Lippincott.

Isaacs A (2001) Mental Health and Psychiatric Nursing, 3rd edn. Philadelphia: Lippincott.

Jones S (1999) Learning disability nursing – holistic care at its best. Nursing Standard 13(52): 61.

Kingston P, Penhale B (1995) Elder abuse and neglect: issues in the Accident and Emergency department. Accident & Emergency Nursing 3: 122–8.

Kingston P, Penhale B (1997) Issues in the sphere of elder abuse and neglect: the role of education. Nurse Education Today 17: 418–25.

Lindsey M (1998) Signposts for Success in the Commissioning and Providing of Health Services for People with Learning Disabilities. London: DoH.

Lindsey M, Russell O (1999) Once a Day. London: DoH.

Malin N, Race D, Jones G (1980) Services for the Mentally Handicapped in Britain. London: Croom Helm.

Mavundla T (2000) Professional nurses' perception of nursing mentally ill people in a general hospital setting. Journal of Advanced Nursing 32(6): 1569–78.

Mayfield D, McLeod G, Hall P (1974) The CAGE Questionnaire: validation of a new alcoholism screening instrument. American Journal of Psychiatry 131: 1121–3.

McConkey R, Truesdale M (2000) Reactions of nurses and therapists in mainstream health services to contact with people who have learning disabilities. Journal of Advanced Nursing 32(1): 158–63.

Meltzer H et al (1995) Surveys of Psychiatric Morbidity in Great Britain Report 1: The Prevalence of Psychiatric Morbidity Among Adults Living in Private Households. London: HMSO.

Mencap (1998) The NHS – Health for All? London: Mencap.

Mental Health Foundation (1997) All About Anorexia Nervosa. London: Mental Health Foundation.

MIND (2001) The prevalence of mental health problems: the Office for National Statistics survey results and evidence from other studies. http://www.mind.org.uk/ (09/07/01): MIND Publications

Ministry of Health (1959) Mental Health Act. London: Ministry of Health.

Molitor L (1996) (ed) Emergency Department Handbook. Maryland: Aspen Publishers.

Patterson W, Dohn H, Bird J, Patterson G (1983) Evaluation of suicidal patients: the SAD PERSON Scale. Psychosomatics 24(4): 343–9.

Penhale B, Kingston P (1997) Elder abuse: the role of risk management. British Journal of Community Health Nursing 2(4): 201–6.

Polli G, Lazear (2000) Mental health emergencies. In Emergency Nurses Association: Emergency Nursing Core Curriculum. Philadelphia: WB Saunders.

Ramirez A, House A (1998) Common mental health problems in hospital. In Davies T, Craig T (eds) ABC of Mental Health. London: BMJ Books.

Seidel H, Ball J, Dains J, Benedict G (1998) Mosby's Guide to Physical Examination, 4th edn. Missouri: Mosby Year Book.

Selfridge-Thomas J (1995) Manual of Emergency Nursing. Philadelphia: WB Saunders.

Slevin E, Sines D (1996) Attitudes of nurses in a general hospital towards people with learning disabilities: influences of contact, and graduate–non-graduate status, a comparative study. Journal of Advanced Nursing 24: 1116–26.

Social Services Inspectorate (1993) No Longer Afraid. The Safeguard of Older People in Domestic Settings. London: HMSO.

Social Services Inspectorate (1996) Social Services Inspectorate, Assessing Older People with Dementia. Practice Issues for Social and Health Services. London: SSI.

Townsend M (1999) Essentials of Psychiatric/Mental Health Nursing. Philadelphia: FA Davis.

Turner S, Moss S (1996) The health needs of adults with learning disabilities and the health of the nation strategy. Journal on Intellectual Disability Research 40(5): 438–50.

United Kingdom Central Council (1999) Practitioner–Client Relationships and the Prevention of Abuse. London: UKCC.

Walker M (1996) The Makaton Core Vocabulary. Surrey: MVCP.

Ward M (1995) Nursing the Psychiatric Emergency. Oxford: Butterworth Heinemann.

World Health Organisation (1992) ICD 10: International Statistical Classification of Diseases and Related Health Problems (10th Revision). WHO: http://www.who.int/msa/mnh/ems/icd/icd10.htm (09/07/2001).

Wyatt J, Illingworth R, Clancy M, Monro P, Robertson C (1999) Oxford Handbook of Accident and Emergency Medicine. Oxford: Oxford University Press.

Further reading

Abuse, neglect and inadequate care of older adults

Ashton G (1995) Elderly People and the Law. London: Butterworths.

Biggs S, Phillipson C, Kingston P (1995) Elder Abuse in Perspective. Buckingham: Open University Press.

Decalmer P, Glendenning F (eds) (1997) The Mistreatment of Elderly People, 2nd edn. London: Sage.

McCreadie C (1996) Elder Abuse: Update on Research. London: Age Concern and Institute of Gerontology, King's College.

Individuals with learning disabilities

Astor R, Jefferys K (2000) Positive Initiatives for People with Learning Difficulties: Promoting Healthy Lifestyles. London: Macmillan Press.

Brandon D (1989) Mutual Respect: Therapeutic Approaches to Working with People with Learning Difficulties. New Malden: Hexagon.

Burke P, Cigno K (2000) Learning Disabilities in Children. London: Blackwell Science.

Cowen H (1999) Community Care, Ideology and Social Policy. Europe: Prentice Hall.

Department of Health and Social Security (1971) Better Services for the Mentally Handicapped. London: DHSS.

Kerr M (1998) Innovations in Health Care for People with Intellectual Disabilities. Chorley: Lisieux Hall Publications.

Philpot T, Ward L (1995) Values and Visions. Oxford: Butterworth Heinemann.

Thompson T, Mathias P (1998) Standards and Learning Disability: Keys to Competence, 2nd edn. London: Baillière.

Wolfensberger W (1972) The Principles of Normalization in Human Management Services. Toronto: National Institute of Mental Retardation.

Patients with mental health needs

Davies T, Craig T (eds) (1998) ABC of Mental Health. London: BMJ Books.

Green B (ed) (2000) The Assessment of Risk. http://www.priory.com/psych/risk.htm (Posted 13/11/2000).

Kumar P, Clark M (2000) (eds) Acute General Medicine. Oxford: Butterworth Heinemann.

Newell R, Gournay K (2000) Mental Health Nursing: An Evidence-based Approach. London: Churchill Livingstone.

South Eastern Sydney Area Health Service (1998) Training Manual for Non-Mental Health Trained Staff to work with Mental Health Patients in Hospital Emergency Departments. Sydney: Area Mental Health Program, South Eastern Sydney Area Health Service (unpublished).

CHAPTER 4

Sudden death

SUE READ AND JANE JERVIS

Aims

This chapter will:

- consider the practical issues relating to the care and support of the relatives of patients who have died suddenly in the Medical Assessment Unit (MAU)
- explore the personal and professional challenges associated with sudden death
- identify and explore ethical issues in practice
- clarify the impact of both giving and receiving bad news and identify ideas for best practice
- critically discuss environmental factors to promote best practice
- identify and clarify the support needs of relatives bereaved by sudden death
- explore typical responses to bad news from a counselling and support perspective
- explore the need for informal and formal staff support systems
- examine the professional development needs for, and provision of, nursing and medical education and training
- provide a checklist as an indicator of best practice

Introduction

Death is indiscriminate, and will touch each one of us as we diligently progress through life. There are many modes of death, from the debilitatingly slow to the traumatically quick; and there are many factors that might affect the way that any surviving relatives cope with their loss. Such factors include the mode of death; the circumstances around the death; the age of the person who has died; whether it was a public death; whether it involved violence; whether it was an avoidable death and whether it was an expected death (Worden 1991, Machin 1998). Such factors may be multifaceted and accumulative; for example, a young person who dies suddenly and traumatically in a road traffic accident may evoke many emotions and issues within the surviving family – because of both the victim's age and the nature of the death (both sudden and traumatic).

According to Wright (1991), no other event in one's life has the same impact as sudden death. For the individual who has experienced the sudden death of a close relative, that impact may be immeasurable; for those professionals caring for such relatives, the stress of continually being involved in such difficult and sensitive activities can be vast. Health care professionals must remain mindful of the personal and professional challenges involved when dealing with such situations. As Wright (1991) reminds us, professionals 'must be aware of its [sudden death] strength, enormity and complexity' in order for constructive help and professional support to be most effective.

In the MAU, nurses are faced with anxious patients who are referred for assessment, investigation and initial treatment. Relatives, who are often distressed because of the uncertain future of their loved ones and who are also uncomfortable in this unfamiliar environment, often accompany them. Such relatives will have to talk to complete strangers (nursing and medical staff) who have total autonomy over their loved ones. Largely, the nursing and medical staff will be meeting these people for the first time. They have to establish in a very short period of time communication channels in order to nurture trusting relationships with the patient and their relatives. These professionals have to be highly skilled communicators who are competent at dealing with the presenting physical problems whilst simultaneously addressing the interpersonal challenges posed by anxious relatives. MAU nurses are in a front line position, are faced with a plethora of medical conditions, and have to cope with a range of problems resulting from illness or death.

At a time of a sudden death in the MAU, the effects may be multiple, as nurses are supporting relatives and often each other. Dealing with death is often difficult and can affect us in three specific ways (Worden 1991, pp 133/4):

- makes us painfully aware of our own losses
- makes us aware of our potential losses
- makes us aware of our own pending mortality

Dealing with death involves addressing a whole range of issues from an environmental, physical, psychological and sociological perspective. Consequently, when considering sudden death within the MAU, a whole range of factors need to be identified, considered and explored from a practical, emotional and psychological perspective. Such factors range from the ethical dilemmas often presented (for example, with witnessed resuscitation) to supporting the resultant bereaved family. A checklist is offered at the end of this chapter (see Box 4.4) as a good practice guide when dealing with sudden death in the MAU setting.

Ethical and legal issues

Death, by the very nature of its diversity, is surrounded by social and cultural traditions and superstition. This contributes to the complex arena that is health care, in which many moral and ethical questions provide continuous debate. In the past, death could be defined as the absence of breathing and a heartbeat. However, advances in medical technology have caused great debate as to the modern definition of death (Stanley 1987, Gillon 1990, Chaloner 1996). Within critical care settings, advances (e.g. mechanical ventilation and drug therapies) have increased the number of ethical questions surrounding the definition of death as technology can now sustain the heart and lungs even when the brain can no longer perform these functions. Ultimately, this leads to such ethical dilemmas as withdrawal of treatment, brain death and organ donation.

For a nurse in an MAU, the most common ethical dilemmas encountered relating to death and bereavement are those involving cardiopulmonary resuscitation (CPR). These tend to relate to resuscitation decisions (e.g. 'do not resuscitate' (DNR) orders and advance directives), but also include the patient's right to refuse life-saving treatment and relative-witnessed resuscitation (see Chapter 5 – Cardiac arrest).

CPR was originally introduced as a method to resuscitate the victim of a witnessed catastrophe or trauma such as drowning or electrocution (Page and Meerabeau 1996). Its use has increased in recent times so that anyone who has a cardiopulmonary arrest may receive CPR. It is important then to consider the first ethical question that arises: is it appropriate to give CPR in all cases of cardiopulmonary arrest? It is possible to glimpse the moral and ethical minefield that surrounds CPR decisions from this one question alone.

All ethical decisions are guided by the four principles of beneficence, non-maleficence, justice and respect for patient autonomy. These principles are also the basis on which resuscitation decisions are made. The principle of beneficence relates to the need to take deliberate actions in order to do good and non-maleficence refers to a person's duty to do no harm. These two principles are often linked together and when related to nursing practice can be applied to clauses 1 and 4 of the UKCC Code of Professional Conduct (UKCC 1992). This states that each nurse must 'act always in such a manner as to promote and safeguard the interests and well-being of patients' and 'ensure that no action or omission ... is detrimental to the interests, condition or safety of patients'.

Respect for patient autonomy involves the MAU nurse respecting the patient's right to make personal treatment decisions regardless of professional opinion. 'Autonomy is by far the most significant value which has been promoted by contemporary medical ethics. The concept which has dominated medical ethics more than any other over the final four decades of the twentieth century is that the individual should have control over his own body, should make his own decisions relating to his medical treatment and should not be hindered in his search for self-fulfilment' (Mason and McCall-Smith 1999, p 6). Therefore, the principle of autonomy must take into account patients' rights when making resuscitation decisions. Although providing a guide to decision making, these rights can be the cause of even more ethical and moral questions since:

- having rights does not mean that one is bound to exercise them
- having rights does not mean that their exercise is unlimited
- negative rights are in general stronger than positive ones (Thompson et al 1988, p 133)

The third point is particularly relevant when discussing resuscitation decisions as it relates to the patient's right to refuse life-saving treatment. Take, for example, the patient who has taken a drug overdose. Although this is often thought of as an action taken by young people, the highest suicide rate in the UK is in the older population due to chronic illness or pain, social isolation or financial problems (Toulson 1996). What then happens if these patients refuse treatment or do not want to be resuscitated? Should the age of the patient bear any relevance to the actions of the health care team in this case? The right to refuse treatment is virtually absolute in law and treating a patient against their will can technically be considered a criminal assault. However, in these circumstances the patient must demonstrate to the medical team that they are mentally competent to make this decision at this time. This also applies to other vulnerable members within society, such as people with learning disabilities or mental health problems (see Chapter 3). The giving of non-consensual treatment to involuntary patients with mental health problems applies to treatment for the mental condition only and does not include any intervention for any other health problem. If the patient is not competent to make the decision, then the doctor is obliged to make any clinical decisions based on the best interests of the patient.

Do not resuscitate (DNR) orders

One of the main ethical issues in society today is that of consent. Therefore, questions such as when to make resuscitation decisions and who should make them are of ethical concern not only to patients, relatives, medical and nursing staff, but also to society as a whole. CPR is a highly invasive procedure, which is not appropriate for all patients. As it has been found to be effective in only one in five patients (De Vos et al 1999), it is important to consider whether each individual patient would benefit from this intervention.

The decision to resuscitate or not must not be considered as a 'black and white' question, where resuscitation is seen as good as it restores life, and the DNR order is seen as bad as it symbolises defeat through death. Using this idea, the principles of non-maleficence and beneficence could change this view to its opposite. For the terminally ill patient, refusal to consider a DNR order may negate that patient's right to receive palliative care, even in acute settings such as MAU and 'palliative care is, ethically, a mandatory part of the care of the dying' (Gordon and Singer 1995). Forcing resuscitation on those who do not want it only achieves a prolonged death and often the exclusion of relatives at the end of life. 'The philosophical acceptance of dying, combined with support for what valuable life remains, have to be incorporated into clinical practice if unnecessary suffering at life's end is to be avoided' (Gordon and Singer 1995, p 165).

As an aid to good practice and uniformity throughout the NHS, guidelines for making decisions related to CPR are available in a Joint Statement from the British Medical Association (BMA), the Resuscitation Council (UK) (RCUK) and the Royal College of Nursing (RCN) (1999). In this paper a number of circumstances are identified as the precursors of DNR orders and decisions. These include:

- where the patient's condition indicates that effective CPR is unlikely to be successful
- where CPR is not in accord with the recorded, sustained wishes of the patient who is mentally competent
- where CPR is not in accord with a valid applicable advance directive (anticipatory refusal or living will). A patient's informed and competently made refusal, which relates to the circumstances which have arisen, is legally binding upon doctors
- where successful CPR is likely to be followed by a length and quality of life that it would not be in the best interests of the patient to sustain (BMA, RCUK and RCN 1999)

These guidelines stress that it is best practice where possible to discuss resuscitation with the patient and/or their relatives and that any discussion should be documented clearly in the patient's notes and regularly updated in accordance with hospital policy. No one has the legal right to make a resuscitation decision for another adult, except that person's doctor when there is no anticipatory decision known and the person is deemed mentally incompetent. At this time, the doctor is legally responsible to advocate for the patient and to make clinical decisions which are in the best interests of that patient. This includes adults with mental health problems and those with learning disabilities. People with a mental health problem and/or a learning disability have the same rights as any other individual and, therefore, any resuscitation decision should be made in the same way as for any patient. This is the same as when dealing with the elderly as age should not be the main factor for a DNR order.

Where possible the patient should be consulted about their views and whether they wish to be resuscitated as failure to involve the patient may neutralise the principle of patient autonomy. This is rarely possible in the MAU environment. Therefore, for the doctor to make a valid resuscitation decision, information from relatives is invaluable in gaining an insight into the patient's views and previous health status.

Effective interpersonal skills are required when discussing resuscitation decisions with relatives as a number of variables affect the family's decision. These include (Blatt 1999, p 220):

- functional role in the family
- emotional dependence
- family problem-solving style
- ethnicity and religion

These factors identify potential differences within families. For example, different religions hold different traditions about death and dying. Likewise, family dynamics can affect their ability to make a unified decision. Some may communicate their feelings in a non-blaming, open and flexible way whilst others may mistrust the health care team and be unable to express feelings without showing anger or distress (Blatt 1999). In order to gain an informed decision from relatives, information must be given in an honest and jargon-free way. There is evidence to suggest that both patients and relatives frequently overestimate the effectiveness of CPR (Mead and Turnbull 1995, Schonwetter et al 1991).

Advance directives

Advance directives are written instructions from mentally competent patients to their family and health care professionals that detail their wishes in relation to future treatment if they become unable to express themselves. This could either be the request not to receive CPR or for all life-sustaining measures to be initiated. Although the advance directive is legally binding to doctors, it remains a controversial subject for a number of reasons in various health care settings. Firstly, there are questions relating to the interpretation and usage of terminology and language within the directive. Secondly, the directive must be available to medical staff. Thirdly, the authenticity of the directive must be ascertained. These issues are a particular problem in an area such as MAU where the health care team does not know the patients and where there is often no immediate access to their medical notes. As patients are admitted with a degree of urgency, the relatives may have forgotten the directive in their hurry to get to the hospital. For these and other reasons it is often suggested that the advance directive should be seen as indicative of the patient's wishes, not absolute (Mason and McCall-Smith 1999).

Critical thinking – ethical complexities

Three short vignettes illustrate the potential ethical complexities involved in the MAU. Discuss them with your colleagues.

Ethical dilemmas relating to treatment and diagnosis in the MAU have been identified. Once the professional team have explored various medical options, informing the patient and relatives and involving them in the future management of the presenting condition and ultimate decision making is vital. Consequently, the manner of breaking such news is crucial to this process.

Vignette 1

Mr Hicks, a 46-year-old with profound learning disabilities, is referred to the MAU with pneumonia. On examination, his condition is critical. He is hypotensive, pyrexial and desaturates without 100% oxygen. Over the past five years Mr Hicks has had recurrent admissions with pneumonia and on each admission he has required more aggressive treatment. The doctor thinks that admission to an intensive therapy unit or CPR in the event of cardiac arrest would not be appropriate owing to his past history, futility of the interventions and the patient's quality of life. However, his family does want active treatment to be given.

How would your health care team approach this situation? Does your hospital policy provide adequate guidelines relating to these circumstances?

Vignette 2

Mrs Evans, aged 85, is referred following an overdose of diazepam and alcohol. She did leave a note and took steps not to be found. On arrival, she expresses the wish that she does not want to receive treatment and if she stops breathing she wants to be left to die.

What actions should the health care team take? Discuss whether Mrs Evans is competent to make this decision at this time. Now reconsider this question as if Mrs Evans were 22 years old. Would her age affect the decisions made by your team?

Vignette 3

Mr Smith has a history of inoperable cancer of the prostate. He is referred to the MAU with an acute myocardial infarction. Whilst in the MAU he has a VF (ventricular fibrillation) arrest.

Would a DNR order be appropriate in this case? Does Mr Smith currently have a good quality of life? Consider whether or not Mr Smith should be defibrillated. VF is a reversible rhythm. Would the age of the patient make a difference to your decision in this case?

Breaking bad news

Buckman (1984, p 288) describes bad news as '... any news that drastically and negatively alters the patient's view of his or her future'. Consequently, such news could emanate from a whole range of situations – from negative and positive test results, to failing exams to hearing of enforced redundancy. Accepting this broad-based definition indicates that most nurses will be involved in the breaking of bad news on a regular basis and, as such, need to be aware of the factors that might enable, rather than disable, effective communication.

Death is among the most difficult types of bad news to receive, largely because of its negative impact, permanence and irreversibility. Within the MAU, bad news might involve the giving of test results, the acknowledgement and sharing of uncertainty related to undetermined illness, sudden death or the impending death of a patient.

Spall and Callis (1997) suggest that health care professionals may break news badly because they have not been adequately trained or prepared. Contributing factors to this may include their lack of awareness of the importance of effective communication (both verbal and non-verbal skills), their own feelings of self-consciousness, the general business of their work, issues around personal mortality and fears around responses.

According to Buckman (1992) individuals may dread breaking bad news for a whole range of professional and personal factors:

- Social factors – where, in our society, great emphasis is placed upon health, wealth and youth. Anything that detracts from these values is likely to be frowned upon. Consequently severe ill health, and the practical, emotional and financial losses that often accompany injury or illness may affect the individual and their family most significantly.
- Patient factors – such as the stigma associated with certain phrases or conditions (e.g. cancer). Some patients might grudgingly accept a diagnosis of a 'tumour' but become distraught at the confirmation of 'cancer'. Some illnesses that may be self-inflicted (e.g. drug or substance abuse) often carry social stigma that surviving relatives may have difficulty accepting or coping with.
- Professional factors – these include:
  - fear of causing pain
  - sympathetic pain
  - fear of being blamed
  - fear of the untaught

- fear of eliciting a response
- fear of admitting what we don't know
- fear of expressing our emotions
- personal fears

Some of these identified fears may be contrary to the perceived role of health care professionals (e.g. causing pain, being blamed, admitting that one does not know the answers) and hence, may affect individual skill performance. Some fears may result purely from lack of training and perceived expertise. However, Kaye (1995) advocates that effectively breaking bad news is important to both professionals and patients in order to:

- maintain trust between patients and professionals
- reduce uncertainty
- allow appropriate adjustment (practical and emotional) so that the patient can make informed decisions
- prevent a conspiracy of silence which may destroy family communication and prevent mutual support (Kaye 1995, p 3)

What is clear is that breaking bad news is an unenviable task that many nurses and doctors would avoid given the chance. It cannot be avoided. Breaking bad news effectively can promote patient autonomy, avoid collusive relationships and maintain open, honest and professional relationships and as such is an important aspect of the health care professional's repertoire of skills. Communication is the key to delivering news in a caring, clear, sensitive and accurate way that does not add to, or detract from, the heavy burden of the content.

Breaking bad news for the first time can be fraught with anxiety for the MAU nurse, as they may be unsure as to how the relative or patient might respond. All professionals should be given the opportunity to explore the potential challenges associated with breaking bad news in a safe, multidisciplinary and supportive environment and to explore the need for effective communication within this sensitive context.

A framework for effective communication

Many authors have explored breaking bad news from a process perspective, and offer frameworks or models to guide professional practice (Buckman 1992, Kaye 1995, Spall and Callis 1997). Such models may be seen as practice guidelines by which professionals can gather cues or reference points to aid the bad news process. An easy to use and easy to remember guide is that offered by Buckman (1992), which comprises six steps:

1. Getting started. Getting the physical context right (Where should the news be broken? Who should be there? How does the professional begin?)
2. Finding out how much the patient knows (language and knowledge)
3. Finding out how much the patient/relative wants to know
4. Sharing the information (aligning and educating)
   - Decide on your agenda (diagnosis, treatment)
   - Start from the patient's/relatives' starting point (aligning)
   - Educating:
     – give information in small chunks
     – use English not medical jargon
     – check reception frequently and clarify
     – reinforce the information frequently and clarify
     – check your level (are you staying with the patient/relative?)
     – listen for their agenda
     – try to blend your agenda with theirs
5. Responding to the patient's/relatives' feelings (acknowledging and identifying their reactions)
6. Planning and follow through:
   - organising
   - making professional contact and following through

Such a simple, yet realistic, framework can help the health care professional to deliver the news in a systematic and meaningful way. Some professionals may dislike the use of a framework in this context for fear of such an important personal process becoming mechanical. In the authors' experience, people are unique individuals who deal with any confronting challenges in individual and unique ways and would be unlikely to become processed by the use of guidelines. Such guidelines should be perceived as a professional tool that can act as meaningful guidance for those who need it. Professionals must also remain aware of the different perspectives of illness from a patient and/or relative versus the professional viewpoint. For example, news about a condition that may, to professionals, seem relatively common and easy to overcome and treat might feel overwhelming to the patient and relatives who have little experience of such conditions.

Guidelines also offer indicators of ways in which practice might be improved; for example, when considering the environment in which difficult news is given. Breaking bad news in a corridor with little privacy or in the midst of distracting and busy activities is not recommended but may be unavoidable. The work compiled by the British Association for Accident and Emergency Medicine (BAAEM) in conjunction with the RCN (1995) offers many salient recommendations that could be usefully translated into MAU practice. The environment is important and rooms designed for relatives must offer accessibility yet privacy and comfort, without creating a sense of foreboding or isolation. Informal terms (e.g. sitting room) help to humanise these facilities and such rooms should be designed to seat a minimum of eight people comfortably. Toilet facilities should be close by and the room should be bright and well lit. In addition to comfortable chairs and tables, tissues, ashtrays, a direct line telephone, wash-basin and toiletries, toys and books for children should be available (BAAEM and RCN 1995). Issues regarding the environment are incorporated within the checklist at the end of this chapter (Box 4.4).

Responding to bad news

When giving someone news that they do not want to hear, MAU nurses should be prepared for a whole range of responses. Wright (1991) identified nine emotional responses often exhibited by people receiving news of a sudden death. These nine emotions are identified in descending order of difficulty for nurses (Box 4.1).

Box 4.1. Possible emotions displayed by people receiving bad news (Wright 1991, p 88)

- Withdrawal
- Denial
- Anger
- Isolation
- Bargaining
- Inappropriate responses
- Guilt
- Crying, sobbing and weeping
- Acceptance

Withdrawal is identified as being the most difficult response to deal with by health care staff since it renders them impotent and unable to offer practical help. Sitting next to someone who has physically, emotionally and psychologically withdrawn is extremely difficult and the nurse needs a wealth of patience and understanding to sit and be with the person at this difficult time.

Acceptance, crying and weeping are probably the easiest to cope with because many professionals anticipate such a response. Anger is a natural response, and professionals need to hear this anger, acknowledge it, help the person to focus and reflect their understanding of such anger back to them in a clear and comprehensive way. Wright's work (1991) could help to prepare MAU nurses to anticipate reactions from relatives and illustrates where support may be needed most from a bereavement perspective. It also serves to indicate development needs of the professionals involved.

Support for relatives

'In human society the loss of one who is dearly loved brings great emotional pain and grief. Some suggest that this pain has significance for the species – that it serves the function of binding the social group, the group essential for survival' (Raphael 1984, p 3). Bereavement is described as the loss of a significant other person in one's life, which typically triggers a reaction we call grief, which is manifest in a set of behaviours we call mourning (Stroebe et al 1993). Whilst the patient's needs are seen to end at death, the needs of associated family members are just beginning (Warren 1997) and MAU nurses need to be alert to these needs in order to respond effectively.

For those people for whom loss is imminent, Hampe (1975) and Breu and Bacup (1978) identify the needs of a relative anticipating loss (Box 4.2).

Box 4.2. The needs of relatives anticipating loss

- To be with the dying person
- To be helpful to the dying person
- To be assured that the dying person is comfortable
- To be kept informed of the dying person's condition
- To know of the impending death
- To experience and express emotions
- To comfort and support family members
- To be accepted, supported and comforted by health care professionals
- To be relieved of anxiety

Wright (1993) identified that relatives who have been suddenly bereaved want clear and concise messages and information about the death; welcome confirmation and affirmation about the circumstances; value the opportunity to ask questions and discuss major issues; need opportunities to spend time with the deceased; and finally, welcome a further chance to clarify the circumstances surrounding the death before they leave the hospital.

Such attention may be time-consuming for MAU nurses but may help relatives both in the initial coming to terms with the enormity of the loss and in the long-term accommodation of their loss (Dubin and Sarnoff 1986). Offering choices to bereaved relatives at this time may help them to begin to accept the death of their loved one. Such choices might involve offering bereaved relatives the opportunity to participate in performing the last rites; the choice to see the deceased and to be with them in private surroundings; the choice about which other relatives should be informed about the death; the choice to instruct others (or participate themselves) in the differing cultural and spiritual rituals surrounding death (Neuberger 1987, Lothian Racial Equality Council 1992, Green 1993). Of course, being able to respond positively to such choices is important and systems need to be in place to ensure that this happens. For example, if the MAU offers relatives 24-hour access to the mortuary to view their loved one, it must be able to honour this option before the information is given to the bereaved relatives.

Nurses need to listen and to hear the concerns of both the patient (if sufficiently aware) and the family (Intensive Care Society (ICS) 1997) and to involve them as much as possible (and as much as they wish to be involved) in the care and decision making of the patient. Medical staff and nurses may play a major role in these initial stages of grief as they often 'become trusted confidants (who) provide a tangible link with the dead person, and talking over the death with those who knew what happened helps to make the loss real' (Parkes et al 1996, p 132).

Whilst every death is unique and everyone grieves in their own unique way, certain circumstances may affect the way that the individual responds to their loss. The ICS Guidelines for Bereavement Care in Intensive Care Units (1997) have identified several factors that potentially indicate a high risk of intense bereavement reaction:

- unexpected loss – if the patient is less than 65 years of age, with no history of serious or chronic disease and no previous life-threatening illness

- sudden loss – the relative has had no preparation for the death
- the relative perceives their family as unsupportive
- the bereavement is traumatic
- the relationship between the deceased and the relative is ambivalent – often manifesting as anger, dependency or guilt
- the relative has a life crisis other than bereavement, e.g. financial (ICS 1997, p 9)

Sudden death issues in MAU run through many of the above indicators (for example, unexpected, sudden and sometimes traumatic death) and may affect how the relatives react to their loss. Bereaved people respond to their loss in many different and unique ways – emotionally, physically, behaviourally and psychologically. Worden (1991) identified typical responses to grief (Box 4.3).

Box 4.3. Typical grief responses

Emotional	*Physical*	*Behavioural*	*Psychological*
Sadness	Hollowness in the stomach	Sleep disturbance	Disbelief
Anger	Tightness in the chest	Appetite disturbance	Confusion
Guilt	Tightness in the throat	Absent-mindedness	Preoccupation
Self-reproach	Over-sensitivity to noise	Social withdrawal	Sense of presence
Anxiety	A sense of depersonalisation	Dreaming	Hallucinations
Loneliness	Breathlessness	Searching	
Fatigue	Muscle weakness	Crying	
Helplessness	Lack of energy	Sighing	
Shock	Dry mouth	Restless over-activity	
Yearning		Visiting old haunts	
Relief			
Numbness			

Knowledge of these reactions will enable the MAU nurse to anticipate possible responses from bereaved relatives and develop potential support strategies. In the MAU, it would be helpful if nurses attend at least a basic, preferably multidisciplinary, bereavement course, during which personal and professional responses to grief can be explored in a constructive way.

Bereavement follow-up support is also important and the MAU must have formal guidelines regarding professional responsibilities in relation to:

- written information offered regarding local or national support groups
- communicating with the patient's GP
- liaising with the local coroner and mortuary

Dealing with death regularly may be particularly draining, and one must not forget the effect that this might have on health care professionals and the ongoing support needs of those involved.

Support for staff

Saines' (1997) phenomenological study identified the following four chronological themes of nurses' experiences of sudden death:

- encountering (e.g. suddenness, unacceptability, individuality)
- facing (e.g. related to self, physical reality, emotional reality)
- dealing with (e.g. witnessed resuscitation, professional competence, grief reactions, advocacy, emotional labour, cultural, religious, legal and gender issues, control and conflicts)
- reflecting upon sudden death (e.g. emotional release, support, time element, conclusion, experience)

Hence, involvement in a sudden death incident is likely to evoke many feelings, thoughts and emotions within the nurses involved. Acknowledging the personal and professional difficulties in dealing with sudden death by encouraging and providing regular access to peer support, professional counselling agencies and the constructive provision of critical incident debriefing (Wright 1989) is crucial in this area. A critical incident is described by Wright (1993, p 189) as 'any situation, faced by emergency personnel, that causes them to experience unusually strong emotional reactions. These feelings have the potential to interfere with their ability to function at the time or later'. Wright (1993) goes on to identify debriefing, defusing and demobilisation as useful frameworks to alleviate the stress of such incidents. Clinical supervision will play an active, useful role, but more immediate measures that can be called upon at short notice should also be routinely available. Such mechanisms enable professionals to constructively reflect on practice from a technical, practical, social, political and economic and self perspective (Clarke et al 1996), thus supporting and promoting the development of professional expertise.

In recognition of its importance, some services (for example, Gloucestershire Royal NHS Trust 1997) have created written documentation regarding bereavement debriefing after a sudden death. Such guidelines are invaluable to both health care professionals and the relatives with whom they are in contact. Indeed, the ICS (1997) recommend that all intensive care units should have a written policy for bereavement care. They also recommend the provision of follow-up bereavement services, that all staff should have access to bereavement training, that staff support systems should be in place and that a named nurse should be responsible for training in bereavement care (ICS 1997, p 3). Although these recommendations are intended for intensive care units, they can be equally applied to MAUs given that they often deal with sudden death and its aftermath.

Professional development needs

The BAEEM and RCN (1995) identify the need for appropriately trained staff 'to provide optimum care for the deceased person and their relatives'. The continuing professional development needs of MAU nurses in respect of sudden death have been highlighted throughout this chapter. Such areas to be addressed include ethical awareness, giving and receiving psychological support (both personally and professionally), communication and counselling skills, dealing with difficult news and bereavement. Not all MAU nurses will have specialist skills in all of these areas but the nursing team needs to be aware of the actual and desirable skill mix of those involved in order to identify skill deficits. Similarly, all individuals need to be aware of their own personal development needs and how these could be met by academic or skills-based education.

Practice development

To identify the skills, environmental features and practical issues associated with sudden death in the MAU, a checklist has been developed based on the issues raised within this chapter (Box 4.4). This checklist is not intended to be a prescription for what every MAU needs to address but it does identify a number of realistic issues that should be considered when dealing with sudden death. The checklist consists of five sections, incorporating 61 indicators, which might be used to:

- highlight issues for discussion by the MAU team
- measure existing baseline resources and act as an indicator of future developments
- help identify professional training and development issues

Box 4.4. Dealing with sudden death – a checklist for positive practice

Tick the appropriate indicators if they are currently available within the MAU
environment.

1. Environmental factors:

1.1   Is the MAU clearly signposted? ❑

1.2   Is the name of the relatives' room/sitting room informal and friendly? ❑

1.3   Is the sitting room within earshot of the main treatment area? ❑

1.4   Is the relatives' room easily accessible for disabled and non-disabled people? ❑

1.5   Does the relatives' room offer comfort and privacy? ❑

1.6   Does the relatives' room seat eight people comfortably (if not, is there potential
      for temporary extension)? ❑

1.7   Can relatives easily access toilet facilities? ❑

1.8   Does the relatives' room contain basic necessities (chairs, tables, tissues,
      telephone, ashtrays, wash-basin and toiletries)? ❑

1.9   Does the sitting room have a window? If so, are there blinds fitted? ❑

1.10 Is the relatives' room child friendly (books and toys)? ❑

1.11 Are there concrete methods (books, photographs) to support individuals who
      may have cognitive difficulties in understanding the complexities of death (for
      example, children, people with learning disabilities or elderly, confused or
      demented people)? ❑

1.12 Is there a visiting room where relatives can view their deceased? ❑

1.13 Is the visiting room en-suite with the sitting room? ❑

1.14 Do the relatives have to walk through public areas to view the deceased? ❑

1.15 Is there anything further that could be done to the sitting room, that would
      provide more comfort, privacy and dignity? ❑

2. Psychological support:

2.1   How many of the staff team have attended any counselling courses? ❑

2.2   Is there a formal staff support system in place? ❑

2.3   Do team members have access to confidential counselling? ❑

2.4   Is there a critical incident debriefing system operating? ❑

2.5   Are members of the team actively encouraged to talk about death on the
      MAU? ❑

2.6   Do the staff wear uniforms which are easily identifiable to the general public? ❑

2.7   Is a named nurse allocated to the relatives for the duration of time that they are
      in the MAU? ❑

2.8   Is there an up-to-date bereavement package available for bereaved relatives? ❑

2.9   Is there a bereavement follow-up service in operation? ❑

2.10 Is there a nominated person to lead the bereavement developments within the
      staff team? ❑

2.11 Does the staff team have good relations with appropriate outside agencies
      (e.g. local bereavement services, the Coroner's Court, medical illustration)? ❑

2.12 Are there any members of the staff team who are identified as being specialist
      in the area of bereavement? ❑

2.13 Are relatives given the choice of seeing the deceased/witnessing
      resuscitation/performing the last offices with their loved ones? ❑

2.14 Are there guidelines regarding multicultural aspects of death? ❑

2.15 Is there an up-to-date directory of religious leaders within the local area? ❑

2.16 Can the staff team contact spiritual leaders of different denominations
      throughout the 24-hour period? ❑

(continued)

Box 4.4. continued

2.17 Are the staff team aware of the different cultures and associated rituals in your
     geographical area?   ❏

2.18 Is there appropriate literature (e.g. information on the Coroner's Court, death
     notification and registration, funeral directors) available to bereaved relatives?   ❏

2.19 Are members of the staff team adequately equipped to deal with initial contact
     with relatives, preparing relatives for news of the death, breaking bad news and
     answering difficult questions?   ❏

2.20 Can the MAU team arrange for deceased patients to be viewed in the
     mortuary throughout the 24-hour period by relatives who may have to travel
     long distances?   ❏

3. Policy and procedure:

3.1 Does the hospital have a policy on resuscitation?   ❏

3.2 Does the hospital or MAU have a policy on care of the bereaved and breaking
    bad news?   ❏

3.3 Is there guidance on requests for organ donation?   ❏

3.4 Does the resuscitation policy contain clear guidelines regarding DNR orders
    and advance directives?   ❏

3.5 Who ensures that the patient's computer records are updated following death?   ❏

3.6 Who informs the patient's GP?   ❏

3.7 What happens to the belongings of the deceased patient?   ❏

3.8 What is the policy for contacting relatives if the patient is unaccompanied to
    the MAU?   ❏

3.9 What are the MAU team expected to do if they are unable to contact any
    next of kin?   ❏

4. Professional development:

4.1 Are there opportunities for multidisciplinary training?   ❏

4.2 How many of the MAU team have attended multidisciplinary sessions to
    explore issues such as ethics and breaking bad news?   ❏

4.3 How many of the staff team have attended multidisciplinary sessions to
    explore bereavement and loss?   ❏

4.4 How many of the team have attended multidisciplinary opportunities to
    explore sudden death?   ❏

4.5 Is research actively encouraged within the MAU?   ❏

4.6 Have any of the MAU team had work published in reputable journals?   ❏

4.7 Is there a personal review system in place?   ❏

4.8 Are there regular team meetings on the MAU?   ❏

4.9 How many of the staff team are familiar with the multicultural dimensions of
    death and dying?   ❏

4.10 Are there training opportunities for all members of the team?   ❏

4.11 Are members of the team adequately prepared for asking difficult questions
     (e.g. relating to organ donation)?   ❏

5. Service development:

5.1 Are there regular reviews of the service?   ❏

5.2 Are there regular reviews of skill mix?   ❏

5.3 Is a feedback system from the patients, relatives and staff in operation?   ❏

5.4 Is there a formal feedback system incorporating the results of such reviews?   ❏

5.5 Is there an audit of how sudden death is managed within the MAU?   ❏

5.6 Are checklists available on the MAU to guide positive, consistent practice?   ❏

The checklist is offered as a practical guide and may be photocopied for professional use. It has been based upon other existing checklists (BAEEM and RCN 1995, ICS 1997, Gloucestershire NHS Trust 1997). Readers are guided to these documents for additional information.

Summary

This chapter has considered the practical issues often associated with the care and support of patients and relatives involved in sudden death situations in the MAU, from a nursing perspective. Personal and professional challenges have been identified through the sensitive exploration of breaking difficult news from both the giver and receiver perspective. The clarification and analysis of ethical issues in practice is provided through case related vignettes. The importance of having an appropriate environment has been highlighted and suggestions for the development of professional guidelines have been introduced. In acknowledgement of the identified and resultant support and developmental needs of both clinicians and families, a checklist has been introduced to audit current practice and to identify future developments required in the MAU setting from a sudden death perspective. Whilst such checklists and guidelines are an aid to promoting good practice, professionals need to be mindful of the uniqueness of every situation involving death and of the importance of individual and sensitive professional responses at this difficult time.

References

Blatt L (1999) Working with families in reaching end-of-life decisions. Clinical Nurse Specialist 13(5): 219–23.

Breu C, Bacup K (1978) Helping the spouses of critically ill patients. American Journal of Nursing 78: 51–3.

British Association for Accident and Emergency Medicine and the Royal College of Nursing (1995) Bereavement Care in A&E Departments: Report of the Working Group. London: BAAEM/RCN.

British Medical Association, the Resuscitation Council (UK) and the Royal College of Nursing (1999) Decisions Relating to Cardiopulmonary Resuscitation. A Joint Statement. London: Resuscitation Council (UK).

Buckman R (1984) Breaking bad news: why is it so difficult? British Medical Journal 297: 1597–9.

Buckman R (1992) How to Break Bad News: A Guide for Health Care Professionals. London: Papermac.

Chaloner C (1996) The final frontier. Nursing Times 92(33): 26–9.

Clarke B, James C, Kelly J (1996) Reflective practice: reviewing the issues and refocusing the debate. International Journal of Nursing Studies 33(2): 171–80.

De Vos R, Koster R, De Haan R, Oosting H, Van Der Wouw P, Lampe-Schoenmaeckers A (1999) In-hospital cardiopulmonary resuscitation: prearrest morbidity and outcome. Archives of International Medicine 159: 845–50.

Dubin W, Sarnoff J (1986) Sudden and unexpected death: interventions with the survivors. Annals of Emergency Medicine 15(1): 54–7.

Gillon R (1990) Death. Journal of Medical Ethics 16: 3–4.

Gloucestershire Royal NHS Trust (1997) Bereavement Debriefing Service Following a Sudden Death. Gloucester: Gloucestershire Royal NHS Trust.

Gordon M, Singer P (1995) Decisions and care at the end of life. Lancet 346: 163–6.

Green J (1993) Death with Dignity, vol II. London: Nursing Times Publications.

Hampe S (1975) Needs of grieving spouse in a hospital setting. Nursing Research 24: 113–20.

Intensive Care Society (1997) Guidelines for Bereavement Care in Intensive Care Units. London: Intensive Care Society of the United Kingdom.

Kaye P (1995) Breaking Bad News: A Ten-step Approach. Northampton: EPL Publications.

Lothian Racial Equality Council (1992) Religions and Cultures: A Guide to Patients' Beliefs and Customs for Health Service Staff. Edinburgh: Lothian Racial Equality Council.

Machin L (1998) Looking at Loss: Bereavement Counselling Pack, 2nd edn. Brighton: Pavilion Publishing.

Mason J, McCall Smith R (1999) Law and Medical Ethics, 5th edn. London: Butterworths.

Mead G, Turnbull C (1995) Cardiopulmonary resuscitation in the elderly: patients' and relatives' views. Journal of Medical Ethics 21: 39–44.

Neuberger J (1987) Caring for Dying People of Different Faiths. Lisa Sainsbury Foundation series. London: Austin Cornish.

Page S, Meerabeau L (1996) Nurses' accounts of cardiopulmonary resuscitation. Journal of Advanced Nursing 24: 317–25.

Parkes C, Relf M, Couldrick A (1996) Counselling in Terminal Care and Bereavement. Leicester: British Psychological Society.

Raphael B (1984) The Anatomy of Bereavement: A Handbook for the Caring Professions. London: Routledge.

Saines J (1997) Phenomenon of sudden death: Part 1. Accident & Emergency Nursing 5: 164–71.

Schonwetter R, Teasdale T, Taffet G, Robinson B, Luchi R (1991) Educating the elderly: cardiopulmonary resuscitation decisions before and after intervention. Journal of the American Geriatric Society 39: 372–7.

Spall B, Callis S (1997) Loss, Bereavement and Grief: A Guide to Effective Caring. Cheltenham: Stanley Thornes.

Stanley J (1987) More fiddling with the definition of death? Journal of Medical Ethics 13: 21–2.

Stroebe M, Stroebe W, Hansson R (eds) (1993) Handbook of Bereavement. Cambridge: Cambridge University Press.

Thompson I, Melia K, Boyd K (1988) Nursing Ethics, 2nd edn. Edinburgh: Churchill Livingstone.

Toulson S (1996) The right to die: the dilemma for A&E nurses. Professional Nurse 11(7): 435–6.

UKCC (1992) Code of Professional Conduct. London: UKCC.

Warren N (1997) Bereavement care in critical care settings. Critical Care Nursing Quarterly 20(2): 42–7.

Worden W (1991) Grief Counselling and Grief Therapy: A Handbook for the Mental Health Practitioner, 2nd edn. London: Routledge.

Wright B (1989) Critical incidents. Nursing Times 85(19): 34–6.

Wright B (1991) Sudden Death: Intervention Skills for the Caring Professions. London: Churchill Livingstone.

Wright B (1993) Caring in Crisis: A Handbook of Intervention Skills. Edinburgh: Churchill Livingstone.

Further reading

Joint Working Party between the National Council for Hospice and Specialist Palliative Care Services and the Ethics Committee of the Association for Palliative Medicine of Great Britain and Ireland (1997) Ethical Decision Making in Palliative Care: Cardiopulmonary Resuscitation (CPR) for People Who Are Terminally Ill.

CHAPTER 5

Cardiac arrest

CAROLE DONALDSON, IAN WOOD
AND MICHELLE RHODES

Aims

This chapter will:

- describe a systematic approach to assessment, treatment and post resuscitative care in peri-arrest and cardiac arrest scenarios
- discuss the role of the MAU nurse at cardiac arrests
- discuss issues relating to witnessed resuscitation

The chapter is based on the Resuscitation Council (UK) (RCUK) Guidelines for Adult Cardiopulmonary Resuscitation (RCUK 2000a).

Introduction

Effective management of a cardiac arrest requires rapid recognition and response from an efficient and well-organised team. For the arrested patient to be given their best chance of survival, the optimum time from recognition of a shockable rhythm to the initiation of the first shock is 3 minutes. As many health care professionals will know, this is the sublime and not the reality, given that the overall survival rate from in-hospital cardiac arrest to discharge from hospital is approximately 17% (Gwinnutt et al 2000). However, with the advent of nurse-led cardiac defibrillation, this poor survival rate may improve.

Early warning signs of cardiac arrest

MAU nurses will recognise that many patients in their care have the potential to 'arrest'. However, signs and symptoms will usually alert the nurse to deterioration in a patient's condition and their predisposition to cardiac arrest. Although nurses often intuitively recognise this, an understanding of 'early warning' vital signs (Box 5.1) can assist in alerting the team to the possibility of cardiac arrest.

Box 5.1. Early warning signs of possible cardiac arrest

- Diminished level of consciousness – due to under-perfusion of the brain
- Diaphoresis – due to the release of adrenaline (epinephrine) and noradrenaline (norepinephrine), causing vasoconstriction and increased sweating
- Altered respiratory rate (either increased or decreased), oxygen desaturation, use of accessory muscles to breathe
- Altered heart rate (either bradycardia, tachycardia or irregular heart rate) – may be due to a variety of reasons such as conditions affecting the conduction system, congenital abnormalities, poisoning, dehydration, heart failure, neurological conditions and sepsis
- Hypotension – usually due to diminished cardiac output. Sometimes the blood pressure may be unrecordable. A useful tool in these circumstances is to estimate the blood pressure by palpating pulses. If a radial pulse is palpable then it can be assumed that the systolic pressure is >80 mmHg. If the radial pulse is absent but the femoral is palpable then the systolic pressure is around 70 mmHg. If only the carotid pulse is palpable then the systolic pressure is >60 mmHg (Merrick 1994)
- Chest pain – may be due to many causes (cardiac, pleuritic or musculoskeletal)
- Reduced urine output – may be due to dehydration or hypovolaemia. Not measured routinely in MAUs unless there is a reason for urinary catheterisation

---

It is important to remember that no single sign or symptom is an indicative precursor to cardiac arrest. The patient must be assessed accurately and holistically to enable their clinical need to be prioritised. The RCUK (2000b) advocate that all hospital staff should undergo regular resuscitation training to a level compatible with their expected clinical responsibilities. Given the acute condition of patients referred to MAUs and the consequent possibility of cardiac arrest, all MAU nurses should be trained in advanced life support (ALS) skills in order to give patients their best chance of survival.

Peri-arrest arrhythmias

Definition: Peri-arrest arrhythmias are potentially serious arrhythmias that may precede cardiac arrest or follow successful resuscitation.

Cardiac arrhythmias are well-recognised complications of myocardial infarction and other common conditions such as hypoxia and tricyclic antidepressant overdose (see Chapter 7 – Altered consciousness, Chapter 8 – Shortness of breath, and Chapter 9 – Chest pain). It is essential that all nurses working in an MAU are able to recognise peri-arrest arrhythmias such as profound bradycardias, broad complex and narrow complex tachycardias. Early recognition of these potentially life-threatening arrhythmias will enable effective medical intervention to improve the patient's chances of returning to an adequately perfusing rhythm. Early detection of peri-arrest arrhythmias can only occur if the patient is monitored haemodynamically (non-invasive blood pressure and continuous cardiac monitoring).

The assessment of arrhythmias has two objectives: firstly, to identify the rhythm correctly and, secondly, to determine if the patient is symptomatic. Once this assessment has been made, there are three routes of action available:

• anti-arrhythmic drugs (or other drugs as appropriate)
• cardioversion
• cardiac pacing

Treatment

1. Treatment of symptomatic arrhythmias

A patient is defined as being 'symptomatic' when there is clinical evidence of shortness of breath, 'low cardiac output, leading to pallor, diaphoresis, hypotension and/or impaired consciousness' (RCUK 1998). Before commencing treatment, monitor the patient through leads via a defibrillator and secure intravenous (IV) access to allow for rapid ALS management should the patient arrest before or during treatment. In order to gain a true appreciation of the rhythm, record a 12-lead electrocardiograph (ECG).

2. The treatment of broad complex tachycardia

Definition: Broad complex tachycardia or ventricular tachycardia (VT) is characterised by the presence of regular broad QRS complexes with a rate >150 bpm.

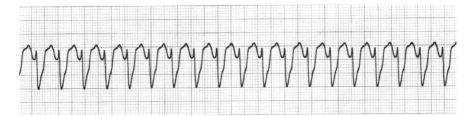

Example of broad complex tachycardia

If this rhythm is present, check the patient's carotid pulse. If the pulse is absent, initiate the pulseless VT branch of the ALS algorithm (see Figure 5.6). If, however, the patient has a broad complex tachycardia with a pulse, is conscious and symptomatic (see Box 5.1), administer 100% oxygen, secure IV access and seek expert help as cardioversion may be required. (Cardioversion is the use of increasing joules of electricity to convert a symptomatic tachycardia to a perfusing rhythm.) In this case, the patient will require a short-acting general anaesthetic. Cardioversion is performed using a manual defibrillator, switched to synchronised mode, thus ensuring that the counter shock is not delivered during the repolarisation phase ('T' wave) as this could induce ventricular fibrillation (VF). As the defibrillator is set to synchronise, there will be a delay from the discharge of the machine to the delivery of the shock. Synchronised shocks should commence at 100 J, increasing to 200 J and then 360 J or their equivalent biphasic energy. In conjunction with cardioversion, the use of IV potassium 30 mmol/hour (in pre-existing hypokalaemia) and IV amiodarone 150 mg may be used for refractory tachycardias (Figure 5.1, page 98). Amiodarone should be diluted in 20 ml of 5% dextrose and may be given into a peripheral vein in an emergency (RCUK 2000a).

If the patient has VT but is asymptomatic, the initial management may be with amiodarone 150 mg IV over 10 minutes or lidocaine (lignocaine) 50 mg IV over 5 minutes, repeated to a maximum dose of 200 mg. Potassium replacement may be considered if the levels are known to be low. Cardioversion may also be used if pharmacological preparations alone are unsuccessful.

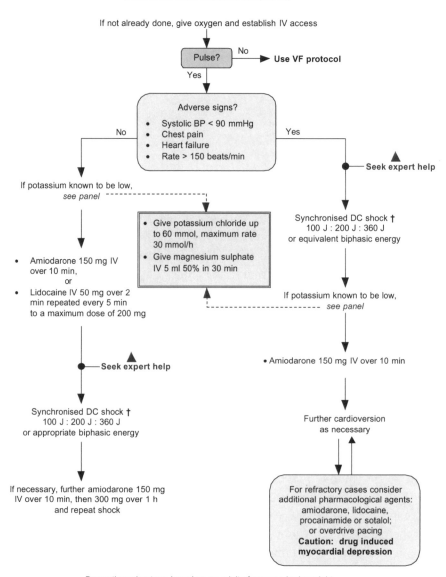

Figure 5.1. Broad complex tachycardia algorithm. Reproduced with permission from the Resuscitation Council UK (2000a) *The Guidelines 2000 for CPR and Emergency Cardiovascular Care.* London:Resuscitation Council (UK).

3. Treatment of narrow complex tachycardias

Definition: Narrow complex tachycardia or supraventricular tachycardia (SVT) is characterised by the presence of narrow, usually regular, QRS complexes, with a ventricular rate often exceeding 200 bpm. The presence of P waves is difficult to determine.

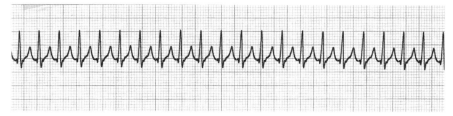

Example of narrow complex tachycardia

The first-line treatment of SVT (having excluded atrial fibrillation (AF)) includes the administration of 100% oxygen, IV access, vagal manoeuvres and/or adenosine 6 mg IV. If the patient is symptomatic then cardioversion may be required along with anti-arrhythmic agents such as IV verapamil or amiodarone (Figure 5.2, p 100). The Resuscitation Council (RCUK 2000a) now recognise that atrial fibrillation may also be a contributing factor to cardiac arrest and have developed a specific algorithm for its treatment (see Figure 5.3).

The most commonly used vagal manoeuvres are carotid sinus massage (see Figure 5.2 for contraindications) or Valsalva manoeuvre (forced expiration against a closed glottis). These stimulate the vagus nerve and induce a reflex that will slow the heart rate. When adenosine is administered the patient must always be monitored via a defibrillator and be informed of its potential for short-acting but alarming side effects, in particular, chest pain, momentary difficulty in breathing, nausea and hot flushing. Adenosine must be used with caution in patients who suffer from Wolff–Parkinson–White syndrome (potential for increasing the ventricular rate) and patients who are taking theophylline-related medications as they block the effect of adenosine.

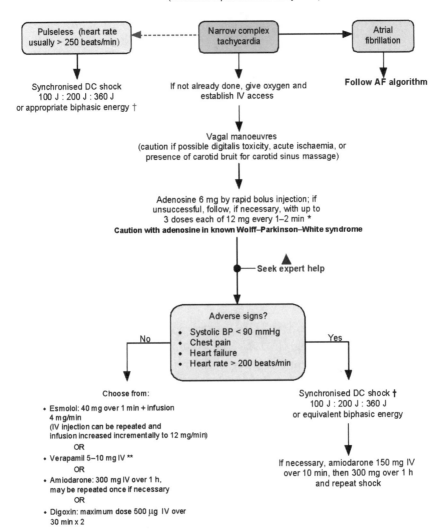

Figure 5.2. Narrow complex tachycardia algorithm. Reproduced with permission from the Resuscitation Council UK (2000a) *The Guidelines 2000 for CPR and Emergency Cardiovascular Care.* London: Resuscitation Council (UK).

4. Treatment of atrial fibrillation (AF)

> Definition: Atrial fibrillation (AF) is characterised by the presence of irregular QRS complexes with no visible P waves and a variable ventricular rate.

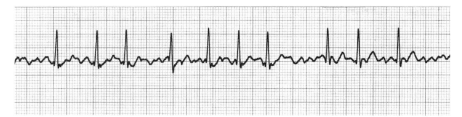

Example of atrial fibrillation

The algorithm for AF is divided into high-risk, intermediate and low-risk categories (Figure 5.3, p 102). The degree of risk centres on the nature of the patient's symptoms, their perfusion status and heart rate. The high-risk patient who is symptomatic with a heart rate >150 bpm is treated with cardioversion and anticoagulation followed by amiodarone 300 mg IV in one hour. Treatment of the intermediate-risk patient, who has poor perfusion and a heart rate of 100–150 bpm, depends on whether they have pre-existing heart disease and if the onset of AF was within the previous 24 hours. Depending upon the answer the patient will be treated with either cardioversion and anticoagulation therapy or IV/oral medication. The "routine" use of IV/oral digoxin is no longer accepted practice in this peri-arrest situation.

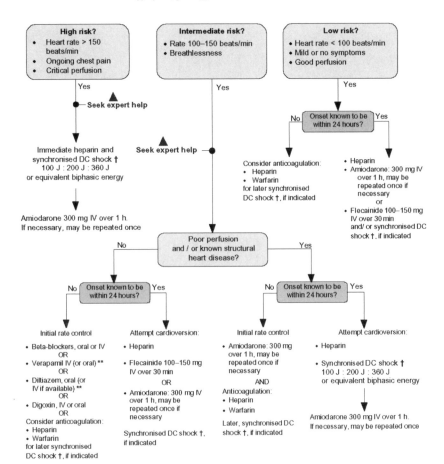

Figure 5.3. Atrial fibrillation algorithm. Reproduced with permission from the Resuscitation Council UK (2000a) *The Guidelines 2000 for CPR and Emergency Cardiovascular Care.* London: Resuscitation Council (UK).

5. Treatment of symptomatic bradycardia

> Definition: Bradycardia is characterised by a ventricular rate of less than 60 bpm, which may be either regular or irregular.

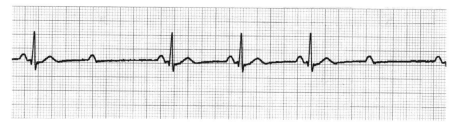

Example of Mobitz type II
Note: – Intermittent loss of QRS complex, causing reduction in ventricular rate.

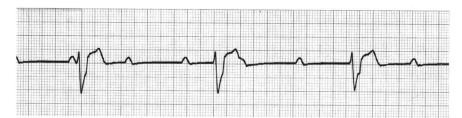

Example of complete heart block
Note: – Complete dissociation between P waves and QRS complexes and slow ventricular rate.

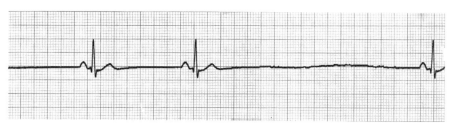

Example of pause
Note: – Temporary loss of any electrical activity.

In patients with poor cardiac function, ventricular rates of <60 bpm may cause symptoms. If the patient is symptomatic, assess the possibility of them developing asystole. The risk of asystole is present if the presenting rhythm is Mobitz type II (second degree), complete (third degree) heart block or if there is a pause of more than 3 seconds on the ECG.

Mobitz type II heart block manifests as sudden unpredictable failure of atrioventricular nodal conduction, resulting in a dropped QRS complex with no preceding changes in the PR interval (Nolan et al 1999). Complete (third degree) heart block presents with complete dissociation between atrial and ventricular activity and usually with broad, regular QRS complexes.

The immediate treatment of symptomatic bradycardia requires the administration of 100% oxygen along with atropine 500 μg IV to block the restraining effects of the vagus nerve, and therefore increase the ventricular rate. Repeat doses of atropine may be given to a maximum dose of 3 mg. Consider urgent referral to the cardiology team, as transvenous cardiac pacing may be necessary. In the presence of clinical signs of diminishing cardiac output (systolic blood pressure <90 mmHg) or pre-existing heart failure, consider external (transcutaneous) cardiac pacing and the use of adrenaline (epinephrine) 2–10 μg/min IV (Figure 5.4).

Non-invasive transcutaneous pacing (external cardiac pacing) should only be used as a temporary measure. Before commencing external cardiac pacing, ensure that the chest is dry and free from combustible substances (such as glyceryl trinitrate (GTN) patches). In some circumstances, the chest hair may need to be clipped (not shaved) in order to provide a good contact with the two pacing pads. Pacing is usually delivered from a multifunction pacing–defibrillator system. During cardiac arrest, it is most convenient to place the pads anteriorly, with one just below the right clavicle and the other in the left mid-axillary line lateral to the nipple. If the system is limited to pacing only, place the pads in the anterior–posterior positions, so that they do not interfere with the positioning of defibrillation paddles. The patient must be continually monitored and reassessed throughout the process. A palpable pulse confirms that pacing is producing a cardiac output.

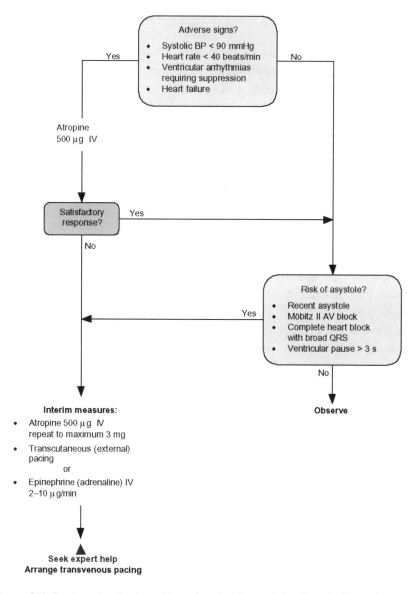

Figure 5.4. Bradycardia algorithm. Reproduced with permission from the Resuscitation Council UK (2000a) *The Guidelines 2000 for CPR and Emergency Cardiovascular Care.* London: Resuscitation Council (UK).

Management of cardiac arrest

Assessment

The recognition of cardiac arrest is based on clinical assessment. The patient presents in a collapsed state with absent respirations and no major pulse. In patients who are undergoing cardiac monitoring it is important to confirm the absence of respirations and pulse rather than simply relying on what is displayed on the monitor. Remember to 'treat the patient and not the monitor'. Other clinical signs may also be present such as diaphoresis and skin mottling but their presence should not detract from the initial assessment of the patient's airway, breathing and circulation. Upon finding a patient collapsed, adopt the sequence of assessment and management set out below.

Initial assessment

Check responsiveness

Shake the patient gently by the shoulders and shout their name or a command such as 'Can you hear me?' If the patient responds verbally then they are obviously not in cardiac arrest. If the patient is unresponsive, sound the emergency bell and shout for help. Lay the patient flat, if not so already, and remove the bed-head if present. When help arrives, the second person should collect the defibrillator as soon as possible and attach the monitoring leads to the patient, while the first person continues with the assessment. This will then allow for rapid defibrillation should the patient be in VF or pulseless VT.

Airway

Gently tilt the patient's head slightly, look inside their mouth and clear any obstructions with the use of suction. When the mouth is clear, open the airway with a head tilt and chin lift. This manoeuvre moves the tongue from the posterior pharynx and opens the airway. If there is the slightest suspicion that a neck injury may be present (consider the mechanism of injury if the patient has suffered any trauma), do not use the head tilt. An alternative manoeuvre in these circumstances is the jaw thrust. If available, insert an oropharyngeal or nasopharyngeal airway.

Breathing

Check for signs of respiratory effort for no longer than 10 seconds using the 'look listen feel' technique. Get close to the patient's mouth, listen and feel for breathing and simultaneously look at their chest for signs of movement. If no breathing is present after 10 seconds, give the patient two slow breaths using a bag-valve-mask device with reservoir (e.g. Ambu bag) connected to oxygen with a flow rate of 15 litres/min. Apply just enough pressure to the bag until a rise of the chest is seen. This usually equates to a tidal volume between 700–1000 ml. Any further pressure could lead to gastric insufflation with the consequent risk of vomiting and aspiration with an unprotected airway. If the patient does vomit, tilt the bed-head down and use suction.

Circulation

Palpate the carotid artery for no longer than 10 seconds to assess if cardiac output is present whilst simultaneously assessing for movement, swallowing or any other signs of life. Although 10 seconds may seem an excessive amount of time, Moule (2000) and Cummins and Hazinski (2000) revealed that on average health care professionals took 30 seconds to determine the absence of a carotid pulse. In 10% of these cases, the health care professional stated that a pulse was present when in fact it was not. For this reason, in 2000, the RCUK recommended that non-health care professionals no longer be taught to palpate a pulse to determine if cardiac output is present.

If a pulse is absent and the monitor shows VF or VT, defibrillate as soon as possible. If a defibrillator is not immediately available, commence external cardiac compressions at a rate of 100 per minute. If a pulse is present, continue to ventilate the patient using a bag-valve-mask with 15 litres/min of supplementary oxygen at a rate of approximately one breath every 6 seconds. Similarly, ventilate the patient if they are making insufficient respiratory effort. Reassess the pulse after one minute of ventilation. If a pulse is not present, combine 15 chest compressions with two ventilations at a rate of 100 compressions per minute (Figure 5.5).

It is important to remember that even when chest compressions are delivered optimally, only 30% of the normal cerebral perfusion is achieved. Therefore, in a hospital environment, basic life support (BLS) should always be delivered in conjunction with airway adjuncts (oropharyngeal or nasopharyngeal airways, bag-valve-mask) and high concentrations of supplementary oxygen. The purpose of BLS is to maintain ventilation and circulation until ALS can be initiated. The priority with any patient suffering cardiac arrest is prompt and effective defibrillation.

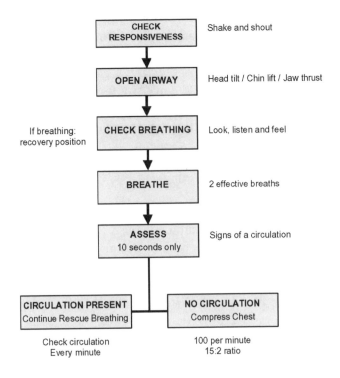

Figure 5.5. BLS algorithm. Reproduced with permission from the Resuscitation Council UK (2000a) *The Guidelines 2000 for CPR and Emergency Cardiovascular Care*. London: Resuscitation Council (UK).

Advanced life support (ALS)

The ALS protocol contains algorithms for shockable and non-shockable rhythms (Figure 5.6). In adults, the commonest primary, shockable arrhythmia at the onset of cardiac arrest is VF (Deluna et al 1989) and the majority of eventual survivors come from this group (Tunstall-Pedoe et al 1992). The other arrhythmia considered in the algorithm of shockable rhythms is pulseless VT. It must be remembered that a pulse can accompany VT and it is therefore imperative to determine the absence of

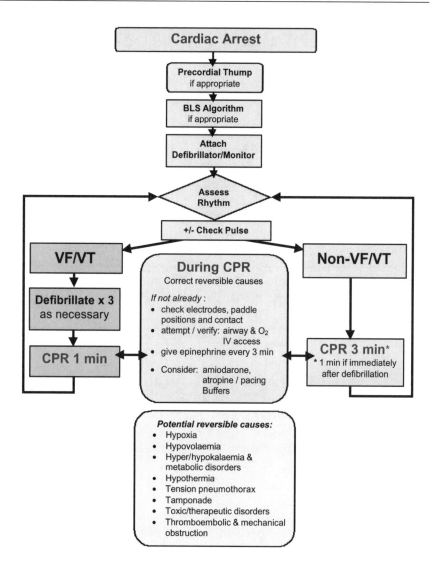

Figure 5.6. ALS algorithm. Reproduced with permission from the Resuscitation Council UK (2000a) *The Guidelines 2000 for CPR and Emergency Cardiovascular Care*. London: Resuscitation Council (UK).

a pulse before proceeding with the algorithm. If a pulse is present and the patient is conscious, go to the peri-arrest algorithm for broad complex tachycardia. The definitive treatment for both pulseless VT and VF is direct current (DC) defibrillation. Probably the greatest advance in the treatment of fatal ventricular arrhythmias came in the 1960s when defibrillation became common practice (Safar and Bircher 1988). Despite much refinement in defibrillation technology, the fact remains that patients who do not respond to the first three shocks have a low survival rate (Nolan et al 1999). The algorithm for non-shockable rhythms includes the management of non-VF/VT (i.e. pulseless electrical activity (PEA) and asystole).

After the diagnosis of cardiac arrest and the delivery of a precordial thump in a witnessed or monitored arrest, initiate BLS and summon the ALS team. Monitor the patient (preferably on a defibrillator) as soon as possible in order to determine the presenting rhythm and to allow the correct side of the treatment algorithm to be followed.

Treatment of VF/pulseless VT

Definition: Ventricular fibrillation (VF) is characterised by the presence of irregular chaotic fibrillation. No P, QRS or T waves are visible.

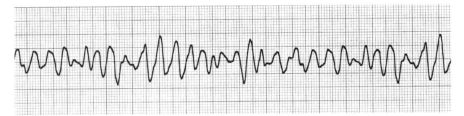

Example of ventricular fibrillation

The aim is to deliver the first shock within 3 minutes of the arrest occurring. Nothing should prevent this, not even the establishment of a secure airway. As nurses are often the first to find a patient in cardiac arrest, there is a very strong argument in support of nurse-led defibrillation in order to improve the patient's survival (Coady 1999). The first two DC shocks are delivered at 200 J with no pulse check between shocks, unless the rhythm changes to one compatible with a cardiac output or the morphology of the rhythm changes. The third shock is delivered at 360 J. The aim is to deliver three shocks (if necessary) within one minute with no interruptions (including BLS). To prevent burning of the skin, and to enhance delivery of electrical energy to the myocardium, gel defibrillation pads are used. Place one pad to the right of the patient's sternum in the mid-clavicular line. Place the second pad over the patient's lower left ribs in the mid-anterior axillary line. Place the defibrillator paddles on these pads and apply firm, even pressure. Paddles should never be placed over breast tissue. The polarity of the paddles is unimportant (Weaver et al 1993) although they are usually labelled 'sternum' and 'apex'. For safety reasons, the chest should be clear of GTN patches, vomit, free-flow oxygen and any other combustible material before delivering shocks. The team member operating the defibrillator is responsible for its safe use. A loud 'stand clear' should be stated and a visual check that nobody (including the operator themselves) is touching the patient or any equipment in contact with the patient. After the first cycle of shocks, carry out one minute of cardiopulmonary resuscitation (CPR). During this time, the team should attempt to gain both IV access and a secure airway with an endotracheal (ET) tube. Tracheal intubation should only be attempted by a competent practitioner. Alternatives to this method of airway management are the laryngeal mask airway (LMA) or Combitube.

As soon as IV access is established, administer 1 mg of adrenaline (epinephrine) 1:10 000 followed by a 20 ml saline flush to expedite its entry into the circulation. If IV access is not possible, give adrenaline (epinephrine) via the ET tube. In this case, give 2–3 mg diluted up to 10 ml with sterile water. The administration of first-line cardiac arrest drugs via the ET tube remains a second-line approach due to impaired absorption and unpredictable pharmacodynamics. The insertion of central lines is not recommended during CPR as the risks associated with their insertion can be life-threatening. Adrenaline is thought to improve both cerebral and myocardial perfusion. Consequently, it is the first drug of choice in cardiac arrest and should be administered every 3 minutes. Evidence that it improves survival or neurological recovery in humans is limited (RCUK 1997). Following a minute of CPR, reassess the rhythm. If VF or pulseless VT persists, deliver all subsequent shocks at 360 J, unless there has been a cardiac output, in which case the algorithm reverts to the beginning with a shock of 200 J. Consider amiodarone 300 mg IV in 20 ml of dextrose as early as before the fourth shock in VF/pulseless VT. A further dose of 150 mg IV may be given followed by an infusion of 1 mg/min over 6 hours if the resuscitation is successful. Give IV magnesium 8 mmol for refractory VF if hypomagnesaemia is known or suspected.

After delivering a DC shock, there is often a delay of a few seconds before an ECG display of diagnostic quality is obtained. Successful defibrillation is followed usually by a few seconds of true asystole (electrical stunning) or temporary impairment of myocardial contractility (myocardial stunning). For this reason, the RCUK recommend that only one minute of CPR is administered before reassessing the rhythm. In this case, withhold adrenaline (epinephrine) in case the rhythm reverts to one that is shockable.

Advances in technology have now produced defibrillators with alternative waveforms, most commonly biphasic. The optimal energies for this type of waveform have yet to be determined. However, repeated biphasic shocks at less than 200 J have been revealed to have equivalent or higher success rates for defibrillation than monophasic waveforms of increasing energy (RCUK 2000a).

Treatment of non-VF/non-VT

The rhythms under this heading are asystole and pulseless electrical activity (PEA) (formerly referred to as electromechanical dissociation (EMD)). These rhythms carry a less favourable prognosis unless a possible cause can be found and treated.

> Definition: Asystole is characterised by a wandering baseline with no visible electrical complexes.

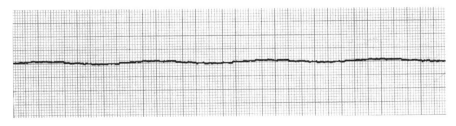

Example of asystole

When observing apparent asystole on the monitor:

- check the patient
- check that the monitoring electrodes are still in position
- check that the size of the ECG waveform (gain) on the defibrillator is turned up in order to discount the presence of fine VF

These actions should take no longer than 10 seconds. If there is still any doubt as to whether the rhythm is fine VF or asystole, treat it as VF as the prognosis is much better. If the rhythm is confirmed as asystole, commence 3 minutes of CPR. During this time, gain IV access and secure the patient's airway as in the VF/pulseless VT algorithm. Give 1 mg of

1:10 000 adrenaline (epinephrine) IV every 3 minutes. The use of a once only dose of atropine 3 mg is recommended for asystole on the basis that there may be increased vagal tone which would contribute to the development of this arrhythmia (Nolan 1998). Evidence of its value in this condition is limited and equivocal. The use of pacing in asystole is also questionable but is advocated when P waves are present (ventricular standstill). When pacing is considered but there is a delay in its delivery, external cardiac percussion should be attempted (repeated precordial blows). Few patients who present in asystole survive except those whose arrest was due to special circumstances such as profound hypothermia.

Where PEA is the primary rhythm, the detection and treatment of potentially reversible causes becomes relatively more important. PEA is recognised by the presence on a monitor of a rhythm that would normally be compatible with a cardiac output but the carotid pulse is not palpable and the patient is lifeless. It is relatively common for the team to linger too long trying to diagnose the rhythm instead of recognising quickly that there is no cardiac output despite QRS complexes being present. The treatment is the same as for asystole with the addition that during the 3 minutes of CPR, the team is considering the possible cause. Consider atropine 3 mg IV if the underlying rhythm is below 60 bpm.

There are broadly eight potentially reversible causes of PEA listed by the RCUK and, for ease of recollection, these are known as the 4Hs and 4Ts (Box 5.2).

Box 5.2. Eight potentially reversible causes of PEA

Hypoxia
Hypovolaemia
Hyper/hypokalaemia, hypocalcaemia and acidaemia
Hypothermia

Tension pneumothorax
Toxic/therapeutic disturbances
Thromboembolic
Tamponade

Hypoxia

This is a common cause of cardiac arrhythmias and subsequent cardiac arrest. Always assume its presence, even in the light of remarkably normal arterial blood gas results. The best treatment is early advanced airway management with ventilatory support and high percentages of supplementary oxygen. The ALS algorithm does highlight the use of buffers (for example, sodium bicarbonate). However, the role of buffers is still uncertain as they can compound acidosis, and arterial gas tensions may be misleading, bearing little relation to the internal cerebral and myocardial intracellular values (Capparelli et al 1989).

Hypovolaemia

Blood/fluid loss leads to underperfusion of vital organs with resultant hypoxia and loss of haemodynamic stability. A high index of suspicion for hypovolaemia should be given to any patient presenting to the MAU who has a recent history of surgery, haemorrhage, trauma, dehydration or heat-related illnesses. Treatment is to replace volume with either a crystalloid (such as 2 litres of 0.9% saline) or colloid (such as Haemaccel or Gelofusine) solution to restore adequate cardiac filling and output.

Hyper/hypokalaemia, hypocalcaemia and acidaemia

Cardiac arrest due to electrolyte abnormalities is uncommon except in the case of hyperkalaemia. Renal failure is a common cause of hyperkalaemia, while dehydration and long-term use of diuretics may cause hypokalaemia. In an MAU environment, clinicians may not have access to urea and electrolyte results; therefore, an estimation of probable values may be made based on the presenting complaint and previous medical history. If an ECG has been obtained before the cardiac arrest, then the presence of 'tented' T waves, small P waves and a prolonged PR interval can be indicative of hyperkalaemia. Treatment is with 10 ml of 10% calcium chloride IV. The presence of inverted T waves, small QRS complexes and large P waves may be indicative of hypokalaemia. This is treated with magnesium 8 mmol IV. The use of sodium bicarbonate 50 mmol can be considered if cardiac arrest is due to tricyclic overdose or hyperkalaemia as there is likely to be a metabolic acidosis in these circumstances.

Hypothermia

Hypothermia inhibits the movement of electrolytes across cell membranes and, therefore, affects the polarity of myocardial cells. Patients rarely present to MAU with hypothermia as a primary condition. However, there is a risk that patients who are intoxicated, elderly or present in a collapsed state could be hypothermic (core temperature <35°C). The hypothermic heart may have a reduced response to pacemaker stimulation, defibrillation and cardioactive drugs. The latter may accumulate to toxic levels. Consequently, modify and prolong the ALS resuscitation until the core temperature rises above 35°C. Active rewarming with heaters, warmed IV fluids or warm peritoneal lavage are the treatments of choice. Extracorporeal bypass can also be performed but this is rare in an MAU.

Tension pneumothorax

This is a rare cause of PEA and is usually diagnosed with a high index of suspicion due to the patient's presenting problem before cardiac arrest. Once the patient's airway has been secured with an ET tube, diagnosis may become easier as there will be increased resistance to ventilation and absence of air entry either unilaterally or bilaterally as the tension (pressure) within the thoracic cavity increases. Tension pneumothorax should always be considered in the young asthmatic patient who is in PEA. Immediate treatment is with needle decompression (i.e. placing a large bore needle or cannula in the second intercostal space, mid-clavicular line on the affected side or bilaterally if indicated). Follow this with the insertion of a chest drain if the resuscitation is successful.

Toxic / therapeutic disturbances

Cardiac arrest due to toxic substances is not uncommon; indeed, toxic substances are the second most common cause of cardiac arrest in 18–35-year-olds (ILCOR 1997). The basic principles of restoring circulation and oxygenation apply here, along with the identification of the toxic substance (e.g. opiate drugs, illegal substances) and the prevention of further absorption. Naloxone, the antidote to opiate medications, may be given intramuscularly (IM) and IV if overdose is suspected. As the half-life of naloxone is relatively short, the IM dose is given to ensure that therapeutic levels are maintained when the IV dose loses its effectiveness.

Thromboembolic

A large pulmonary embolus or cerebrovascular accident is the usual cause. Treatment is limited and the prognosis is poor. The use of anticoagulants or thrombolytic agents in this situation requires further research.

Tamponade

Cardiac tamponade can occur with as little as 10 ml of fluid occupying the pericardial space. This leads to malfunctioning of the heart's pumping action. In an MAU, the most common cause of tamponade is rupture of the ventricular free wall following acute myocardial infarction (Nolan et al 1999). Cardiac tamponade is usually diagnosed by Beck's triad of symptoms. In usual circumstances, the three symptoms of muffled heart sounds, distended neck veins and hypotension are indicative of cardiac tamponade but in the cardiac arrest situation they are not present. As tamponade is so difficult to diagnose and treat, it is usually considered last in the potentially reversible causes of cardiac arrest. The exception to this is when chest trauma is involved. Successful resuscitation in these circumstances is very rare. Treatment with thoracocentesis (needle aspiration) requires a confident approach, skill and accuracy that is almost impossible when CPR is in progress.

Delivery of compressions and ventilations

The 2000 RCUK guidelines for ALS now advocate that, once the airway has been secured by advanced techniques (such as ET intubation, LMA or Combitube), chest compressions and ventilations should be unsynchronised. Research by Kern et al (1998) indicates that continuous chest compression, without interruptions for ventilation, maintains higher mean coronary artery perfusion pressures. Consequently, once the patient has been intubated, chest compressions continue uninterrupted at a rate of 100/min (except for defibrillation or pulse checks when indicated) and ventilations continue at approximately 12 breaths/min. Intubation should only be attempted by a competent practitioner. If correctly positioned, a Combitube should allow for unsynchronized compressions and ventilations. If an LMA has been used, monitor the degree of gas leakage around the cuff during unsynchronized CPR. If continuous compressions cause excessive leakage, revert to the usual ratio of 15 chest compressions to two ventilations.

The MAU nurse's role in the management of a cardiac arrest

Traditionally, nurses have adopted a subservient role within the resuscitation team, whereby they initiate BLS and then 'slip into the background', allowing medical colleagues to lead the resuscitation attempt and conduct the more technical procedures. The advent of multi-disciplinary ALS courses has led to a standardised approach to cardiac arrest management in which nurses and doctors make equal contributions to improving patient outcome. *The Scope of Professional Practice* (UKCC 1992), government strategies (DoH 1999, 2000) and the RCN Guidelines on Clinical Governance (RCN 1998) have enabled nurses to become autonomous decision-makers in cardiac arrest situations and to undertake roles that have previously been medically led. The MAU nurse's role in cardiac arrest situations comprises several components, described below.

1. Early defibrillation

As they have a continuous presence in the unit, MAU nurses are more likely to discover or witness a patient in cardiac arrest than a member of the medical team. They are ideally placed to initiate the first link in the hospital 'chain of survival' (Spearpoint et al 2000) whereby defibrillator paddles/pads are immediately attached to the patient upon recognition of cardiac arrest. Studies conducted by Soar and McKay (1998) and Spearpoint et al (2000) indicate that the majority of in-hospital survivors of cardiac arrest were in VF and had early defibrillation carried out by nursing staff. As a first responder in this way, the appropriately trained MAU nurse can promptly administer the first counter shock to patients who display VF/pulseless VT. This is of paramount importance as the chances of successful defibrillation decline by around 5% with each minute that passes. The commencement of BLS, as would traditionally have been the case, can only slow and not reverse this process of decline (Nolan 1998).

Defibrillation is arguably the most important enhanced role for MAU nursing staff if they are to increase the chances of survival of the arrested patient. There are, however, issues associated with the use of manual defibrillators, in that the operator requires skill in cardiac rhythm interpretation. Unless practised on a regular basis, the skill in recognising cardiac rhythms may decline (Soar and McKay 1998). With regular updates on rhythm interpretation and safety aspects of defibrillation as recommended by the RCUK (2000b), this potential problem can be overcome. The use of automated external defibrillators (AED) is advocated for health care professionals who deal infrequently with cardiac arrests as the operator requires no rhythm interpretation skills and the system uses the safer 'hands off' approach. First responders in pre-hospital settings often use AEDs and training requirements are approximately 4 hours per year. Mancini et al (1995) and Soar and McKay (1998) also concluded that overall retention of knowledge in the use of AEDs is greater than that of manual defibrillators. In the MAU setting, a manual defibrillator is the equipment of choice because of its ability to display a rhythm and its versatility in lead selection and external pacing facilities.

2. Airway management

The RCUK ALS Provider courses are now more easily accessible and, in conjunction with regular updates from hospital-based resuscitation training officers (RTO), the whole concept of the nurse's role in cardiac arrest management is changing. MAU nurses must be competent in the sizing and insertion of oropharyngeal and nasopharyngeal airways and the use of bag-valve-masks. In addition, it may be appropriate for some MAU nurses to develop skills in advanced airway management with the use of LMAs and Combitube and, in some cases, ET intubation. If the latter is the case, regular skills updates may be required if the skill is not practised frequently.

3. Venous access

Many hospital-based nurses working in acute areas are trained to perform cannulation and to collect blood samples. Consequently, many have more expertise in this respect than their junior doctor colleagues. Cannulation should ideally be performed in the pre-arrest phase of the patient's care when superficial veins are more likely to be visible or palpable. Having assessed the patient as requiring one, the MAU nurse is ideally placed to insert and flush a venous cannula as part of the initial management.

4. Continuity of care

As well as being in a position to lead cardiac arrest situations, MAU nurses are also required to maintain continuity of care. This continuity comprises issues within and outwith the arrest scenario. Within the arrest, ensuring that the correct drugs are prepared and ready at the appropriate place in the algorithm helps continuity. The nurse responsible for the drugs can prompt the team leader when the next dose is due and maintain a record of the times and doses of the various drugs that have been administered. During and after the arrest, continuity of care for the patient's relatives must be maintained. A nurse should be allocated to liaise with the family and to keep them informed as to their relative's progress. Similarly, important information can be gathered from relatives with regard to the patient's previous medical history and medications. This liaison role continues in the post-resuscitation phase. Even though the family have no legal right to decide to terminate further medical intervention (RCUK 2001), their views about the further management of their loved one's condition should be sought and considered by the team.

Post-resuscitation care

If the outcome of the resuscitation is successful, post-resuscitative care decisions need to be made. MAU nursing staff must take an active role in monitoring for peri-arrest arrhythmias and recording vital signs. Specific knowledge of indications, contraindications and dosages of medications used to support the patient's cardiac function is required. The MAU nurse may perform post-resuscitation procedures such as recording an ECG, taking venous and arterial blood samples and ordering a chest X-ray. The patient may have a urinary catheter inserted and may require the insertion of central venous and arterial lines. The MAU nurse will also have a contribution to make to the patient's safe transfer to either an intensive therapy unit (ITU), coronary care unit (CCU) bed or a medical ward.

During the post-resuscitation phase, the MAU nurse has an important role as a channel for communication between the resuscitation team and the patient's family. As previously mentioned, a nurse should be allocated to liaise with the family during the resuscitation attempt. The same nurse should continue this role on conclusion of the resuscitation – be it favourable or otherwise.

Should the resuscitation attempt be unsuccessful, a nurse (and if necessary, a doctor) should inform the family as soon as possible. All the literature pertaining to 'breaking bad news' advocates a direct approach, using accurate wording that cannot be misinterpreted. The environment in which relatives are told of the death of a loved one must have all the resources at hand to provide for their needs. The nurse liaising with the family should provide written as well as verbal information to the relatives regarding hospital procedures for post mortem, registration of death and the provision of support groups or bereavement liaison officers. Each family member is unique in the way that they react to distressing news and the nurse delivering this news should be prepared for this (see Chapter 4 – Sudden death). The nurse should be prepared to provide the family with details of treatments given as this will help them to gain a more complete understanding of the events leading to their relative's death.

Witnessed resuscitation in MAUs

An important aspect of caring for the relatives of patients being resuscitated is whether relatives should be offered the opportunity to witness the resuscitation taking place. This controversial and emotive subject has been discussed with increasing frequency in recent years in nursing and medical literature. Historically, the question of witnessed resuscitation has centred on Emergency Departments (EDs) and ITUs. To date, there is little research pertaining to this subject for MAUs. Traditionally, relatives have been excluded when resuscitation involves adults, but with the increased coverage of these events by the media and TV dramatisations, relatives are more aware of what to expect. This has led to an increased number of requests by relatives to be present during resuscitation (RCUK 1996).

Witnessed resuscitation originated in 1982 at Foote Hospital in Michigan, USA. Following a 9-year survey of family members of recently deceased patients to determine whether they felt a need to be present during resuscitation attempts, Hanson and Strawser (1992) revealed a positive response from the families concerned, with 94% stating that they would like to be present at a resuscitation attempt should it occur again. These positive findings have been reflected in other North American ED studies conducted by Meyers et al (1998, 2000) and in the UK by Robinson et al (1998) and the RCUK (1996).

The literature shows that there is a difference of opinion between the public and health care professionals in this matter. In most hospitals, the goal is to save human life and within this culture, relatives may be viewed as a hindrance in resuscitation attempts (Albarran and Stafford 1999). From the family's perspective, the time that they have with their loved one during the resuscitation process may be the last contact before that individual's death. Hanson and Strawser (1992), Meyers et al (2000) and Eichhorn et al (1996) suggest that witnessed resuscitation assists relatives with the grieving process and many relatives believe it to be a positive experience. Findings suggest that relatives should be given the opportunity to touch and speak to their loved one and to ensure that they are not 'alone' in death. Similarly, the family's presence enables the medical team to view the patient as part of a loving family and less as a clinical challenge. However, despite the literature suggesting the benefits of providing the option of family presence during resuscitation, there are arguments against this. Medical and nursing opinions vary considerably, but the main concerns expressed by staff are as follows:

- increased stress to staff
- increase in relatives' distress
- presence of relatives may influence the decision to stop resuscitation
- relatives may try to interfere in the resuscitation attempt
- distressed relatives may influence clinical performance of the teams
- litigation
- patient confidentiality

There is little evidence to support any of these concerns and many can be disputed. Experiences from North America suggest a small decline in litigation where relatives have been present during resuscitation (Hadfield-Law 1999). This may be because of open communication with relatives who can observe that every intervention has been attempted. It is interesting to note that at Foote Hospital, where the biggest study of witnessed resuscitation took place, there were no incidences of relatives interfering whilst resuscitation activities were carried out (Hanson and Strawser 1992). On the occasions when relatives became faint or hysterical, the support person played a vital role in escorting them from the resuscitation area and assisting them with their physical and emotional needs. By so doing, they enabled the resuscitation to continue smoothly.

It cannot be assumed that patients would consent to relatives witnessing their treatment (Stewart and Bowker 1997). However, few patients who have survived resuscitation have been involved in this debate (Hadfield-Law 1999). Certainly, confidentiality issues need consideration and patients who require resuscitative measures should be afforded the same rights to confidentiality as everyone else. By the very nature of their condition, it is not possible to ask patients whether they would wish their relatives to witness their treatment, and in such situations, the legal and confidentiality issues are generally outweighed by humane considerations (McLauchlan 1997). Clearly these issues require much further debate and discussion in order to provide doctors and nurses with clear evidence on which to base future practice.

All other areas of concern may be addressed by the development and introduction of witnessed resuscitation guidelines within the MAU. These guidelines can be developed around the following principles (Eichhorn et al 1996):

- assessing the needs of the family
- preparing the family for the resuscitation environment
- supporting the family during and after resuscitation

The RCUK (1996) also address these issues in their guidelines (Box 5.3) and advocate the presence of an appropriately trained and experienced nurse or member of the clergy to accompany the relatives during the resuscitation. Effective preparation and training is of prime importance to ensure the success of this supportive role.

Box 5.3. Guidelines on the principles of enabling witnessed resuscitation (RCUK 1996)

These guidelines are generalised but can be adapted to most circumstances. It is important to remember that every situation is unique and every person different. The carer must be able to:

- Acknowledge the difficulty of the situation. Ensure that the relatives understand that they have a choice whether or not to be present during resuscitation. Avoid provoking feelings of guilt whatever their decision.
- Explain that they will be accompanied by someone specifically to care for them, whether or not they enter the resuscitation room. Make sure introductions are made and names are known.
- Give a clear and honest explanation of what has happened in terms of the illness or injury and warn them of what they can expect to see when they enter the room, particularly the procedures they may witness.
- Ensure that they understand that they will be able to leave and return at any time, and will always be accompanied.
- Ask the relative not to interfere for the good of the patient and their own safety. They will be allowed the opportunity to touch the patient when it is safe to do so.
- Explain the procedures as they occur in terms that the relatives can understand. Ultimately, this will mean being able to explain that the patient has failed to respond and has died and that the resuscitation has had to be abandoned.
- Advise that once the relative has died, there will be a brief interval while equipment is removed after which they can return to be with the deceased in private. Under some circumstances, the coroner may require certain tubes to be left in place.
- Offer the relatives time to think about what has happened and give them the opportunity to ask further questions.

The literature supporting the inclusion of families within the resuscitation room far outweighs the concerns of the medical and nursing staff. With the implementation of strong guidelines and with appropriately trained staff, MAU nurses can alleviate the loss of control experienced by relatives when isolated from their loved one at such a critical time. By excluding families from a dying patient's resuscitation as a matter of routine, death is portrayed merely as a clinical event. By so doing, we devalue the importance of death as a profound human event that touches the lives of others, we protect and perpetuate our own myth of control (Van der Wong 1997), and as a medical team, we allow our own insecurities to compound the grief of the dying patient's relatives.

Summary

This chapter has outlined practice guidelines for the management of cardiac arrest and peri-arrest situations. MAU nurses' roles in recognising and responding to cardiac arrests are fundamental in ensuring that these guidelines are effectively implemented, thereby offering the patient their best chance of survival. Despite the fact that many MAUs have a constant presence of medical personnel, nurse-led cardiac arrest management and defibrillation would further improve the care of this patient group. Similarly, the development of a unit policy on the issue of relatives witnessing resuscitation is recommended.

References

Albarran J, Stafford H (1999) Resuscitation and family presence; implications for nurses in critical care areas. Advancing Clinical Nursing 3(1): 11–19.

Capparelli E, Chow M, Kluger J, Fieldman A (1989) Differences in systolic and myocardial blood acid–base status during cardiopulmonary resuscitation. Critical Care Medicine 17: 442–4.

Coady E (1999) A strategy for nurse defibrillation in general wards. Resuscitation 42:183–6.

Cummins R, Hazinski M (2000) Guidelines based on fear of type 11 (false negative) errors. Why we dropped the pulse check for lay rescuers. Resuscitation 46(1–3): 439–42.

Deluna A, Courrel P, Ledercq J (1989) Ambulatory sudden cardiac death; mechanisms of production of fatal arrhythmia on the basis of data from 157 cases. American Heart Journal 117: 151–9.

Department of Health (1999) Making a Difference; Strengthening the Nursing, Midwifery and Health Visiting Contribution to Health and Health Care. London: Department of Health.

Department of Health (2000) The NHS Plan – a Plan for Investment, a Plan for Reform. London: Department of Health.

Eichhorn D, Meyers T, Thomas G, Guzetta C (1996) Opening the doors: family presence during resuscitation. Journal of Cardiovascular Nursing 10(4): 59–70.

Gwinnutt C, Columbo M, Harris R (2000) Outcome after cardiac arrest in adults in UK hospitals: effect of the 1997 guidelines. Resuscitation 47: 125–35.

Hadfield-Law L (1999) Do relatives have a place in the resuscitation room? Care of the Critically Ill 15(1):19–22.

Hanson D, Strawser D (1992) Family presence during cardiopulmonary resuscitation – Foote Hospital Emergency Department's nine year perspective. Journal of Emergency Nursing 18(2): 104–6.

International Liaison Committee on Resuscitation (ILCOR) (1997) Special resuscitation situations. Resuscitation 34:129–49.

Kern K, Hilwig R, Berg R, Ewy G (1998) Efficiency of chest compressions only BLS CPR in the presence of an occluded airway. Resuscitation 39:179–88.

Mancini M, Kaye W, Giuliano K, Richards N, Nagid D, Marker C, Sawyer-Silva S (1995) Strengthening the in-hospital chain of survival with rapid defibrillation by first responders using automated external defibrillators; training and retention issues. Annals of Emergency Medicine 25(2):163–8.

McLauchlan C (1997) Letter in British Medical Journal 314: 1044.

Merrick C (1994) Pre Hospital Trauma Life Support Provider Manual, 3rd edn. St Louis: Mosby Year Book.

Meyers T, Eichhorn D, Guzetta C (1998) Do families want to be present during CPR? – A retrospective survey. Journal of Emergency Nursing 24: 400–5.

Meyers T, Eichhorn D, Guzzetta C, Clark A, Klein J, Taliaferro E, Calvin A (2000) Family presence during invasive procedures and resuscitation. Advanced Journal of Nursing 100: 32–43.

Moule P (2000) Checking the carotid pulse; diagnostic accuracy in students of the health care profession. Resuscitation 44(3): 195–201.

Nolan J (1998) The 1998 European Resuscitation Council Guidelines for Advanced Life Support. British Medical Journal 316: 1863–9.

Nolan J, Greenwood J, Mackintosh A (1999) Cardiac Emergencies – A Pocket Guide. Oxford: Butterworth Heinemann.

Resuscitation Council UK (1996) Should Relatives Witness Resuscitation? – A Report from a Project Team of the Resuscitation Council UK. London: Resuscitation Council (UK).

Resuscitation Council (UK) (1997) Resuscitation Guidelines for Use in the United Kingdom. London: Resuscitation Council (UK).

Resuscitation Council (UK) (1998) Advanced Life Support Course Provider Manual, 3rd edn. London: Resuscitation Council (UK).

Resuscitation Council UK (2000a) The Guidelines 2000 for CPR and Emergency Cardiovascular Care. London: Resuscitation Council (UK).

Resuscitation Council UK (2000b) Cardiopulmonary Resuscitation Guidance for Clinical Practice and Training in Hospitals. London: Resuscitation Council (UK).

Resuscitation Council UK (2001) Decisions Relating to Cardiopulmonary Resuscitation – A Joint Statement from the British Medical Association, the Resuscitation Council (UK) and the Royal College of Nursing. London: Resuscitation Council (UK).

Robinson S, MacKenzie-Ross S, Campbell Hewson G, Egleston C, Prevost A (1998) Psychological effect of witnessed resuscitation on bereaved relatives. Lancet 352: 614–17.

Royal College of Nursing (1998) Guidance for Nurses on Clinical Governance. London: RCN.

Safar P, Bircher N (1988) Cardiopulmonary Cerebral Resuscitation, 3rd edn. London: WB Saunders.

Soar J, McKay U (1998) A revised role for the hospital cardiac arrest team? Resuscitation 38:145–9.

Spearpoint K, McLean C, Zidemann D (2000) Early defibrillation and the chain of survival in 'in hospital' adult cardiac arrest: minutes count. Resuscitation 44: 165–9.

Stewart K, Bowker L (1997) Might lead to a complaint for breach of confidentiality. British Medical Journal 314: 145.

Tunstall-Pedoe H, Bailey L, Chamberlain D, Marsden A, Ward M, Zideman D (1992) Survey of 3765 cardiopulmonary resuscitations in British hospitals (BRESUS Study). British Medical Journal 304: 1347–51.

UKCC (1992) The Scope of Professional Practice for Nurses, Midwives and Health Visitors. London: United Kingdom Central Council.

Van der Wong M (1997) Should relatives be invited to witness a resuscitation attempt? A review of the literature. Accident and Emergency Nursing 5(4): 215–18.

Weaver W, Martin J, Wirkus M, Vincent S, Litwin P (1993) Influence of external defibrillator electrode polarity on cardiac resuscitation. Pace 16: 285–90.

CHAPTER 6

Shock

JUDITH MORGAN

Aims

This chapter will:

- describe the causes and pathophysiology of shock
- describe the clinical features of patients who present with shock
- outline a systematic approach to the assessment and immediate management of the shocked patient

Introduction

The diagnosis and treatment of shock can be one of the most challenging situations for the medical assessment team. Shock can be defined as a life-threatening condition where tissue metabolism is inadequate and it develops when oxygen supply is inadequate to meet oxygen demand at cellular level (Selfridge-Thomas 1995). Shock can be classified in many ways. However, MAU nurses will mainly deal with four types (Box 6.1).

Box 6.1. Types of shock most commonly seen in the MAU

Hypovolaemic
Cardiogenic
Septic
Anaphylactic

Clinical features of shock

The clinical features associated with the shocked patient vary according to the type of shock present. However, several clinical features are common to all types of shock (Box 6.2).

Box 6.2. Clinical features common to all types of shock

Raised respiratory rate
Tachycardia (in initial stages)
Altered blood pressure
Reduced urine output
Altered consciousness

Initial assessment

An initial assessment, as for any patient in the MAU, must identify life-threatening problems. Assessment of the patient's airway, breathing, circulation and neurological disability are of paramount importance (see Chapter 2 – Initial assessment). Gather a history of the patient's present problem and their previous medical history.

Airway

Ensure that the patient's airway is clear. If necessary, use positioning and suctioning techniques, airway adjuncts or advanced airway management techniques to maintain a patent airway.

Breathing

Respiratory rate is the first physiological parameter to be affected when shock is developing. Count the patient's respiratory rate and note their depth of respiration. Assess the adequacy of their ventilation and note any altered breathing sounds. Check that the patient has bilateral air entry and lung expansion. Record their oxygen saturation levels and commence 100% oxygen therapy to ensure satisfactory saturations.

Circulation

The adequacy of the patient's circulation can be assessed through several physiological parameters: pulse, blood pressure, capillary refill, skin colour, appearance, turgor and texture, urine output and level of consciousness.

Disability (neurological)

Evidence of an altered consciousness level (e.g. irritability, confusion, drowsiness) is a late developing feature of shock caused by reduced cerebral tissue perfusion.

If appropriate, emergency care should be initiated immediately and expert assistance sought from the multiprofessional team (i.e. nurses, physicians, anaesthetists, surgeons, medical emergency team).

Exposure

It is important to undress the patient in order to inspect their skin for rashes that may indicate meningococcal septicaemia.

Immediate management

In suspected cases of shock, the management interventions shown in Box 6.3 can be administered whilst the assessment is being carried out.

Box 6.3. Immediate management of the shocked patient

Administer 100% oxygen
Lay the patient flat to maintain cerebral perfusion (if appropriate)
Insert two large bore (14G) IV cannulae in large veins (ante-cubital fossae)
Consider commencing IV fluids depending on the cause of shock (see later)

Hypovolaemic shock

Causes

There are three main causes of hypovolaemia (Box 6.4). A hypovolaemic state results from a mismatch between fluid intake and fluid loss/output.

Box 6.4. Main causes of hypovolaemia

Haemorrhage
Inadequate fluid intake
Excessive fluid output

Extensive haemorrhage is an important cause of hypovolaemic shock. It is common following a gastrointestinal bleed (e.g. duodenal ulcer, gastric ulcer, oesophageal varices) and from a ruptured or leaking aortic aneurysm.

Inadequate fluid intake can occur in states of unconsciousness, confusion, dysphagia, mental ill health, depression, reduced mobility, loss of thirst, fever, lack of care from carers (Iggulden 1999).

Excessive fluid output can have many causes:

- increased gut motility (e.g. diarrhoea and vomiting)
- diaphoresis (i.e. sweating)
- skin loss with subsequent fluid seepage (e.g. burns, scalds)
- effusions (e.g. capillary leakage or ascites)
- acute haemorrhagic pancreatitis
- endocrine conditions (e.g. diabetes insipidus, diabetes mellitus)
- diuretic therapy or overdose (e.g. furosemide (frusemide))
- excessive fluid removal during renal dialysis

Pathophysiology

In an average 70 kg adult, there are approximately 42 litres of fluid distributed between three compartments: intracellular fluid (within the cells) and extracellular fluid, which is distributed in an intravascular compartment, and an interstitial fluid compartment (Guyton and Hall 1996).

The intravascular compartment comprises 5 litres of blood. Of this, 3 litres is water with the remainder being made up of blood cells and proteins. Interstitial fluid accounts for approximately 11 litres of fluid, mainly of water and electrolytes (e.g. potassium, magnesium, nitrates) with other dissolved substances and urea. The intracellular compartment contains approximately 28 litres of fluid, which consists mainly of glucose with little or no sodium.

When fluid is lost through dehydration or blood loss, it is important to replace the fluid lost from each compartment with the appropriate type in order to maintain an equilibrium (Figure 6.1). In haemorrhage, initial fluid loss can be replaced by using a crystalloid (a substance that is evaporated to crystals when heated) such as 0.9% sodium chloride (normal saline) or Hartmann's solution. If haemorrhage is significant, blood is the preferred replacement fluid as only blood has an oxygen-carrying capacity. In this case, the ideal treatment is to replace like with like (e.g. replace blood loss with blood). In the event of extensive blood loss, the blood pressure can be increased by using gelatine-based solutions (e.g. Haemaccel™, Gelofusine™) or complex carbohydrate solutions (Hesteril™,

Pentaspan™, Hetastarch™). These types of colloid are not intended to replace more than a third of the circulating volume as they remain in the circulation for 12–24 hours (ABPI 1999–2000).

Extracellular fluid		Intracellular fluid
Intravascular compartment	Interstitial compartment	
Crystalloid		
0.9% sodium chloride IV infusion Isotonic solution Replaces fluid and sodium chloride outside the cell		5% glucose IV infusion
Hartmann's solution IV infusion Contains: sodium chloride, potassium chloride and calcium chloride Replaces fluid and electrolytes outside the cell		
0.9% sodium chloride and 5% glucose IV infusion Composed of both dextrose, sodium and chloride Water from the solution will pass into the cell Glucose will cross into the cell Isotonic sodium chloride will remain extracellular		
Colloid		
Plasma substitutes		
Gelofusine or Haemaccel Animal product – gelatine based Large protein molecules which stay in circulation Maximum infusion 2000 ml Haematocrit should not fall below 25% (ABPI 1999–2000)		
Hetastarch or Pentastarch Etherified starch based Large molecules which stay in circulation Supports the circulation for more than 24 hours (ABPI 1999–2000) Maximum dose 20 ml/kg/24 hours (ABPI 1999–2000)		
Dextran 70 Starch-based solution Large molecules which stay in circulation Maximum dosage 20 ml/kg in first 24 hours (BMA/RPSGB 1999)		

Figure 6.1. Fluid replacement suitable for compartments.

Hypovolaemia due to blood loss

Local reaction

Vessel damage causes local vasoconstriction of the damaged area and its surrounding tissue. A platelet plug forms in an attempt to occlude the damage and to arrest bleeding. Blood flow in this area is slowed to prevent the clot from dislodging. If the damage to the vessel is greater than 5 mm, the platelet plug may not be able to form and bleeding will continue.

Systemic reaction

When blood loss reaches a critical level, baroreceptors in the carotid sinus and arch of the aorta detect a drop in blood pressure and a number of compensatory mechanisms are activated via the sympathetic and parasympathetic branches of the autonomic nervous system. This leads to vasoconstriction (increased peripheral vascular resistance) and an increase in heart rate and force of ventricular contraction, which increases stroke volume, cardiac output and blood pressure. Breathing becomes deeper and more rapid to ensure maximum oxygenation of remaining haemoglobin molecules. If bleeding continues and fluid loss is not replaced, there will be a steady increase in the respiratory rate, heart rate, force of ventricular contraction and peripheral vascular resistance. Only when approximately 30% of the normal blood volume is lost will the systolic blood pressure start to drop (American College of Surgeons (ACS) Committee on Trauma 1997). Hypotension has physiological effects on other systems.

Renal effects. Low blood pressure affects the afferent arterioles of the kidney and causes renin production, which splits angiotensinogen (plasma protein) to form angiotensin I. This is then converted to angiotensin II, which is a very powerful vasoconstrictor. In response to the production of angiotensin I and II, aldosterone is released. This causes the renal tubules to retain sodium and water, leading to a reduced urine output, increased circulating blood volume and a rise in blood pressure.

Neurological effects. Hypotension leads to reduced cerebral oxygenation (cerebral hypotension and reduced cerebral blood flow), causing the patient to become progressively confused and, on occasions, aggressive as their conscious level starts to deteriorate.

When the blood loss exceeds 50% of normal circulating volume, the compensatory mechanisms described above are no longer effective and haemodynamic collapse ensues (ACS Committee on Trauma 1997). Some young, fit adults are able to maintain their blood pressure until significantly more blood is lost. However, after this there is a marked drop in systolic blood pressure that can lead rapidly to cardiac arrest.

Hypovolaemia due to dehydration

Dehydration can occur insidiously or acutely. Insidious onset of dehydration frequently occurs in the older person, as they lose ability to concentrate urine adequately (Watson 1996) and may deliberately limit their fluid intake throughout the day so as not to get up at night to urinate. The elderly may also have a reduced sensation of thirst (Watson 1996). This insidious onset can cause hypernatraemic dehydration, as water is lost without some of the salts. This should be suspected when the specific gravity of the urine is at the lower limits of normal (normal range: 1.000 to 1.025). The presenting features of this type of dehydration can be confusion and/or hallucinations (Iggulden 1999) as well as the classic signs of shock (increased heart and respiratory rate with a late drop in blood pressure). Acute dehydration occurs because conditions such as vomiting (with or without diarrhoea) cause hyponatraemia in which both salts and water are depleted. The thirst reflex is absent in this type of dehydration (Watson 1996).

Presenting features

Clinical features of hypovolaemic shock will depend upon the degree of shock present. In addition to the physiological responses outlined in Table 6.1, the patient may be pale, diaphoretic (sweaty), peripherally cold and clammy. As shock progresses, the patient will show signs of cerebral hypoxia, as detailed above.

Immediate management

The immediate management for all causes of hypovolaemic shock is to find the cause and treat it as quickly as possible. The immediate management for the shocked or critically ill adult is outlined in Table 6.2. Aim to titrate warmed IV fluids to ensure that the patient's systolic blood pressure remains at approximately 100 mmHg. This ensures that a rising blood pressure does not dislodge clots that may have formed at bleeding points and is known as 'hypotensive fluid resuscitation'.

Table 6.1. Physiological responses to estimated fluid loss (adapted from ACS 1997)

	Class 1	Class 2	Class 3	Class 4
Fluid/blood loss	Up to 15%	15–30%	30–40%	>40%
Respiration rate	14–20	20–30	30–40	>35
Heart rate	<100	>100	>120	>140
Pulse pressure	Normal or increased	Decreased	Decreased	Decreased
Capillary refill	<2 seconds	>2 seconds (slow)	>2 seconds (slow)	Undetectable
Blood pressure	Normal	Systolic – normal Diastolic – raised	Systolic – decreased Diastolic – raised	Both decreased
Urine output	>30 ml/h	20–30 ml/h	5–15 ml/h	Negligible
Fluid replacement	Crystalloid/ colloid	Crystalloid/ colloid	Crystalloid/ colloid and blood	Crystalloid/ colloid and blood

Table 6.2. Immediate management for the shocked or critically ill patient

Airway	Maintain a patent airway Use suction, adjuncts and advanced techniques as appropriate
Breathing	Administer high flow oxygen (100%) via an oxygen mask with non-rebreathing bag Record respiratory rate, depth and oxygen saturation levels Monitor respiratory effort and equality of ventilation
Circulation	Insert two 14G IV cannulae in ante-cubital fossae Commence warmed IV fluid as appropriate (crystalloid 20 ml/kg or colloid 10 ml/kg) Record pulse rate, volume and regularity manually Note the patient's skin colour Feel the skin for heat and moisture Consider possible causes for hypovolaemia Record a 12-lead ECG Commence continuous cardiac monitoring and observe for arrhythmias Insert a central venous catheter and record central venous pressure (CVP) Insert a urinary catheter and record hourly urine output

Obtain blood samples for group and cross match, urea and electrolytes, clotting screen, full blood count and arterial blood gases. If the patient is bleeding and showing signs of class 3 shock (Table 6.1), order type-specific blood. If class 4 shock is evident, consider administering 'O' negative blood (universal donor). Remember that haemoglobin (Hb) results may be unreliable, as when extensive bleeding occurs, the blood is not diluted immediately. The patient's Hb may remain at a pre-haemorrhage level until fluid from the interstitial space or from the IV infusion dilutes the circulating volume. When this happens the Hb falls, as does the packed cell volume (PCV).

If the patient is suffering from diarrhoea and vomiting, they may need to be isolated until it is known that they are not infectious.

Diagnostic investigations

If the patient is bleeding from the gastrointestinal tract, gastroscopy or sigmoidoscopy may be considered (see Chapter 10 – Abdominal pain and upper gastrointestinal bleeding). Likewise, a patient suffering from diarrhoea and vomiting will need stool samples sent for microscopy, culture and sensitivity.

Ongoing assessment and nursing management

Ongoing assessment is important in determining the cardiovascular state of a patient who may be developing hypovolaemic shock. If untreated, hypovolaemia can progress through four stages (classes) as the patient's condition deteriorates (Table 6.1). Early, accurate assessment and prompt intervention will prevent this happening. When using this classification system of shock, the individual's underlying state of health must be considered. For example: a fit, healthy patient with a normal resting pulse rate of 50 bpm could be considered to be tachycardic even before their pulse rate increases to 100 bpm. A core care plan for the ongoing assessment and nursing management of the shocked or critically ill adult is outlined in Table 6.3.

Cardiogenic shock

Causes

Cardiogenic shock can be defined as severe heart failure with significant hypotension due to left ventricular dysfunction. It usually occurs following an acute myocardial infarction (AMI), but can occur with cardio-myopathy, mitral valve incompetence, arrhythmias, rupture of papillary muscle or ventricular septal defect. Dysfunction of the left ventricle is the cause in 85% of patients who develop cardiogenic shock. Shock occurs when more than 40% of the left ventricle is damaged. Cardiogenic shock may also develop because of cumulative damage to the left ventricle, for example due to a new infarct in a patient with a previous history of AMI

Table 6.3. Core nursing plan for shocked or critically ill patient

Problem or potential problem	Plan of care
Airway Compromise or potential for	Maintain a patent airway. If appropriate use airway adjuncts Use suction as required, exercise care when suctioning endotracheal tubes as oxygen depletion can occur if suctioning extends beyond 15 seconds
Breathing Complications or potential for	Record respiratory rate and depth – initially recordings every 5–10 minutes may be necessary Record oxygen saturations continuously. Set alarms to alert when levels are <90–95% Observe for reduced air entry on either side of chest Titrate oxygen to maintain saturation levels ≥95% Monitor arterial blood gases
Circulatory Insufficiency or potential for	Continuous cardiac monitoring of heart rate and rhythm – if a new arrhythmia presents, record serial ECGs Record heart rate – initially recordings every 5–10 minutes may be necessary Note regularity and strength of pulse Feel the skin for heat and moisture and monitor peripheral perfusion Record blood pressure – initially recordings every 5–10 minutes may be necessary Seek medical help if the systolic pressure falls below 90 mmHg or the mean arterial pressure falls below 60 mmHg Inspect IV cannulae for inflammation and swelling Administer warmed IV fluid and medications as prescribed Measure (manual or transduced) CVP every 15 minutes whilst patient is shocked or has the potential to become shocked Insert a urinary catheter and measure urine output every 15 minutes Record hourly fluid intake and output
Reduced conscious level or potential for	Observe for reduced conscious level or early signs of confusion, agitation or aggression Record neurological observations as indicated by the patient's condition
Dry sore mouth and lips due to oxygen therapy	Offer sips of water or mouth washes frequently Lubricate lips
Potential for pressure sore development	Undertake a pressure sore risk assessment and plan care accordingly Keep skin and bedding as dry as possible
Anxiety	Keep patient informed of what is going to happen, be honest and reassure the patient even when they are confused or have a reduced conscious level With the patient's permission, inform relatives of condition and progress – ensure consent is real as individuals who are shocked can argue that they were not of sound mind when they agreed to an action Reassure and support relatives
Nutrition	Consider how best to meet the patient's nutritional needs

(Hands 1997). In such cases, the prognosis is poor and carries an 80% in-hospital mortality rate (Nolan et al 1998). The remaining 15% of patients have potentially reversible cardiogenic shock due to extensive inferior myocardial infarction, which involves the right ventricle, and carries a mortality rate of 20% (Nolan et al 1998, Thompson 1997a). Rarer causes of cardiogenic shock are those that produce low cardiac output as the heart is prevented from ejecting blood with sufficient force (e.g. cardiac tamponade, tension pneumothorax, pulmonary embolism and aortic stenosis).

Pathophysiology

When the left side of the heart fails to pump blood with sufficient force, the cardiac output drops, with the result that the systolic blood pressure falls to below 90 mmHg. Hypotension triggers an autonomic nervous system response causing increased respiratory rate, increased heart rate with increased ventricular contractility and increased peripheral vascular resistance (vasoconstriction). These responses increase the diastolic blood pressure (afterload) and so, more force is needed to eject blood effectively from the left ventricle. A state of persistent hypotension causes reduced urine output even though there has been no depletion in fluid volume. In the vasculature, pre-capillary vasodilation and post-capillary vasoconstriction result in circulating fluid seeping into the interstitial spaces (Swanton 1994). Hypotension can also cause cerebral underperfusion with the resultant cerebral hypoxia causing confusion, agitation or a reduced conscious level. Poor ejection of blood from the left ventricle causes congestion within the left atrium and pulmonary veins with resultant pulmonary oedema, as the pulmonary circulation tries to empty into an already full left side of the heart. If severe, this will eventually lead to right-sided heart failure due to the high pressure within the pulmonary circulation that the right ventricle has to contract against. Right-sided heart failure subsequently causes back-pressure into the systemic venous circulation. This is characterised by neck vein distension, pitting oedema in the lower limbs or abdominal ascites.

In cardiogenic shock due to right ventricular dysfunction (which may occur when a right ventricular MI accompanies an extensive inferior MI), the pathophysiology is quite different. The right ventricle dilates, leading to a drop in right ventricular pressure and a subsequent fall in cardiac output from the right ventricle. This results in back-pressure into the systemic venous circulation and less blood being pumped to the left ventricle (reduced left ventricular preload). As a result, left ventricular output is reduced and blood pressure falls. Typical features include hypotension and raised neck veins without pulmonary oedema (Nolan et al 1998). The treatment varies considerably from the conventional treatment for cardiogenic shock, and includes reperfusion of the ischaemic myocardium by the early administration of a thrombolytic agent and infusion of IV fluids to increase right ventricular filling pressure. This will improve right ventricular output and, therefore, increase left ventricular filling and cardiac output leading to an increase in blood pressure. Treatments which reduce right ventricular filling pressure, including diuretics and nitrates, must be avoided as they would lead to a further drop in blood pressure (Thompson 1997a). Fluid loading must be done carefully, preferably with invasive haemodynamic monitoring (including pulmonary artery pressure and pulmonary capillary wedge pressure) in either the coronary care unit (CCU) or intensive care unit (ICU). Dobutamine may be introduced to improve right ventricular contractility and dual chamber pacing may be necessary if heart block is present (Thompson 1997a).

Presenting features

A diagnosis of myocardial infarction, based on clinical symptoms and ECG evidence, may or may not have already been made. The patient will usually present with severe chest pain (Box 6.5).

Box 6.5. Presenting features of cardiogenic shock

Chest pain (remember, no pain in silent MI)
Anxiety (feeling of impending doom)
Tachypnoea
Severe dyspnoea (with pink, frothy sputum if acute left ventricular failure)
Tachycardia (more rarely, bradycardia)
Hypotension
Pallor or cyanosis
Cold, clammy skin
Reduced urine output
Pitting oedema

Patients in cardiogenic shock will have severe dyspnoea and tachypnoea. This poor respiratory state will progress to Cheyne–Stokes breathing in the pre-terminal stage. Cardiac arrhythmias may be present. The patient will invariably have a tachycardia or, more rarely, a bradycardia. If bradycardia follows a tachycardia, this is usually a pre-terminal sign (Horvath 2000). Persistent hypotension results in a reduced urine output of <30 ml/h, which will progress to anuria. The patient will look pale or cyanosed, their skin will feel cold and clammy and they may have a delayed capillary refill time. Poor cerebral perfusion will lead to restlessness and irritability. In patients with ensuing right ventricular failure, distended neck veins and pitting oedema in the lower parts of the body (legs, hands or sacral area if sitting) will be present. In the older person the symptoms of cardiogenic shock can progress rapidly (Horvath 2000).

Immediate management

The aim in managing these patients is to reduce cardiac workload by reducing afterload and oxygen consumption, to correct the filling pressures and improve the contractility of the heart whilst reducing fluid overload. This is very complex and the condition is associated with a high mortality rate if symptoms of shock are present for more than 2 hours in patients with underlying left ventricular failure (Swanton 1994). Factors which may be contributing to the hypotension must be excluded (Box 6.6).

Box 6.6. Other factors that may contribute to hypotension (Hands 1997)

Hypovolaemia
Sepsis
Acidosis
Hypoxaemia
Arrhythmias
Narcotics (such as diamorphine)
Nitrates
Beta-blockers
Calcium antagonists

Critically ill patients should be transferred urgently to a CCU or ICU. Here, invasive monitoring and treatment can occur as the best prognosis is achieved through early, aggressive supportive therapy using intra-aortic balloon pumping, right heart catheterisation, ventilatory support and percutaneous transluminal coronary angioplasty (PCTA) (Nolan et al 1998). Echocardiography can help to assess ventricular function and identify specific mechanical problems (Hands 1997).

Specific management includes the following:

- Core management for the shocked or critically ill adult (see Table 6.3).
- If more comfortable, nurse the patient upright or semi-recumbent if pulmonary oedema or air hunger is present.
- If the patient is in pain or has pulmonary oedema, administer an IV opioid (e.g. diamorphine 2.5–5 mg or morphine 5–10 mg). This will act as an analgesic, reduce anxiety and reduce the ventricular preload (increases venous capacity) and afterload (causes mild arterial

vasodilation) of the heart. Combined, these effects should help to reduce the heart's oxygen demand, but may drop the blood pressure.

- Administer an IV antiemetic (e.g. metoclopramide 10 mg for those aged 20 or older (British Medical Association (BMA) and the Royal Pharmaceutical Society of Great Britain (RPSGB) 1999) with the opioid – to counteract the side effects of nausea and/or vomiting (Resuscitation Council (UK) (RCUK) 1998).
- Treat any cardiac arrhythmias. If the heart rate is less than 60 bpm, administer small amounts of atropine IV and titrate them so that a tachycardia is not produced (Moulton and Yates 1999). Temporary transvenous pacing may be required.
- Nitrates may be given (providing systolic blood pressure is 90 mmHg or greater) to relax smooth muscle and dilate the vasculature (especially venous circulation), thus reducing preload (RCUK 1998). One of the common nitrates is IV glyceryl trinitrate (GTN), which should be administered cautiously at a rate of 10–200 μg/min (BMA and RPSGB 1999).
- If the cause of the shock is due to left-sided dysfunction, furosemide (frusemide) 20–120 mg can be administered IV to reduce the ventricular preload (causes venodilation) and pulmonary oedema. Furosemide (frusemide) may itself lower blood pressure and will not work in the presence of severe hypotension (Thompson 1997b). Monitor potassium levels as furosemide (frusemide) causes potassium depletion. Potassium replacement should be given when levels fall below 3.0 mmol/l (Guy's Hospital 1994).
- Inotropes (drugs that increase the contractility of the heart) are usually indicated if the mean arterial pressure falls below 60 mmHg. The two inotropes most commonly used are:
  - dobutamine (2.5–15 μg/kg/min) given IV, increases the contractility of the heart, without significantly increasing the heart rate at lower doses. Dobutamine also causes mild peripheral vasodilation (Swanton 1994).
  - dopamine (1–10 μg/kg/min) given IV. At a rate of 1–5 μg/kg/min, dopamine causes renal vasodilation, improving renal perfusion and inducing a diuresis. At higher infusion rates (2–10 μg/kg/min), dopamine will increase the heart rate and contractility (similar effects to dobutamine). At rates greater than 10 μg/kg/min, dopamine causes widespread vasoconstriction, which is disadvantageous in a failing heart (RCUK 1998) and would be counter-productive (Swanton 1994). When treating cardiogenic

shock, Nolan et al (1998) recommend that both of these drugs are given, dobutamine to increase cardiac output and a lower dose of dopamine ($2.5–5\,\mu g/kg/min$) to improve renal perfusion. Careful observation must be made of heart rate, as any marked increase will increase the myocardial oxygen consumption and may extend the size of the MI (Thompson 1997c).

- Once cardiogenic shock has occurred thombolysis has not been found to improve the prognosis (Nolan et al 1998) and is, therefore, not routinely indicated.

Diagnostic investigations

- Record a 12-lead ECG to check for cardiac abnormalities or indication of pulmonary embolism (see Chapter 9 – Chest pain).
- Take blood samples for full blood count, urea and electrolytes, blood gases, cardiac enzymes and clotting. Serial samples may be needed.
- Obtain a chest X-ray to check for heart size and pulmonary oedema.
- Monitor central venous pressure (CVP). Measurements will be higher than normal (i.e. >10 cm water when measured at a mid-axillary point with a manometer or >8 mmHg with a transducer (Herbert and Alison 1996)).

Ongoing assessment and nursing management

- Core care plan for the shocked or critically ill adult (Table 6.3).
- Repeated regular 12-lead ECG recordings should be made, as well as at every rhythm change.

Septic shock

Causes

Septic shock is a progression from bacteraemia, commonly known as blood poisoning (Guyton and Hall 1996). One-third of patients will develop an infection whilst in hospital and of these, 9% will be nosocomial (hospital acquired) (Xavier 1999). Sepsis occurs in 1% of patients and, of these, up to 40% will develop septic shock (Hudak and Gallo 1994). Patients who have developed septic shock have a mortality rate of up to 60% (Horvarth 2000). Most commonly, sepsis is caused by Gram-negative organisms (e.g. *Escherichia coli*, *Klebsiella*, *Pseudomonas*, *Bacteroides*, *Proteus*)

(Ledingham 1997). Gram-positive organisms (e.g. *Staphylococcus*, *Streptococcus*, *Pneumococcus*), yeasts and fungi also cause sepsis. Approximately 10–20% of patients with septic shock have no organisms identified (Hudak and Gallo 1994). This may be attributed to associations with non-infective inflammatory responses such as severe pancreatitis or trauma (Urban and Porth 1998).

The focus of the infection can be an abscess, a urinary tract infection (especially if urinary catheter in situ), IV cannula site, wound infection, chest infection, uterine infection, pelvic inflammatory disease or rupture of the gastrointestinal tract. When the causative agent is a Gram-positive bacillus (usually *Staphylococcus aureus*), a rare type of septic shock called toxic shock syndrome can occur. Toxic shock syndrome most frequently occurs in those who have had nasal piercing or in menstruating women who use tampons. It can also be found subsequent to surgical and non-surgical infections of the skin, subcutaneous or osseous tissue (Urban and Porth 1998).

Several patient groups are more prone to develop infection owing to their reduced immune response (Hudak and Gallo 1994):

- the older person
- the individual with an underlying mental health problem
- those with nutritional problems (related to drug, alcohol problems or eating disorders)
- those who are immunosuppressed (patients receiving chemotherapy or those with AIDS)

Pathophysiology

Generalised fever is a significant response to localised infection or inflammation. This fever increases the body's basal metabolic rate and its oxygen demand (Herbert and Alison 1996). As a result, there is an increase in respiratory rate and depth. When the infection cannot be contained locally and the body is no longer able to defend itself, a generalised bacteraemia (haematogenous spread) occurs and the organism is widely distributed to many organs in the body. This causes widespread and indiscriminate vascular (arterial and venous) dilation. This dilation leads to fluid leaking from the vessels into the interstitial compartment (third space) with the subsequent hypovolaemia causing reduced tissue perfusion and hypotension (Selfridge-Thomas 1995). This hypotensive state (hypovolaemia) initiates an autonomic nervous system response, which causes an increase in heart rate and cardiac output. If untreated, when the hypovolaemia reaches a critical level, the patient's conscious level will decrease (cerebral hypoxia), and haemodynamic collapse (lack of perfusion to the tissues) and renal failure with oliguria will ensue (Collins 2000). In the early stages, hyperglycaemia is frequently found (increase in gluconeogenesis and insulin resistance which prevent glucose moving into the cell). However, in more advanced states this becomes hypoglycaemia as the glycogen stores become depleted (Hudak and Gallo 1994).

Disseminated intravascular coagulation (DIC) is a serious complication of septic shock and occurs when damaged tissue factor is released into the circulation, causing widespread clotting throughout the body and subsequent consumption of clotting factors. As too few clotting factors remain to sustain normal clotting mechanisms, bleeding occurs (Guyton and Hall 1996).

Presenting features

The patient might present with a history of an infection with purulent discharge, hyperpyrexia (Table 6.4) or hypothermia, rigors, malaise, weakness or fatigue. From the patient's history, they may have had recent examination with instrumentation (e.g. speculum examination of vagina, suction termination of pregnancy, cardiac catheterisation, central venous access), recent surgery or may have a long-term invasive device in-situ (e.g. urinary catheter, venous catheter or tracheostomy tube) (Horvath 2000).

Table 6.4. Grades of pyrexia (Mallet and Bailey 1996)

<30°C	Severe hypothermia
30°C–35°C	Hypothermia
35°C–37°C	Normal temperature range
37°C–38°C	Low grade pyrexia
38°C–40°C	Moderate pyrexia
>40°C	Hyperpyrexia
>41°C	Convulsions can occur
>43°C	Death can occur

The patient can present to the MAU in either of the following progressive stages:

• Hyperdynamic phase: In this presentation, there are no signs of the patient being shocked (Horvath 2000). The patient will present with mild hyperventilation to reduce the metabolic acidosis caused by the bacteraemia (Urban and Porth 1998). Tachycardia with a bounding pulse will be present. The blood pressure will be normal or slightly reduced with a widened pulse pressure (vasodilation causing reduced systemic vascular resistance) (Horvath 2000). A negative CVP may be present (Hudak and Gallo 1994). The skin will be warm, dry and flushed (caused by vasodilation) and the capillary refill time will be normal. A thorough assessment and history may reveal a focus for the infection.

• Hypodynamic phase: As the condition deteriorates, the respiratory rate will increase and the breathing will become more laboured as pulmonary oedema develops. Pink or white frothy sputum may be evident. The heart rate will increase and the radial pulse will become weak and thready (loss of circulating volume as fluid seeps into the interstitial (third) space). The pulse pressure will become narrowed as the diastolic pressure rises and cardiac arrhythmias may occur owing to reduced myocardial oxygenation. CVP will read higher than normal (Hudak and Gallo 1994). The skin will become clammy, pale and mottled with a prolonged capillary refill (circulation insufficient to supply the peripheries) and central cyanosis will be present (reduced oxygenation to tissues).

Immediate management

The aim of immediate management is early detection and treatment to prevent shock developing or progressing. In addition to the immediate core management for the shocked or critically ill adult outlined in Table 6.3, consider the following measures:

• Aggressive fluid management to correct hypovolaemia.
• The patient may require transfer to ICU for ventilatory and circulatory support.
• The circulation may need to be supported by use of inotropes (e.g. adrenaline (epinephrine) or noradrenaline (norepinephrine) by slow IV infusion) to further increase the afterload and promote vasoconstriction (Horvath 2000). Other inotropes such as dopamine may also need to be given. Dopamine is appropriate in the initial management of septic shock as it increases cardiac contractility and maintains oxygen delivery to the tissues (Urban and Porth 1998).
• After taking a blood specimen for blood cultures, early use of broad-spectrum antibiotics is indicated as 20–30% of patients are affected by more than one organism (Hudak and Gallo 1994).

- The patient should be examined to find the source of infection or inflammation.

Diagnostic investigations

- Take blood samples for full blood count (with differential), urea and electrolytes, blood sugar and arterial blood gases. These may need to be repeated frequently. Neutrophil count should be raised but if infection is not the cause or if immunosuppression is present, levels may be low.
- Obtain specimens to find the causative organism. These may include urine, sputum, wound, cervical, high vaginal, penile, throat, skin lesions and any drainage fluid.
- Obtain a chest X-ray to check for heart size and air under the diaphragm.
- Obtain a plain abdominal X-ray to check for intraperitoneal fluid.
- Monitor CVP. Measurements will be higher than normal (i.e. >10 cm water when measured at a mid-axillary point with a manometer or >8 mmHg with a transducer (Herbert and Alison 1996)).
- Specialised radiographic investigations, e.g. computerised axial tomography (CT) scan, magnetic resonance imaging (MRI) scan, radioactive isotopes to tag white blood cells may be indicated to locate an abscess or the focus of infection.

Ongoing assessment and nursing management

Continuing management centres on the core care plan outlined in Table 6.3. In addition, monitor the patient's:

- temperature and note any change
- skin for skin rashes – of particular importance is a petechial rash as seen in meningococcal septicaemia
- response to antipyretics (paracetamol or ibuprofen) that may have been administered

Anaphylactic shock

Anaphylaxis can be defined as an excessive response to a foreign substance (i.e. a severe allergic reaction to an antigen). The severity of an allergic reaction can range from very mild symptoms (e.g. a mild skin reaction) to circulatory collapse and subsequent death.

Causes

Anaphylactic shock refers to the state when a severe allergic reaction causes circulatory collapse. The speed of onset of the shock is related to the route by which the antigen enters the body. The quickest response follows injection of the substance (Henderson 1998). Antigens are substances foreign to the body, for example proteins (such as nuts), drugs (especially antibiotics), latex and insect bites/stings.

Pathophysiology

There are four types of allergic reaction (Tortora and Grabowski 1996):

- type I (anaphylaxis)
- type II (cytotoxic)
- type III (immunocomplex)
- type IV (cell mediated)

Both types I and II provoke an anaphylactic reaction.

Type I occurs when a foreign substance called an antigen enters the body. These antigens bind to antibodies (immunoglobulin – IgE) on the surface of basophils in the blood and mast cells in body tissue. On first encounter, they do not usually cause a noticeable reaction but, in some individuals, a subsequent exposure to the antigen is recognised by the antibodies and an immune response starts. The antigen (now known as an allergen because it causes an allergic reaction) causes the cell membrane of the basophils and mast cells to rupture, thus releasing allergy-producing mediators (e.g. histamine and leukotrienes) (Guyton and Hall 1996, Porth and Dunne 1998). Subsequently, histamine, heparin and other chemical mediators are released that cause an inflammatory allergic response. Histamine causes widespread vasodilation and increased permeability of the capillaries and venules. This increased permeability results in loss of plasma from the circulation, a drop in blood pressure, increased heart rate and oedema. Leukotrienes cause spasm of the smooth muscles of the bronchioles with subsequent stridor and increased vascular permeability (Copstead and Banasik 2000). If the reaction is severe, death can be rapid if untreated.

Type II is known as an anaphylactoid reaction. It results from non-specific degranulation of mast cells that release allergy-producing mediators. This reaction is not an IgE-based sensitivity. It is, however, impossible in an emergency situation to identify which type is presenting and, as the initial management is the same (Ledingham 1997), identifying the type is not relevant in this situation.

Presenting features

Any of the features shown in Box 6.7 may be present or absent depending upon the site and source of the allergen.

Box 6.7. Possible features of anaphylaxis

Cardiovascular collapse with tachycardia, tachypnoea and/or hypotension
Angioedema (deep cutaneous and visceral swelling) (Candioti 1999)
Swelling of the tongue
Laryngeal oedema (with or without drooling or hoarseness of their voice)
Stridor
Tightness of the chest
Wheezing
Urticarial rashes with or without pruritus (itching)
Warm skin that may be erythematous
Abdominal spasm with or without diarrhoea
Extremities could be cold and clammy due to peripheral shut-down

---

Stridor may be especially severe due to bronchospasm that presents as wheezing. In these cases, the patient may only be able to complete short sentences, words only or may even have insufficient expiratory force to produce any sound at all.

Immediate management

The aim is to reduce the allergic response whilst supporting the circulation (Figure 6.2, p 147). In addition to the immediate core management for the shocked or critically ill adult (Table 6.3), consider the following:

- The drug of choice in severe anaphylactic reactions is adrenaline (epinephrine) as it is a bronchodilator and vasoconstrictor. It is quickly absorbed, increases the force of cardiac contraction and suppresses histamine and leukotriene release. Administer a dose of 0.5 mg (0.5 ml of 1:1000 solution) IM to all patients with clinical signs of shock, airway swelling or definite breathing difficulty (Box 6.7). Repeat this dose again if there is no improvement after 5 minutes or if the patient shows any signs of deterioration. The effective half-life of adrenaline (epinephrine) is only approximately 5–10 minutes depending upon the patient's metabolism. Consequently, in some cases several doses may be needed, particularly if improvement is transient.

- IV adrenaline (epinephrine) in a dilution of at least 1:10 000 (never 1:1000) is hazardous and must be reserved for patients with profound shock that is immediately life-threatening and for special indications (e.g. during anaesthesia). In this case, give the injection as slowly as seems reasonable while monitoring the ECG and heart rate. ECG monitoring is mandatory if adrenaline is given IV. A further dilution of adrenaline to 1:100 000 allows more accurate titration of the dose and reduces the risk of adverse effects (RCUK 2001). Beware if the patient is taking beta-blockers as the anaphylactic reaction may be heightened and the effects of the adrenaline reduced (RCUK 2001).
- Administer an antihistamine such as chlorpheniramine (Piriton) 10–20 mg IM or by slow IV infusion.
- If the patient has severe bronchospasm and was non-responsive to other treatment, consider a salbutamol nebuliser (RCUK 2001). Use oxygen rather than air for its administration.
- Nurse the patient in a position comfortable for them. Sitting upright will help breathing difficulties but may be unhelpful if the patient is hypotensive. Raising the legs may aid venous return and help correct hypotension.
- Record the patient's peak expiratory flow (PEF) prior to treatment as long as the patient is not in extremis.
- If the patient has profound hypotension and does not respond to the medications administered, rapid fluid replacement with 1–2 litres of crystalloid is recommended (RCUK 2001).
- Administer IV corticosteroids (e.g. hydrocortisone). As their optimum effect takes 4–6 hours, these should be the last on the list of routine medications to be administered for anaphylaxis (Figure 6.2).

Diagnostic investigations

- Record a 12-lead ECG to check for arrhythmias.
- Obtain blood samples for full blood count, urea and electrolytes and blood gases. These may need to be repeated frequently.
- Obtain a chest X-ray to check for heart size and pulmonary oedema.
- Monitor CVP.

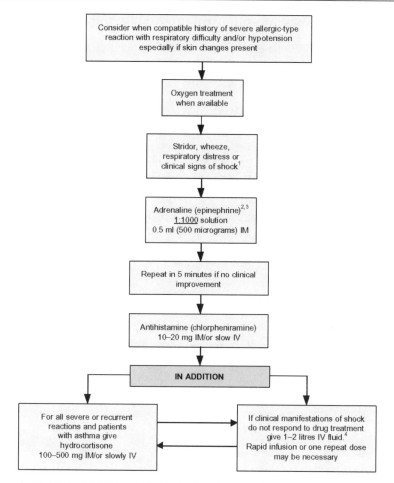

1. An inhaled beta₂-agonist such as salbutamol may be used as an adjunctive measure if bronchospasm is severe and does not respond rapidly to other treatment.

2. If profound shock judged immediately life-threatening give CPR/ALS if necessary. Consider slow IV adrenaline (epinephrine) 1:10 000 solution. This is hazardous and is recommended only for an experienced practitioner who can also obtain IV access without delay. Note the different strength of adrenaline (epinephrine) that may be required for IV use.

3. If adults are treated with an Epipen, the 300 micrograms will usually be sufficient. A second dose may be required. Half doses of adrenaline (epinephrine) may be safer for patients on amitriptyline, imipramine, or beta-blocker.

4. A crystalloid may be safer than a colloid.

Figure 6.2. Anaphylactic reactions: treatment for adults by first medical responders. Reproduced with permission from the Resuscitation Council UK (2001) Update of the emergency medical treatment of anaphylactic reactions for first medical responders and for community nurses. Resuscitation 48: 239–41.

Ongoing assessment and nursing management

In addition to the core care plan for the shocked or critically ill adult in Table 6.3, record PEF every 4 hours or before and after the administration of nebulisers.

Summary

The recognition of the early signs of shock is vital if mortality and morbidity are to be reduced. This chapter has outlined the initial assessment and management of patients who develop shock. It is important to remember that the presenting features of shock can be caused by 'non-medical' conditions (e.g. ruptured abdominal aortic aneurysm) that require 'non-medical' treatment. In this context, it is important for MAU nurses to have a high index of suspicion for both medical and non-medical causes when patients present with signs of shock. Initial assessment and management is only the first component of a successful outcome for the patient. Treatment of the underlying cause of shock is vital and can only be successfully achieved through effective teamwork from all members of the health care team.

References

ABPI (1999–2000) Data Sheet Compendium. London: Datapharm Communications.

American College of Surgeons Committee on Trauma (1988) Advanced Trauma Life Support for Doctors. Chicago: American College of Surgeons.

American College of Surgeons Committee on Trauma (1997) Advanced Trauma Life Support for Doctors, 6th edn. Chicago: American College of Surgeons.

British Medical Association and the Royal Pharmaceutical Society of Great Britain (1999) British National Formulary. London: BMJ Books.

Candioti V (1999) Shortness of breath. In Davis M (ed) Signs and Symptoms in Emergency Medicine. St Louis: Mosby.

Collins T (2000) Understanding shock. Nursing Standard 14(49): 35–41.

Copstead L-E, Banasik J (2000) Pathophysiology: Biological and Behavioral Perspectives. Philadelphia: WB Saunders.

Guy's Hospital (1994) Nursing Drug Reference, 2nd edn. London: Mosby Year Book Europe.

Guyton A, Hall J (1996) Textbook of Medical Physiology, 9th edn. Philadelphia: WB Saunders.

Hands M (1997) AMI: cardiogenic shock. In Thompson P (ed) Coronary Care Manual. New York: Churchill Livingstone.

Henderson N (1998) Anaphylaxis. Nursing Standard 12(47): 49–55.

Herbert R, Alison J (1996) Cardiovascular function. In Hinchliff S, Montague S, Watson R (eds) Physiology for Nursing Practice, 2nd edn. London: Baillière Tindall.

Horvath C (2000) Shock emergencies. In Emergency Nurses Association – Emergency Nursing Core Curriculum, 5th edn. Philadelphia: WB Saunders.

Hudak C, Gallo B (1994) Critical Care Nursing: A Holistic Approach, 6th edn. Philadelphia: JB Lippincott.

Iggulden H (1999) Dehydration and electronic disturbance. Nursing Standard 13(19): 48–56.

Ledingham I (1997) Shock. In Skinner D, Swain A, Peyton R, Robertson C (eds) Cambridge Textbook of Accident and Emergency Medicine. Cambridge: Cambridge University Press.

Mallet J, Bailey C (1996) The Royal Marsden's Manual of Clinical Nursing Procedures, 4th edn. Oxford: Blackwell Science.

Moulton C, Yates D (1999) Lecture Notes on Emergency Medicine. Oxford: Blackwell Science.

Nolan J, Greenwood J, Mackintosh A (1998) Cardiac Emergencies – A Pocket Guide. Oxford: Butterworth Heinemann.

Porth C, Dunne W (1998) Alterations in the immune response. In Porth C (ed) Pathophysiology: Concepts of Altered Health State, 5th edn. Philadelphia: Lippincott.

Resuscitation Council (UK) (1998) Advanced Life Support Course Provider Manual, 3rd edn. London: Resuscitation Council (UK).

Resuscitation Council (UK) (2001) Update of the emergency medical treatment of anaphylactic reactions for first medical responders and for community nurses. Resuscitation 48: 239–41.

Selfridge-Thomas J (1995) Manual of Emergency Nursing. Philadelphia: WB Saunders.

Swanton R (1994) Cardiology: Pocket Consultant, 3rd edn. Oxford: Blackwell Science.

Thompson P (1997a) AMI: Right ventricular infarction. In Thompson P (ed) Coronary Care Manual. New York: Churchill Livingstone.

Thompson P (1997b) AMI: Cardiac failure and pulmonary oedema. In Thompson P (ed) Coronary Care Manual. New York: Churchill Livingstone.

Thompson P (1997c) Inotropic agents. In Thompson P (ed) Coronary Care Manual. New York: Churchill Livingstone.

Tortora G, Grabowski S (1996) Principles of Anatomy and Physiology, 8th edn. New York: Harper Collins.

Urban N, Porth C (1998) Heart failure and circulatory shock. In Porth C (ed) Pathophysiology: Concepts of Altered Health State, 5th edn. Philadelphia: Lippincott.

Watson R (1996) Thirst and dehydration in elderly people. Elderly Care 8(3): 23–6.

Xavier G (1999) Asepsis. Nursing Standard 13(36): 49–53.

Further reading

Cross S (1997) The foundations of allergy. Nursing Standard 12(7): 49–55.

Edwards J (1993) Management of septic shock. British Medical Journal 306: 1161–4.

Gavaghan M (1998) Vascular hemodynamics. Journal of the Association of PeriOperative Registered Nurses (AORN) 68(2): 211–2, 214–9, 222, 224, 228, 230, 235–6.

Lerner J (1997) Complementary therapies: Herbal therapy: there are risks. Registered Nurse 60(8): 53–4.

Molitor L (1999) A 45-year old man with dizziness. Journal of Emergency Nursing 25(1): 67–8.

Moss T (1998) Herbal medicine in the emergency department: a primer for toxicities and treatment. Journal of Emergency Nursing 24(6): 509–13.

Porth C (1998) Heart failure and circulatory shock. In Porth C (ed) Pathophysiology: Concepts of Altered Health State, 5th edn. Philadelphia: Lippincott.

Sommers C (1998) Immunity and inflammation In Porth C (ed) Pathophysiology: Concepts of Altered Health State, 5th edn. Philadelphia: Lippincott.

CHAPTER 7

Altered consciousness

BRENDAN DAVIES, MICHELLE DAVIES,
LORRAINE TAYLOR AND IAN WOOD

Aims

This chapter will:

- describe a systematic approach to the initial assessment and management of patients presenting with altered consciousness in the MAU
- outline the clinical features and immediate management of acute stroke, acute subarachnoid haemorrhage, tonic-clonic status epilepticus and bacterial meningitis
- describe the clinical features and immediate management of hypoglycaemia, hyperglycaemia and diabetic ketoacidosis (DKA) and hyperosmolar non-ketotic hyperglycaemia (HONK)
- describe the clinical features and immediate management associated with common overdoses causing altered consciousness

Introduction

Alteration of conscious level is a common feature of patients referred to an MAU and often presents as a medical or neurological emergency. There are several medical and neurological disorders that may need to be considered and can be partially suspected on the basis of associated clinical features (Table 7.1). The presence or absence of focal weakness, meningeal irritation or previously known premorbid illnesses (e.g. a prior diagnosis of epilepsy) may point towards the underlying aetiology.

Table 7.1. Common causes of altered consciousness and associated clinical features

Causes of altered consciousness	Typical clinical features
Neurological emergencies:	
Stroke/cerebrovascular disease	**Anterior (carotid) circulation** Hemiparesis Hemisensory disturbance Visual field loss Dysphasia Sensory inattention and neglect Eye deviation away from the hemiparesis **Posterior (vertebrobasilar) circulation** Quadriparesis Limb or gait ataxia Dysphagia Bilateral visual loss Diplopia Facial sensory loss Eye deviation towards the hemiparesis
Subarachnoid haemorrhage	Sudden, severe headache Neck stiffness, photophobia – may take hours to develop Nausea and vomiting Epileptic seizure Transient loss of consciousness Coma
Epileptic seizure	Abrupt onset, usually preceded by a warning symptom Tonic-clonic movements affecting all four limbs* Impaired consciousness Incontinence Tongue biting
Meningitis	Acute fever Malaise Worsening headache Neck stiffness, photophobia, nausea Non-blanching skin rash Loss of consciousness
Diabetic emergencies:	
Hypoglycaemia	Shaking Sweating Pins and needles in lips, tongue Hunger Palpitations Double vision Difficulty concentrating Slurred speech Confusion Loss of consciousness

(continued)

Table 7.1. continued

Causes of altered consciousness	Typical clinical features	
Hyperglycaemia and diabetic ketoacidosis (DKA)	Polydipsia Polyuria Smell of 'pear drops' on breath Hunger Fatigue Nausea and vomiting Abdominal pain Confusion	
Hyperosmolar non-ketotic hyperglycaemia (HONK)	Severe dehydration Altered consciousness Seizures	
Overdose of drugs or alcohol:		
Aspirin	Restlessness Tinnitus Sweating Epigastric pain Hyperventilation Dehydration Hypotension Convulsions†	Tachycardia Deafness Blurred vision Nausea/vomiting Hyperpyrexia Confusion Unconsciousness†
Paracetamol	Few if any presenting features Nausea and vomiting (>24 hours after ingestion)	
Tricyclic antidepressants	Dry mouth Drowsiness Muscle twitching Hypertonia/hyperreflexia Hypothermia or hyperpyrexia Excitement/visual hallucinations Urinary retention Depressed respiration† Tachycardia/arrhythmias† Hypotension† Convulsions† Unconsciousness†	Blurred vision Dilated pupils
Alcohol	Slurred speech Loss of inhibitions Aggression Red conjunctivae Smell of alcohol on breath Altered conscious level Hypoglycaemia Gastric irritation Nausea/vomiting Postural hypotension Respiratory depression	Ataxia Loss of judgement Irritability
Narcotic	Altered conscious level Respiratory depression Hypothermia Non-cardiogenic pulmonary oedema Bradycardia Hypotension Pinpoint pupils (miosis)	

*Multiple tonic-clonic seizures lasting >20 min with no recovery of consciousness indicates tonic-clonic status epilepticus.
†Indicates severe toxicity.

The cause of altered consciousness may be better understood and identified if the initial assessment considers the following common presentations:

- Short-lived/transient (seconds to minutes) or episodic impairment of consciousness. This often suggests an episode of syncope, an epileptic seizure or, rarely, other causes (e.g. transient ischaemic attack (TIA) if focal symptoms, cataplexy, or hydrocephalic attacks).
- Persistent and/or worsening impairment of conscious level. This may suggest an intracranial (e.g. meningitis, encephalitis, raised intracranial pressure, cerebral venous sinus thrombosis), systemic (e.g. hypoxic brain injury, substance or alcohol intoxication, hypothermia, septicaemia) or metabolic cause of altered consciousness. Metabolic causes include diabetic coma (e.g. hypoglycaemia, hyperglycaemia with ketoacidosis or hyperosmolar non-ketotic coma) or hyponatraemia.

In studies of patients presenting with persistent impairment of consciousness (i.e. more than 6 hours), the commonest cause is drug overdose or alcohol excess (Bates 1993). The relative frequency of other common causes is shown in Figure 7.1.

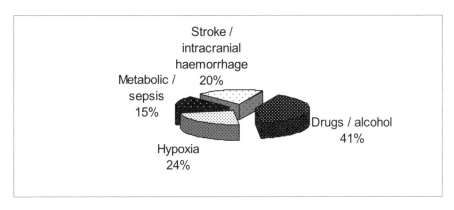

Figure 7.1. Relative frequency of presenting causes of altered consciousness (fits, syncope and hypoglycaemia excluded).

Initial assessment of patients with altered consciousness

Patient management is determined by the underlying cause but an initial ABCDE assessment (see Chapter 2 – Initial assessment) should always be performed to identify and treat any immediately or potentially life-threatening problems.

Airway

Assessment and management of airway problems is of paramount importance in patients who present with altered consciousness.

Listen for stridor/wheeze.
Observe for chest movement.
Observe for and remove foreign bodies in the airway.

Breathing

Assess respiratory rate and depth.
Observe for peripheral and central cyanosis.
Measure oxygen saturations/arterial blood gases.
Smell the breath for unusual odours.

Circulation

Measure the heart rate.
Assess pulse volume and regularity.
Measure the blood pressure.
Observe for signs of haemorrhage.
Feel the patient's skin for warmth and texture.

Disability

Level of consciousness may be apparent when the patient arrives.
Confirm the level of consciousness using AVPU (**A**lert, responds to **V**oice, responds to **P**ain or **U**nresponsive) and/or Glasgow Coma Score (GCS).
Check pupil size and reaction to light.
Observe for obvious signs of facial/postural weakness.

Exposure

> Undress the patient.
> Observe for rashes/puncture wounds/injuries.
> Record the temperature.
> Urinalysis.
> Measure capillary blood sugar (e.g. BM stix).

Initial management of the patient with altered consciousness

- Use appropriate airway management techniques (Chapter 2 – Initial assessment).
- Give high concentration oxygen via non-rebreathing mask or bag-valve-mask.
- Monitor cardiac rate and rhythm.
- Secure intravenous access.
- Consider possible causes of altered consciousness.
- Measure the patient's capillary blood sugar (e.g. BM stix, glucostix).

A. NEUROLOGICAL EMERGENCIES
(Brendan Davies and Michelle Davies)

Stroke/cerebrovascular disease (excluding subarachnoid haemorrhage)

A stroke is a clinical syndrome characterised by symptoms and signs of acute focal, neurological disturbance with loss of function lasting more than 24 hours. It has an underlying vascular cause and is the third commonest cause of death and disability in adults after cancer and ischaemic heart disease. Stroke is distinguished from a transient ischaemic attack (TIA) by the duration of symptoms. A TIA lasts less than 24 hours and usually less than 60 minutes. The clinical distinction between a TIA and mild stroke is important from an epidemiological viewpoint but not particularly useful when considering future prognosis and investigation as both necessitate emergency assessment to minimise the risk of future disabling stroke.

The concept of therapeutic nihilism in stroke care is changing and stroke should now be considered an acute medical emergency. The term

'Brain attack' and the concept of 'Time is brain' are analogous to the commonly accepted notion of 'heart attack' where 'Time is muscle'. These principles become ever more important with therapies emerging that make the time to initiation of treatment for stroke a fundamental consideration (NINDS study group 1995 and 1997, Hacke et al 1998).

Pathophysiology

The pathological subtype of stroke is important because treatment, prognosis and secondary prevention may differ. In general, most strokes are ischaemic (approximately 85%) with the remainder being due to primary intracerebral haemorrhage. The majority of ischaemic strokes occur as a complication of atherosclerosis. There may be artery-to-artery thromboembolism (e.g. from the carotid or vertebrobasilar arteries to the cerebral circulation), embolism from the heart (e.g. cardiac thrombus or endocarditis) or in-situ intracranial small vessel disease and arteriosclerosis. Haemorrhagic stroke usually results from uncontrolled hypertension, rupture of a saccular aneurysm or arteriovenous malformation. Rarely, stroke may occur as a result of venous occlusion due to thrombosis of the cerebral venous sinuses and may reflect an inherited thrombophilic tendency. Cerebral venous occlusion should always be considered as a cause of stroke occurring in pregnancy.

The pathophysiology of stroke may also vary with age, with atherosclerosis the commonest cause of stroke in patients over the age of 45 to 50 years. There are several common reversible risk factors for stroke, including hypertension, smoking, hypercholesterolaemia, and also several irreversible factors including increasing age and male sex. In younger patients, stroke may occur as a result of arterial tearing (dissection), especially following minor trauma, or as a result of cardiac defects (e.g. atrial septal defects) and occasionally genetic inheritance (MELAS – mitochondrial encephalopathy with lactic acidosis and stroke-like-episodes – and CADASIL – cerebral autosomal dominant arteriopathy with subcortical infarcts and leucoencephalopathy) or thrombophilia.

The pathological consequence of stroke is reduced oxygen delivery to the brain and thus cerebral infarction and irreversible tissue damage. The infarction and irreversible tissue damage usually results in clinical disability. In the early stages of cerebral infarction the area of irreversible tissue infarction is surrounded by an area of reversible tissue ischaemia called the 'ischaemic penumbra'. This area of brain may potentially be salvaged with appropriate early and continuing stroke care and thus there is the potential to limit physical disability with appropriate care.

Presenting features

It is difficult to differentiate without brain imaging whether patients have suffered an ischaemic or haemorrhagic stroke (Muir 2001). Patients typically present with acute onset, focal negative symptoms, i.e. loss of function (NB, compared with the slowly spreading positive symptoms of migraine or sensory epileptic seizures). The pattern of symptoms and signs helps differentiate whether the stroke has affected the anterior (carotid) or posterior (vertebrobasilar) circulation. In addition, headache is more common with haemorrhagic and posterior circulation ischaemic stroke. Typical presenting features are outlined in Box 7.1.

Box 7.1. Typical presenting features of anterior and posterior cerebral circulatory dysfunction

Anterior (carotid) circulation
Hemiparesis
Hemisensory disturbance
Visual field loss
Dysphasia
Sensory inattention and neglect
Eye deviation away from the hemiparesis

Posterior (vertebrobasilar) circulation
Quadriparesis
Limb or gait ataxia
Dysphagia
Bilateral visual loss
Diplopia
Facial sensory loss
Eye deviation towards the hemiparesis

Alteration of consciousness with stroke is uncommon unless secondary to an associated pathophysiological cause. Altered consciousness in the context of stroke may thus indicate raised intracranial pressure, involvement of the brainstem, bilateral cerebral hemisphere disease or co-morbid disease. Possible scenarios include:

- large haemorrhagic stroke with secondary raised intracranial pressure
- massive anterior circulation stroke with dense hemiparesis and secondary raised intracranial pressure (usually 2–3 days after onset)
- posterior circulation, brainstem stroke with involvement of the reticular formation
- subarachnoid haemorrhage (see below)

Thus, impaired consciousness in the context of stroke suggests the need for more extensive medical assessment to exclude other metabolic factors and early brain CT to exclude cerebral haemorrhage or alternative intracerebral pathology.

Initial assessment

The initial medical assessment involves detailed history taking of the acute event from the patient (or witness if the patient has dysphasia). A relevant past medical history of hypertension, diabetes mellitus, ischaemic heart disease or atrial fibrillation should be sought in addition to any family history of stroke. A smoking, alcohol and drug history may be relevant. In younger patients, a history of recent drug ingestion may identify illicit drugs that can cause stroke (e.g. cocaine, amphetamine). In addition, a recent history of neck trauma or rotational injury may suggest arterial dissection as a potential cause of stroke in young patients.

General examination should specifically include an assessment of ABCDE, temperature, pulse rate, rhythm and arterial blood pressure (in both arms if pulse asymmetry) and heart auscultation, in addition to a more general assessment of the patient's condition. The initial neurological assessment should include Glasgow Coma Scale, speech (for dysarthria or dysphasia) and orientation.

Neurological examination should characterise visual fields, oculomotor abnormalities, pupil size and reactivity, swallowing ability and the pattern and severity of focal weakness and/or sensory loss both in the cranial nerves and in limbs. Walking ability or disturbances of co-ordination and balance should preferably be included in the assessment. A capillary blood sugar measurement and urine dipstick test should be an extension of the examination of patients presenting with stroke.

Immediate management and investigations

Following clinical assessment, CT brain imaging should be performed as soon as possible to exclude haemorrhagic stroke and differentiate stroke from non-vascular brain disorders (Muir 2001). Basic screening tests for the cause of stroke should be performed on admission and should include a full blood count, clotting studies, erythrocyte sedimentation rate (ESR), glucose, urea and electrolytes (U&E), ECG and cholesterol (if within 12 hours of symptom onset).

Aspirin (75–300 mg) should be given within 48 hours of the diagnosis of suspected ischaemic stroke. This should be stopped if primary intracerebral haemorrhage is confirmed on brain CT scanning. Combined data from three trials (Chen et al 2000) indicate that early initiation of aspirin:

- prevents early recurrence of stroke
- reduces death and disability at 3–6 months
- increases the proportion making a full recovery at the expense of a small increase in intracranial and extracranial haemorrhage risk

There is also increasing evidence that intravenous (IV) thrombolysis is efficacious in acute stroke and produces a highly significant increase in the proportion of patients making a full recovery if used within 3 hours in appropriately selected patients (NINDS study group 1995). Logistical difficulties currently preclude its routine use in the UK.

There is now good evidence to show that all stroke patients benefit from direct admission and subsequent multidisciplinary input on a Stroke Unit. Thus, direct admission should be arranged at the earliest opportunity following stabilisation in the MAU. Evidence from systematic reviews has illustrated that inpatient care in discrete Stroke Units is superior to domiciliary or general medical ward care with respect to long-term survival and disability (Stroke Unit Trialists' Collaboration 1997). Current service organisation and infrastructure in the UK limits the availability of this facility for all patients, although the *National Service Framework for Older People* (Department of Health 2001), which incorporates stroke care, emphasises Stroke Unit development as an important factor in improving outcome.

Patients with a TIA and non-disabling stroke may be suitable for urgent outpatient assessment only if appropriate investigations and rehabilitation services can be accessed promptly.

Ongoing assessment and treatment

The long-term clinical outcome and increased mortality of stroke can be adversely affected by several physiological variables that need monitoring within an MAU setting and, subsequently, on transfer to a Stroke Unit/Ward. High body temperature, low diastolic blood pressure, hyperglycaemia and hypoxia have detrimental effects on stroke outcome and should be monitored and treated accordingly.

Continued assessment of neurological status is imperative, with treatment of secondary stroke complications such as seizures (2% of strokes at onset), infection (e.g. aspiration or hypostatic pneumonia) and early involvement of appropriate paramedical services (i.e. occupational therapy and physiotherapy).

Subarachnoid haemorrhage

Subarachnoid haemorrhage (SAH) accounts for 3% of all strokes and 5% of all stroke deaths. It is a common neurological emergency and has an approximate incidence of 11 per 100 000 person years and appropriate recognition is important to avoid a potentially fatal outcome (van Gijn and Rinkel 2001).

Pathophysiology

Subarachnoid haemorrhage most commonly occurs as a result of rupture of an intracranial saccular aneurysm and less commonly an arteriovenous malformation. Such aneurysms are not congenital but develop during life, usually at the bifurcation of cerebral arteries. It is largely unknown why different individuals develop an aneurysm but smoking, hypertension and excess alcohol consumption are all risk factors. In some cases an abnormality of connective tissue in the blood vessel wall may play a role (e.g. Ehlers–Danlos type IV). In addition, there may be a genetic element in some families either independent of other diseases or as part of an inherited disease affecting other organs (e.g. autosomal dominant polycystic kidney disease, neurofibromatosis type I).

Presenting features

The classic history of SAH consists of sudden onset (within seconds), severe (worst ever) headache. This may be the only initial presenting feature as meningism (neck stiffness and photophobia) may take several hours to develop; vomiting, although often present, can also be associated with other conditions that may mimic SAH. Less commonly, an epileptic seizure may occur at onset in up to 16% of cases and the presence of an unusually severe headache following a first seizure should raise the suspicion of SAH. Presentation with an acute confusional state is less frequent (1–2%) but transient loss of consciousness of more than 1 hour's duration is reported in more than 50% of patients in case series. There is often no complaint of focal weakness and in its mildest form (Grade I SAH), there is only headache with otherwise intact neurological status. Massive SAH may cause coma and extensive focal neurological deficits and 25% of patients die within the first 24 hours of onset.

Initial assessment

Initial assessment should ensure adequate assessment and stabilisation of patient ABCDE and subsequent confirmation of an appropriate history for SAH. The presence of co-morbid illness that may be associated with aneursymal SAH should be sought and any recent history of trauma or drug ingestion recorded to exclude a provoked cause for SAH.

Examination should record baseline GCS, neuro-observations and vital signs (e.g. pulse, blood pressure, respiratory rate and temperature). The presence/absence of neck stiffness, photophobia, focal neurological deficit, conjunctival haemorrhage should be noted.

Immediate management and investigations

Appropriate supportive care is needed to avoid secondary brain insults following SAH and minimise the risk of subsequent vasospasm. Patients should be nursed in dimmed light, in a quiet environment with complete bed rest to avoid the risk of early rebleeding. General measures should include IV hydration (at least 2.5–3.5 litres/24 hours of 0.9% saline), avoidance of hypotension and adequate analgesia (e.g. paracetamol or codeine phosphate). Specific treatment should be aimed at limiting vasospasm and secondary ischaemia and reducing the rebleed risk (e.g. nimodipine orally/nasogastric or IV).

CT brain imaging should occur at the earliest opportunity after the onset of symptoms to confirm radiological evidence of SAH. In addition, this enables prompt management decisions about future angiography in confirmed SAH.

CT scanning may be negative in 2% of patients with subsequent confirmed SAH even when it is performed within the optimum time of 12 hours from headache onset. In patients whose CT scan is negative, lumbar puncture (LP) is mandatory to detect or exclude the presence of xanthochromia in suspected SAH before a diagnosis can be confirmed or refuted (van der Wee et al 1995). Lumbar puncture if needed should not be performed less than 12 hours after the onset of headache as xanthochromia takes time to develop and earlier LP may produce a false negative result (Vermeulen and van Gijn 1990). Xanthochromia represents the breakdown products of red blood cell haemoglobin (i.e. bilirubin and oxyhaemoglobin) in the cerebrospinal fluid (CSF). It can only be detected reliably in vivo 12 hours following SAH. The introduction of blood into the subarachnoid space can occur by a difficult to perform, and thus traumatic, tap. Similarly, xanthochromia can develop in vitro if CSF samples are allowed to stand after LP for several hours without appropriate analysis. Thus, it is imperative to differentiate SAH related xanthochromia from traumatic or in-vitro xanthochromia using the following steps. The CSF sample should be processed by the laboratory at the earliest opportunity and centrifuged immediately after LP in order to test for xanthochromia properly and avoid a false positive diagnosis of SAH as the 3-tube test for a traumatic tap is unreliable. Immediate centrifugation avoids the in vitro development of xantho-chromia as a result of a traumatic tap (van Gijn and Rinkel 2001).

Ongoing assessment and treatment

Patients with confirmed SAH should be transferred to specialist neurological/neurosurgical care promptly following diagnosis. Cerebral angiography should be instituted at an early stage to plan neurosurgical management and limit the risks of morbidity and mortality that can result from rebleeding. Continued monitoring of the GCS and pupillary responses allows detection of clinical change and directs the need for reassessment and investigation. The continuing assessment of neurological status permits the early detection of secondary complications of SAH (e.g. early rebleeding, intracerebral haematoma, hydrocephalus, secondary ischaemia due to vasospasm).

Epileptic seizures

Patients presenting to an MAU with an apparent epileptic seizure are a common clinical problem. They may present with an isolated first seizure which may be symptomatic, provoked (e.g. due to alcohol intoxication/ withdrawal or head injury) or have no apparent cause. The episode may be a seizure in the context of established epilepsy. Alternatively, patients may present with an increasing frequency of seizures or even status epilepticus. Each of these circumstances necessitates structured assessment and management. The main purpose of treatment is to prevent cerebral damage and patient morbidity caused by uncontrolled seizure activity. The following relates predominantly to tonic-clonic status epilepticus.

Pathophysiology

The physiological status of the brain is markedly disturbed in status epilepticus. In the initial stages, there are compensatory mechanisms for increased seizure activity with matching of the brain energy requirements by increased cerebral blood flow and cerebral auto-regulation and increased autonomic activity. This initially protects the brain from the damaging effects of hypoxia, acidosis and hypoglycaemia and, if seizure activity is terminated at this stage, there is unlikely to be long-term cerebral damage. With continued seizure activity, particularly for more than 60 minutes, these compensatory mechanisms start to fail with consequent brain-tissue hypoxia and inability to maintain brain metabolism homeostasis. This leads to secondary effects on the systemic control of other body organ systems. This ultimately results in impaired brain metabolism and function from continuing seizure activity and the increasing risk of permanent, irreversible brain damage and even death. The loss of autonomic control due to continued seizure-induced brain dysfunction may cause worsening systemic metabolic changes (e.g. hypoglycaemia, acidosis, tissue hypoxia, hypothermia, disseminated intravascular coagulation). This may cause progressive multi-organ failure with respiratory failure, hypotension and hepato-renal failure in addition to cerebral oedema and death (Shorvon 2001).

The recognition of early status epilepticus and initiation of appropriate therapy therefore provides a window of opportunity to avoid the potentially fatal consequences.

Presenting features

The commonest presentation to an MAU is following one or more tonic-clonic seizures. The first and most important issue is whether the patient's episode was a definite epileptic seizure rather than an alternative paroxysmal episode such as syncope (vasovagal, cardiac or drug induced), cataplexy (as part of narcolepsy), migraine or, rarely, a TIA (if other focal, usually brainstem symptoms).

Typically with a tonic-clonic seizure there is an abrupt onset, sometimes with a preceding warning that may be brief (e.g. an uncomfortable epigastric sensation or sensation of deja vu in focal epilepsy originating from the temporal lobe). In generalised seizures, tonic-clonic movements affect all four limbs and occur with associated impaired consciousness. Incontinence and severe (especially lateral) tongue biting may be seen. Tonic-clonic seizures usually have duration of 1–3 minutes before self-termination. Following a tonic-clonic seizure there is usually post-ictal confusion that may be prolonged and recovery to the patient's normal state may be slow in contrast to the rapid recovery following syncope. Less commonly transient, focal weakness following a generalised tonic-clonic seizure may occur (e.g. Todd's paresis). Prolonged impairment of consciousness following seizures is uncommon unless there have been multiple seizures.

If multiple tonic-clonic seizures occur with no recovery of consciousness (arbitrarily defined as lasting more than 20 minutes), this is termed 'tonic-clonic status epilepticus' and constitutes a neurological emergency.

Acute symptomatic seizures account for up to one-third of all new onset seizures and are not classified as epilepsy. In such patients, several causes may be apparent. Equally precipitants may induce seizures in patients with known epilepsy and include:

- alcohol (intoxication and/or withdrawal)
- drugs (illicit and pro-convulsant prescribed drugs)
- central nervous system (CNS) or systemic infection
- trauma
- stroke
- acute metabolic disorder (e.g. hypoxia, hyponatraemia, hypocalcaemia, hypomagnesaemia)

The annual incidence of tonic-clonic status epilepticus is 18–28 cases per 100 000 persons and occurs most commonly in children, individuals with learning disability and patients with intracranial structural pathology. Most cases of 'status' develop without a prior history of epilepsy and can also be caused by all the conditions described above (Shorvon 2001). In patients with established epilepsy, drug withdrawal, intercurrent illness or metabolic disturbance are the commonest provoking factors. The possibility of non-epileptic seizure disorder should always be considered in patients with a past history of psychiatric disorder, particularly if there are atypical features or the patient presents with status epilepticus.

Important conditions to differentiate from isolated seizures include syncope (both vasovagal and cardiac), hypoglycaemic attacks, postural hypotension and, rarely, cataplexy or intracranial disorders that cause intermittent obstructive hydrocephalus. Patients in ventricular fibrillation may also exhibit twitching or signs of convulsion.

Syncope is the commonest missed diagnosis and is characterised by presyncopal symptoms (e.g. feeling light-headed, hot, sweaty, blurring or dimming of vision and tinnitus before loss of consciousness) and subsequent short-lived loss of consciousness with rapid recovery without confusion. Some patients who experience syncope may exhibit short-lived tonic-clonic or myoclonic involuntary limb movements that may be mistaken for epileptic seizures. This is termed 'convulsive syncope'

(Lempert et al 1994). Incontinence can also occur with syncope and thus does not discriminate between a seizure and syncope.

Initial assessment

Initial ABCDE assessment aims to identify immediate and potentially life-threatening problems with subsequent history taking confirming the likelihood of a seizure. As the patient usually has no recollection of events, an account of the events should be sought from witnesses. This is imperative for the adequate recognition of a seizure.

Recording of vital signs and GCS (especially pupillary responses and motor function) are important. Similarly, it is important to evaluate whether there is evidence of head trauma, skin rash (especially if non-blanching – indicative of meningococcal septicaemia), meningism, venous puncture wounds or abnormal breath odour (e.g. alcohol, ketones). Identify any mouth trauma (e.g. bitten tongue or inner cheeks) and the presence or absence of urinary/faecal incontinence. Gain IV access, check blood sugar and perform a cardiovascular assessment including an ECG to exclude possible alternative causes of transient of loss of consciousness.

Immediate management and investigations

With patients presenting in status epilepticus, once the ABCDEs have been managed, give appropriate IV or rectal medication to stop the fit. Nasopharyngeal airways are particularly well suited for use during a convulsion as they are easily inserted and are well tolerated. Administration of high flow oxygen is beneficial. If the patient suffers a convulsion, ensure they are safe by removing/padding equipment that may cause injury. The treatment of status can be divided into three stages (Shorvon 2001) and is outlined in Figure 7.2. Continuing generalised tonic-clonic status epilepticus increases the risk of irreversible brain damage and systemic decompensation; thus aggressive intervention and step-up therapy should occur within the first 2 hours of presentation with status epilepticus. This is the period when the patient is usually managed within an MAU environment.

In conjunction with the emergency management outlined above, consider performing the following investigations:

- blood glucose, sodium, calcium and magnesium
- renal and hepatic function
- full blood count and clotting studies

Stage 1

Early status epilepticus
0–30 min since seizure onset

Lorazepam bolus 4 mg IV bolus or Diazemuls 10 mg IV or rectally (given over 2–5 min) Repeated once only after 15 min if no cessation of seizures

If continued seizures

Stage 2

Established 'status'
30–60 min since seizure onset

IV infusion of phenytoin (15 mg/kg at a rate of 50 mg/min) (Approx. 1000 mg in an average adult over 20 min) or (and) IV infusion of phenobarbital 10 mg/kg at a rate of 100 mg/min (Approx. 700 mg in an average adult over 7 min) or IV fosphenytoin 15 mg/kg at a rate of 100 mg/min (Approx. 1000 mg in an average adult over 10 min)

If continued seizures

Stage 3

Refractory 'status'
60 min or more following seizure onset
without recovery

With EEG monitoring to identify burst-
suppression pattern

Intensive care/anaesthetic support Treat with general anaesthesia Either: Propofol 2 mg/kg IV bolus followed by infusion according to local/national protocols to control seizures Or Thiopental 100–250 mg IV bolus and subsequent induction regime until seizures are controlled and then maintenance regime with IV infusion until a burst suppression pattern is seen on the EEG Both anaesthetic drugs should be slowly withdrawn 12 hours after the last seizure

Figure 7.2. Emergency drug treatment for patient presenting with continuing seizure activity in status epilepticus.

- blood anticonvulsant drug levels (if appropriate medications are being taken)
- toxicology screening (blood and urine)
- arterial blood gases (for hypoxaemia and acidosis)
- ECG
- saved sera (for subsequent virology if needed)

Correct metabolic abnormalities if present. Administration of IV glucose and thiamine should be considered if there is a possibility of hypoglycaemia or alcoholism.

Ongoing assessment and treatment

If tonic-clonic seizures continue despite initial drug treatment, early anaesthetic review and subsequent transfer to an intensive care unit (ICU) is needed. An EEG needs to be performed for three reasons: firstly, to confirm the clinical impression of generalised electrical status, particularly if there is any suspicion of non-epileptic pseudo-status in patients with tonic-clonic motor activity; secondly, in comatose and ventilated patients where motor activity has ceased but electrical status may be continuing; and thirdly, to identify burst suppression on the EEG and assess the response to anticonvulsant treatment.

When the patient has been stabilised, and in cases of refractory status, CT brain imaging as well as lumbar puncture needs to be performed to identify the aetiology of status epilepticus when the cause is not readily apparent.

If patients fail to respond to therapy, reassessment is needed to ensure that:

- sufficient anticonvulsant drug dosages have been used
- maintenance anticonvulsant drug therapy has been initiated
- co-morbid medical conditions have been treated, especially the underlying cause
- there is no persisting metabolic problem provoking seizures
- the diagnosis is correct and the patient is not having 'pseudoseizures'.

Meningitis

Few clinical conditions merit more prompt assessment and immediate treatment than bacterial meningitis. There are several recognised causes of meningitis but an infective cause (i.e. bacterial meningitis) is the most common aetiology with at least 900 adult cases per year in the UK (Moller and Skinhoj 2000). It is a neurological emergency that should always be considered in anyone presenting with headache and fever. Any delay in the recognition and treatment of this condition is always associated with a poor prognosis. One in four adults with bacterial meningitis will die or sustain significant neurological deficit even with early treatment.

Infective meningitis represents an inflammatory response to an infection of the leptomeninges and sometimes the brain parenchyma (known as meningo-encephalitis). It can be caused by both bacterial and viral agents. The former can prove rapidly fatal whereas the latter may have a more benign prognosis. The remainder of this section will concentrate on acute bacterial meningitis and will not consider viral, tuberculous, fungal or auto-immune meningitis.

Pathophysiology

The commonest bacterial pathogens responsible for acute bacterial meningitis vary according to different age groups in society. The recently implemented vaccination programme in the UK for some of these agents (e.g. *Haemophilus influenzae* (type B) and *Neisseria meningitidis* (type C)) may change the relative incidence of infection in the future. Currently meningococcal infection in UK adults is caused in equal measure by serotype B and C organisms, with no vaccination available against the B strain. Pneumococcal infection is an equally common bacterial pathogen in adults. *Staphylococcus aureus, Listeria monocytogenes, Streptococcus pyogenes, Escherichia coli* and other organisms are less common but may affect certain patient groups (e.g. post neurosurgical procedures or penetrating head injuries (*Staphylococcus aureus*), pregnant women and the elderly (*Listeria monocytogenes*) and children (*E. coli, Haemophilus, Streptococcus pyogenes*).

The organisms responsible for meningitis often colonise the host's (i.e. the patient's) mucosal surfaces (e.g. nasal mucosa, sinuses, mastoids) before spreading either locally from adjacent structures or as a complication of bacteraemia from a more distant source of infection. Meningitis may also result from a localised collection within the skull (e.g. a subdural empyema or cerebral abscess).

Table 7.2 sets out the commonest bacterial pathogens according to age and immunocompetence (e.g. pregnancy, immunocompromised secondary to hereditary or acquired causes).

Table 7.2. Age at presentation and bacterial pathogens commonly responsible for bacterial meningitis

Clinical setting and age	Likely organism	Drug sensitivity
Children and adults	*Neisseria meningitidis* *Streptococcus pneumoniae*	IV benzyl penicillin or 3rd generation cephalosporin ± rifampacin
Head trauma (e.g. penetrating skull injury/fracture)	Staphylococci Gram-negative bacteria *S. pneumoniae*	Vancomycin ± rifampacin
Immunocompromised and pregnancy	As above for adults plus *Listeria monocytogenes* Opportunistic organisms, e.g. *Nocardia asteroides*	Ampicillin and 3rd generation cephalosporin As per local protocol
Neonates (less than 3 months old)	Group B streptococcus *Escherichia coli (E. coli)* *Listeria monocytogenes*	Ampicillin and 3rd generation cephalosporin (e.g. ceftriaxone/cefotaxime)

Presenting features

Patients with acute bacterial meningitis usually present with an acute (hours to a few days) fever, malaise, worsening headache (often occipital or generalised) associated with meningism (neck stiffness, photophobia and nausea). Abnormal mental states with confusion and disorientation are often seen (80% of patients) and patients may sometimes present hyper-acutely with acute onset, severe headache resembling acute SAH but with a high fever. Coma with high fever is also a recognised presentation. A characteristic non-blanching rash on the skin may be a 'tell-tale' sign of meningococcal infection and should provoke high diagnostic suspicion in conjunction with the appropriate history. Approximately 15% of patients (especially the elderly) may complain of focal neurological symptoms and up to 50% may have seizures during the course of their illness, particularly in pneumococcal meningitis.

Important conditions that may sometimes mimic bacterial meningitis include viral encephalitis and intra-cerebral focal infection (e.g. a cerebral abscess or subdural collection). The former often follows a prodromal viral illness and often has confusion, impaired consciousness, dysphasia and focal seizures as prominent parts of the history in conjunction with fever, headache and meningism. Focal infection in the brain often produces rapidly progressive focal neurological deficits often associated with seizures and high fever.

Initial assessment

A rapid assessment of ABCDE precedes appropriate history taking. For those patients with headache and fever, carry out a rapid assessment looking for meningism, rash and depressed conscious level using the GCS. Evaluate the patient's orientation, alertness and speech. Note cardiovascular signs of sepsis or instability (e.g. sinus tachycardia, arterial hypotension) and act promptly. An initial low baseline GCS and the presence of double vision, ocular motility dysfunction and focal signs in the limbs may suggest a more severe pathological disease process and raise the possibility of alternative diagnoses. Establish IV access at an early stage. The occurrence of seizures warrants early appropriate intervention to control them (see Figure 7.2).

In suspected bacterial meningitis, the initial assessment should be brief so that antibiotic therapy can be initiated at the earliest opportunity, with further clinical information gained later to avoid delayed antibiotic therapy. Ideally, pre-hospital antibiotics will have been given by the patient's GP prior to their arrival in the MAU. The individual who accepts the patient should suggest this when receiving the referral call from the GP.

Immediate management and investigations

If bacterial meningitis is suspected, empirical antibiotics should always be given pending later confirmation of the diagnosis using nationally/locally agreed antibiotic protocols for meningitis. These should take into account local microbiology advice and knowledge of local drug resistance. A suggested general management plan based on a consensus statement on the treatment of adult bacterial meningitis is shown in Figure 7.3. The role

Patient with suspected bacterial meningitis

Pre-hospital antibiotics   IV or IM benzyl penicillin 1200 mg (2 mega units) by GP with
                                        subsequent transfer urgently to hospital (cefotaxime or ceftriaxone 1g
                                        if penicillin allergic)

On arrival in hospital   Brief clinical assessment and supportive care as above
                                        Immediate blood sampling for:
                                        • cultures
                                        • basic haematology and clotting studies
                                        • serological blood testing for bacterial organisms with PCR
                                        • rapid initiation of appropriate antibacterial treatment

                                        IV 2.4 g benzyl penicillin 4-hourly
                                             or
                                        IV 2 g ceftriaxone 12-hourly
                                             or
                                        IV 2g cefotaxime 6-hourly
                                        ± IV 2 g ampicillin 4-hourly

                                        Early brain imaging (CT scan) once patient stabilised
                                        Exclude other causes
                                        Lumbar puncture
                                        If no contraindications to establish/confirm diagnosis
                                        Identify organism responsible (Gram stain and PCR)
                                        Nasal and posterior pharyngeal wall swabs

                                        Early involvement of ICU/HDU if problems with:
                                        • cardiovascular or respiratory instability
                                        • seizures and impaired conscious level
                                        • septicaemia (especially meningococcal)

                                        Consider steroids: dexamethasone 4–6 mg 6-hourly (Coyle 1999) in
                                        adults with:
                                        • impaired consciousness, focal signs or
                                        • evidence of raised intracranial pressure

Figure 7.3. Management of bacterial meningitis (adapted from Begg et al 1999).

of steroids in the treatment of adult bacterial meningitis remains unclear (Coyle 1999). In children, there is good evidence to support steroid use at an early stage as long-term complications (e.g. hearing loss) after meningitis are reduced. An ongoing double-blind, placebo-controlled European multicentre trial examining the role of steroids in the acute treatment phase of bacterial meningitis may soon answer this important question in adults.

The early involvement of specialist infectious disease, neurology and anaesthetic specialty care should be encouraged to advise on management, particularly if complications are apparent. Seizures, hydrocephalus, raised intracranial pressure, acidosis, coagulopathy and any other co-morbidity should be treated conventionally.

Ongoing assessment and treatment

Following stabilisation, patients should be transferred to specialised care (Infectious diseases or Neurology) for continued bacterial chemotherapy and monitoring. The relevant Consultant in Communicable Disease Control (CCDC) should be informed of the diagnosis without delay. This enables contact tracing and chemoprophylaxis to be arranged for recent close contacts if appropriate to prevent secondary meningitis cases. General principles of fluid balance monitoring and intervention should be continued. Changes in alertness, worsening GCS and the development of new neurological deficit or focal seizures should prompt further review, including brain imaging to look for secondary complications of meningitis (e.g. hydrocephalus, localised subdural empyema, stroke and cerebral venous sinus thrombosis).

B. DIABETIC EMERGENCIES
(Lorraine Taylor)

Introduction

Diabetes mellitus is a medical condition in which malfunction of the pancreas interrupts insulin secretion (Forbes 2001). There are two main types of diabetes. Insulin dependent diabetes mellitus (IDDM) (also known as type 1 or juvenile-onset) can occur at any age but is most commonly diagnosed between the ages of 5 and 20 years. It affects approximately 10% of patients with diabetes. Non-insulin dependent diabetes mellitus

(NIDDM) (also known as type 2 or mature-onset) occurs in later years and affects 90% of diabetics. IDDM is characterised by the inability of pancreatic beta cells to produce any insulin. This is thought to result from the auto-immune destruction of the beta cells in the islets of Langerhans (Mandrup-Poulson 1998). NIDDM is caused by peripheral insulin resistance, secondary to defective insulin secretion. This may be due to a deficiency in the insulin receptors on the target cells (Harris and Zimmet 1992).

The management of diabetes mellitus requires compliance, understanding and some degree of self-control by the patient in order to preserve glycaemic equilibrium. Patients may present to the MAU with a number of diabetic emergencies including hypoglycaemia, hyperglycaemia and diabetic ketoacidosis (DKA), and hyperosmolar non-ketotic coma (HONK).

Hypoglycaemia

Hypoglycaemia (defined as a blood glucose less than 4 mmol/l) is one of the main complications of IDDM and is a major concern for this group of patients (BDA 1993). The onset of hypoglycaemia is often rapid, occurring within 30 minutes, and can be quickly reversed if treated promptly (McDowell 1991, Forbes 2001). The causes of hypoglycaemia include alterations to lifestyle, increased amounts of exercise or activity, infections and alterations to insulin or oral hypoglycaemic drug regime (the latter can be deliberate or accidental) (Lewis 1999).

Pathophysiology

During a hypoglycaemic event, the body's normal response to a sharp fall in blood glucose is the production of more glucose by the liver. In addition, hormones (e.g. adrenaline, cortisol and glucagon) are released into the bloodstream. Glucagon stimulates the conversion of glycogen stored in the liver and muscles to glucose (glycogenolysis). The production of glucose from amino acids and other substances in the liver (gluconeogenesis) also takes place (Lewis 1999).

Presenting features

Most patients receive adequate warning of impending hypoglycaemia, enabling them to take preventative measures. Early warning signs (Box 7.2) include shaking, sweating, pins and needles in lips and tongue, hunger and palpitations. Neuroglycopenic features include double vision, difficulty in concentrating and slurred speech. When the blood sugar level falls below 3 mmol/l cerebral dysfunction starts to occur, below 2 mmol/l confusion is typical and below 1 mmol/l coma will result (Lewis 1999).

Box 7.2. Presenting features of hypoglycaemia

Shaking
Sweating
Pins and needles in lips and tongue
Hunger and palpitations
Double vision
Slurred speech
Difficulty in concentrating
Confusion
Coma

Initial assessment and management

When assessing patients who present to the MAU with suspected hypoglycaemia, initial assessment should include ABCDE (see Chapter 2 – Initial assessment). Assessment of conscious level is particularly important. Administer high concentration oxygen (100%) via a non-rebreathing mask, secure intravenous (IV) access quickly and measure capillary blood glucose.

The treatment of hypoglycaemia has three aims: firstly, to increase blood glucose quickly; secondly, to prevent blood glucose reducing subsequently; and thirdly, to identify and treat any underlying cause (Tattersall and Gale 1990). Give oral glucose as 25 g (or 3–4 lumps of sugar) dissolved in 150 ml of water and repeat as necessary after 10–15 minutes. If the patient is unconscious, administer 100 ml of 20% glucose IV. Response to this treatment is usually immediate but if not, a further dose can be given. If prolonged hypoglycaemia occurs, consider commencing an IV glucose infusion. Once the patient has recovered sufficiently, take a history to identify any causative factors.

Hyperglycaemia and diabetic ketoacidosis (DKA)

Any illness suffered by a diabetic patient may cause their blood glucose levels to rise. History of recent surgery, inappropriate reduction in insulin, myocardial infarction, infection and emotional stress are all recognised as precipitating factors causing hyperglycaemic states. Classic signs of hyperglycaemia include increased thirst (polydipsia), urinary frequency (polyuria), increased hunger (polyphagia) and general fatigue. Once the cause of the raised blood glucose has been established and treatment commenced, patients usually recover quickly. If untreated, however, hyperglycaemia can lead to the patient developing DKA.

Pathophysiology

DKA is a life-threatening condition with a significant morbidity and mortality rate. The most common causes are underlying infection, missed insulin (either accidental or intentional), newly diagnosed diabetes, drugs and excessive use of alcohol (Snorgaard et al 1989). DKA may be defined as a blood glucose above 12 mmol/l, the presence of ketonuria and an arterial blood pH less than 7.35 (Singh et al 1997). As such, it is a metabolic disorder consisting of three concurrent abnormalities: hyperglycaemia, hyperketonaemia and metabolic acidosis. It develops in people with either an absolute deficiency of insulin or a relative deficiency caused by an excess of counter-regulatory hormones (e.g. glucagon) (Kitbachi and Wall 1995). In the absence of insulin, tissues such as muscle are unable to take up glucose. Counter-regulatory hormones (e.g. adrenaline, cortisol, glucagon) lead to the breakdown of body fat into fatty acids with these then being broken down in the liver to form ketoacids. The formation of glucose by the liver (gluconeogensis) is enhanced in response to tissue glucose deprivation and this, in turn, contributes to further production of ketoacids. Blood pH falls due to the formation of these acids, ketones are excreted in the urine and, consequently, osmotic fluid loss increases with resultant loss of sodium, potassium, magnesium and phosphates. This degree of fluid loss can lead to hypovolaemia with resultant hypovolaemic shock if not treated. Respiratory compensation for this metabolic acidosis leads to deep, laboured respirations (Kussmaul's breathing). Ketones are excreted through the lungs as well as in the urine, giving the patient's breath a characteristic 'pear drops' smell. In short, the body's metabolism in DKA shifts from a normal well-fed state, whereby carbohydrate is metabolised, to a fasting state in which body fats are broken down, thereby causing metabolic acidosis (Lewis 2000).

Presenting features

In some patients, DKA can take more than 48 hours to develop (Padmore 1998) and, in other cases, it may be the initial presentation of a previously undiagnosed diabetic. The classic features (Box 7.3) include a raised blood sugar level, nausea and vomiting, abdominal pain, thirst, hunger, increased urinary frequency, dehydration, fatigue, weakness and confusion. Symptoms of an underlying infection may be present (Lewis 2000, Miller 1999).

Box 7.3. Presenting features of hyperglycaemia and DKA

Nausea and vomiting
Abdominal pain
Thirst
Hunger
Increased urine output
Dehydration
Fatigue
Weakness
Confusion

Initial assessment and management

On admission to the MAU, the patient should be assessed according to the ABCDE framework. Measure the capillary blood glucose promptly to give an indication of the degree of hyperglycaemia. Administer high concentration oxygen (100%) and monitor respiratory function continuously. Monitor cardiovascular status carefully as hypovolaemia may be evident (see Chapter 6 – Shock). Monitor heart rate and rhythm continuously as cardiac arrhythmias may be present due to hypokalaemia. Establish IV access and take venous blood for full blood count (to identify the white cell count), urea and electrolyte levels (especially serum potassium), blood glucose (for an accurate serum glucose level) and blood cultures (to indicate any infection). Arterial blood gas analysis is required to establish the degree of metabolic acidosis present. Check the patient's breath for the smell of 'pear drops' and check the patient's urine by dipstick for the presence of ketones. Use the GCS to assess the patient's conscious level every 15 minutes.

Once a raised blood glucose level has been identified, give the patient 10 units of soluble insulin IV (Advanced Life Support Group (ALSG) 2001) whilst fluids are prepared. Fluid replacement is one of the critical elements in the treatment of DKA (Kumar and Clark 1998). Commence IV fluids (e.g. 0.9% saline) as prescribed (e.g. 1 litre over 30 minutes as a fluid challenge), especially if the patient is hypotensive. IV fluids aid the replacement of intra- and extravascular fluid, and electrolyte losses (particularly potassium and chloride). Replacing ongoing losses and correcting dehydration will quickly restore the circulating blood volume. Once IV fluids have been started, an infusion of short-acting insulin (e.g. Actrapid) should be commenced. A solution of 50 units of soluble insulin in 50 ml of 0.9% saline at a rate of 6 ml/hour is suggested (ALSG 2001). This will usually lower the blood glucose by approximately 5 mmol/hour. Consider IV potassium supplements depending upon the patient's serum potassium level.

Hyperosmolar non-ketotic hyperglycaemia (HONK)

Hyperosmolar non-ketotic hyperglycaemia (HONK) is a diabetic emergency that presents mainly in elderly patients with NIDDM.

Pathophysiology

HONK is characterised by hyperglycaemia, hyperosmolality and severe dehydration in the context of absent or minimal metabolic acidosis (Charalambous et al 1999). Hyperglycaemia and dehydration develop in a similar manner to DKA. The presence of residual insulin inhibits excessive metabolic acidosis but not hyperglycaemia. Ketonuria, if present, is usually mild and lactic acidosis may occur secondary to tissue hypoperfusion and renal insufficiency.

Initial assessment and management

Assessment is again based on ABCDE principles. Blood sugar levels are usually very high, often up to 80–100 mmol/l and 30% of cases are thought to arise in previously undiagnosed diabetics (Lewis 2000). Clinical features are the same as in DKA. However, fluctuations in consciousness, seizures and neurological deficits are more frequent whilst hyper-ventilation and abdominal pain are unusual. The main characteristic of HONK compared to DKA is the much higher degree of hyperglycaemia present, with only slightly raised or absent ketonuria.

Treatment of HONK differs from that of DKA in three ways. The average patient has an approximate 25% deficit in their total body water. They are sensitive to insulin; therefore, lower infusion rates (i.e. 3 ml/hour of soluble insulin) should be used to avoid rapid falls in blood glucose. Seizures caused by hyperosmolarity may require anticonvulsant treatment. Finally, these patients are at risk of thromboembolic events and, thus, prophylactic anticoagulation treatment with heparin is essential unless there are contraindications (Charalambous et al 1999).

Patient education

Evidence suggests that effective control of blood glucose levels in diabetic patients improves their health, reduces admissions to hospital and delays the onset of long-term complications. The Diabetes Control Complications Trial (1993) found that tight control of blood glucose prevents or delays the development of serious complications such as blindness, kidney failure, an increased risk of stroke and coronary heart disease. Most diabetic emergencies are preventable but occur as a result of complex situations that arise in patients' lives (Padmore 1998). Nurses are in a unique position to supervise and support diabetic patients and their families. Patient education is, therefore, an important aspect of MAU nursing practice. The MAU nurse has an important role to play in raising awareness of the symptoms of a diabetic emergency, so that patients seek medical attention much earlier. Encouraging the patient to check their blood glucose regularly gives them the potential to adjust their treatment and promote self-management.

C. DRUGS AND/OR ALCOHOL AS A CAUSE OF ALTERED CONSCIOUSNESS
(Ian Wood)

As previously indicated (Figure 7.1), 41% of the presenting causes of altered consciousness (excluding fits, syncope and hypoglycaemia) relate to the effects of drugs or alcohol. Therefore, overdose of drugs and/or alcohol should be considered as a potential cause in any patient who is unconscious. Patients may be referred to an MAU as a result of an overdose that may have been a deliberate or accidental act. The taking of a deliberate overdose may relate to the patient's pre-existing psychological problems in an attempt to cause self-harm or may be a spontaneous attempt to gain help. Accidental overdoses can occur when a patient unwittingly takes more than their usual dose of medication but it is important to remember that non-accidental overdoses occur when patients are deliberately given excessive amounts of medication (e.g. Munchausen's syndrome by proxy). The number of drugs that can cause an alteration in conscious level is immense. For this reason, this chapter focuses on those agents that are most commonly associated with overdose and that may be referred to the MAU. These are overdoses of:

• aspirin (salicylates)
• paracetamol

- tricyclic antidepressants
- alcohol
- narcotics

Detailed information regarding poisons is available from National Poisons Centres (www.doh.gov.uk/npis.htm).

Initial assessment

Assess all patients who have taken an overdose according to ABCDE principles. In most cases referred to an MAU, initial assessment, treatment and investigations will have been carried out in the A&E department. It is important, however, for MAU nurses to understand the importance of accurate history taking in cases of overdose. History should include details about the substance, how much was taken, when it was taken, whether it was taken with any other substances (e.g. alcohol) and why it was taken. Some patients will freely volunteer such information whilst others will deliberately withhold information or may deliberately try to mislead the history taker. All patients who have taken an overdose should receive a psychiatric referral to allow expert assessment of their mental health status.

Overdose of aspirin (salicylates)

Four categories may be used when assessing the potential severity of an acute, single event, non-enteric-coated, salicylate ingestion (Kreplick 2001):

- less than 150 mg/kg – no toxicity to mild toxicity
- from 150 to 300 mg/kg – mild to moderate toxicity
- from 301 to 500 mg/kg – serious toxicity
- greater than 500 mg/kg – potentially lethal toxicity

Pathophysiology

Salicylates cause disruption of cellular function leading to catabolism secondary to the inhibition of ATP-dependent reactions with the following physiological results:

- increased oxygen consumption
- increased carbon dioxide production
- depletion of hepatic glycogen
- hyperpyrexia

Acid–base disturbances vary depending on the patient's age and the severity of the intoxication. Initially, a respiratory alkalosis develops secondary to direct stimulation of the respiratory centre. This may be the only consequence of a mild overdose. The kidneys excrete potassium, sodium and bicarbonate, resulting in alkaline urine. A severe metabolic acidosis with compensatory respiratory alkalosis may develop with severe overdose. Excretion of hydrogen ions produces acidic urine (Kreplick 2001).

Presenting features

Clinical features that may be evident when a patient has ingested an overdose of aspirin are shown in Box 7.4

Box 7.4. Presenting features of aspirin (salicylate) overdose

Restlessness	Tachycardia
Tinnitus	Deafness
Sweating	Blurred vision
Epigastric pain	Nausea/vomiting
Hyperventilation	Hyperpyrexia
Dehydration	Confusion
Hypotension	Unconsciousness*
Convulsions*	

* Indicate severe toxicity.

Immediate management and investigations

Consider gastric lavage if >10 g has been ingested and the patient attends within 1 hour of ingestion. Give 50 g activated charcoal orally or via gastric tube after lavage. If the patient has features of salicylate toxicity, give further doses of 12.5 g activated charcoal every hour to a total dose of 150–220 g (West Mercia Guidelines Partnership (WMGP) 2001). If the patient has taken <10 g of aspirin, simply give 50 g of activated charcoal. Activated charcoal acts by absorbing drugs but only absorbs 10% of its own weight (i.e. 50 g of charcoal will absorb 5 g of drug).

Results of investigations will determine further treatment. Take blood samples for U&E, creatinine, glucose and salicylate levels. Measure arterial blood gases and urine pH. If plasma salicylate levels are

≤3.6 mmol/l, rehydrate with oral fluids or IV if vomiting. If levels are >3.6 mmol/l, consider alkaline diuresis provided renal function is within normal limits (creatinine 150 μmol/l) and heart failure or shock are not present. Consider alkaline diuresis if altered consciousness and/or acidaemia co-exist with raised salicylate levels (WMGP 2001).

Overdose of paracetamol

In England and Wales, on average approximately 130 deaths per year can be directly attributed to paracetamol alone (Paracetamol Information Centre 2001). It is a relatively common presenting complaint to A&E departments but figures are unavailable for referrals to MAUs.

Pathophysiology

The maximum dose of paracetamol is 4 g per day in adults. In these therapeutic doses, the drug is mostly metabolised by the liver, although 5% is excreted by the kidney. In cases of overdose (>12 g or 150 mg/kg body weight), the normal metabolic processes within the liver become saturated, causing depletion of hepatic glutathione and the production of toxic metabolites. These metabolites cause hepatocellular death and subsequent centrilobular liver necrosis (Farrell 2001, Jenkins and Braen 2000).

Presenting features

Many people mistakenly believe that an overdose of paracetamol will cause unconsciousness. It does not; indeed, it causes few, if any, presenting features. Nausea and vomiting may be present if a hepatotoxic dose has been ingested but these features usually occur more than 24 hours after ingestion. Serious liver complications of an overdose usually occur 3–4 days after an overdose. Occasionally, patients may present even later with complications such as hypoglycaemia, bleeding and cerebral oedema (Moulton and Yates 1999).

Immediate management and investigations

Gastric lavage is no longer indicated for paracetamol overdose, as activated charcoal is more effective at reducing absorption. If the patient has taken >12 g or 150 mg/kg within the previous hour, give 50 g activated charcoal either orally or via a nasogastric tube (WMGP 2001). Collect blood samples for paracetamol levels 4 hours after ingestion. This time can be extended up to 16 hours after ingestion if the patient has

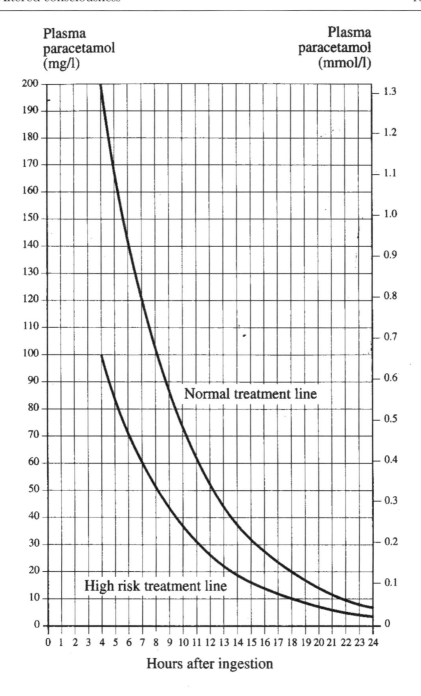

Figure 7.4. Treatment graph for paracetamol overdose.

delayed their presentation to hospital. Compare levels with the treatment graph in Figure 7.4. Treat patients whose levels are above, on or even slightly below the treatment line with IV N-acetylcysteine in 5% glucose. The treatment regime is as follows:

150 mg/kg in 150 ml 5% glucose over 15 minutes followed by
50 mg/kg in 500 ml 5% glucose over 4 hours followed by
100 mg/kg in 1000 ml 5% glucose over 16 hours (WMGP 2001).

Patients who are referred more than 8–15 hours after a potentially dangerous overdose should be given N-acetylcysteine immediately whilst awaiting the results of paracetamol levels.

Ongoing management of all patients who have taken significant paracetamol overdoses includes measurement of their INR (international normalised ratio), liver function tests, creatinine and blood glucose.

Overdose of tricyclic antidepressants (TCAs)

Overdose of TCAs can be dangerous, with over 20% of fatal ingestions involving this category of drug (e.g. dothiepin and amitriptyline). An overdose of 35 mg/kg is the median lethal dose for an adult (Moulton and Yates 1999).

Pathophysiology

When taken in therapeutic doses, TCAs are rapidly absorbed from the gastrointestinal tract. In the case of overdose, however, absorption is thought to be slowed by delayed gastric emptying (Shannon 2000). Toxic levels of TCAs have peripheral and central anticholinergic effects and cause cardiac depression due to sodium channel blockade. The latter leads to delayed myocardial conduction with prolonged PR, QRS and QT intervals on the ECG. Progressive toxicity leads to tachycardia, ventricular bigeminy and ventricular fibrillation.

Presenting features

The effects of a TCA overdose usually occur within 12 hours of ingestion. Presenting features are varied (See Box 7.5, page 183).

Immediate management and investigations

Consider gastric lavage if the patient presents within 1 hour of ingestion and if the overdose is potentially serious (>750 mg). Give 50 g of activated charcoal orally or via a nasogastric tube. Monitor the patient and record a 12-lead ECG. Measure arterial blood gases and correct metabolic acidosis if accompanied by hypotension.

Box 7.5. Presenting features of tricyclic antidepressant overdose

Dry mouth	Blurred vision
Drowsiness	Dilated pupils
Muscle twitching	Hypertonia/hyperreflexia
Hypothermia or hyperpyrexia	Excitement/visual hallucinations
Urinary retention	Depressed respiration*
Tachycardia/arrhythmias*	Hypotension*
Convulsions*	Unconsciousness*

* Indicate severe toxicity.

Overdose of alcohol (ethanol)

Ingestion of alcohol is a common cause of altered consciousness. Alcohol may be taken in isolation but may also accompany ingestion of other substances. It may also be associated with a head injury.

Pathophysiology

Ethanol has sedative–hypnotic effects on the CNS, which cause many of the features below. It is rapidly absorbed by the gastrointestinal tract and is metabolised by the liver to form water and carbon dioxide. Alcohol also suppresses gluconeogenesis in the liver, which leads to hypoglycaemia.

Presenting features

The features of alcohol ingestion depend upon the amount taken and how well the patient tolerates its physiological effects. Presenting features are shown in Box 7.6.

Box 7.6. Presenting features of alcohol overdose

Slurred speech	Ataxia
Loss of inhibitions	Loss of judgement
Aggression	Irritability
Red conjunctivae	Smell of alcohol on breath
Altered conscious level	Hypoglycaemia
Gastric irritation	Nausea/vomiting
Postural hypotension	Respiratory depression

It is important to remember that the smell of alcohol on a patient's breath does not necessarily mean that they are intoxicated. Other causes of altered consciousness must be considered, especially if there is a head injury.

Immediate management and investigations

Management is based on ABCDE principles. In the patient with altered conscious level, ensure that their airway is maintained and supplemental oxygen given if tolerated. Ensure that breathing and circulatory status are satisfactory. Measure capillary blood glucose and send blood samples for laboratory investigation. Record the patient's GCS regularly, especially if a head injury is suspected. If wounds are present, check the patient's anti-tetanus status.

Overdose of narcotics

Narcotics can be divided into opiates (e.g. morphine and codeine), semi-synthetic (e.g. heroin) and synthetic substances (e.g. methadone). Narcotics, which can be taken by oral or IV routes, may result in overdose following therapeutic administration or recreational use.

Pathophysiology

Narcotic agents have effects on neurotransmission in the CNS and peripheral nervous system (PNS). Physiological effects include analgesia, euphoria, respiratory depression, pinpoint pupils and sedation (Stephens 2001).

Presenting features

Features of narcotic overdose (Box 7.7) usually appear within minutes of IV administration or within 20–30 minutes if taken orally (Shannon 2000).

Box 7.7. Presenting features of narcotic overdose

Altered conscious level	Respiratory depression
Hypothermia	Non-cardiogenic pulmonary oedema
Bradycardia	Hypotension
Pinpoint pupils (miosis)	Reduced gut motility

Immediate management and investigations

Management of the patient's airway, breathing and circulation is particularly important as the support of breathing with a bag-valve-mask and oxygen will be required if respiratory depression is evident. Administration of naloxone 2–4 mg IV rapidly restores CNS and cardiopulmonary functions. The IV dose should be supplemented with an equivalent amount given intramuscularly to ensure that blood levels are maintained. In cases of severe narcotic intoxication, a naloxone infusion may be required (Shannon 2000).

Summary

This chapter has focused on a range of conditions that may cause an alteration in the patient's conscious level. In some cases, identification of the underlying condition may be relatively simple whilst in others, there may be no obvious cause. It is important to reiterate that whatever the cause of the altered conscious level, assessment and management of the patient's airway, breathing, circulation and neurological disability are of paramount importance. Similarly, once a diagnosis has been made and treatment given, management of the patient's ABCDEs must continue until definitive care is given.

References

Advanced Life Support Group (2001) Acute Medical Emergencies – The Practical Approach. London: BMJ Books.

Bates D (1993) The management of medical coma. Journal of Neurology Neurosurgery and Psychiatry 56: 589–98.

Begg N, Cartwright K, Cohen J, Kaczmarski E, Innes J, Leen C, Nathwani D, Singer M, Southgate L, Todd W, Welsby P, Wood M (1999) Consensus statement on diagnosis, investigation, treatment and prevention of acute bacterial meningitis in immunocompetent adults. Journal of Infection 39: 1–15.

British Diabetic Association (1993) Approach to the Management of Recurrent Symptomatic Hypoglycaemia. London: British Diabetic Association.

Charalambous C, Schofield I, Malik R (1999) Acute diabetic emergencies and their management. Care of the Critically Ill 15(4): 132–5.

Chen Z, Sandercock P, Pan H (2000) Indications for early aspirin use in acute ischaemic stroke: a combined analysis of 40 000 randomised patients from the Chinese acute stroke trial and the international stroke trial. On behalf of the CAST and IST collaborative groups. Stroke 31: 1240–9.

Coyle P (1999) Glucocorticoids in central nervous system bacterial infection. Archives of Neurology 56: 796–801.

Department of Health (2001) National Service Framework for Older People London: Department of Health (www.doh.gov.uk/nsf).

Diabetes Control Complications Trial Research Group (1993) The effect of intensive treatment of diabetes on the development and progression of long-term complications. New England Journal of Medicine 329: 977–86.

Farrell S (2001) Acetaminophen toxicity. www.emedicine.com/emerg/topic819.htm

Forbes C (2001) Managing diabetic hypoglycaemia. Journal of Community Nursing 15(1): 14–18.

Hacke W, Kaste M, Fieschi C and the Second European-Australasian Acute Stroke Study Investigators (1998) Randomised double-blind placebo controlled trial of thrombolytic therapy with intravenous alteplase in acute ischemic stroke (ECASS II). Lancet 352: 1245–51.

Harris M, Zimmet P (1992) Classification of diabetes mellitus and other categories of glucose intolerance. In Alberti K (ed) International Textbook of Diabetes Mellitus. Chichester: Wiley.

Jenkins J, Braen G (eds) (2000) Manual of Emergency Medicine. Philadelphia: Lippincott Williams & Wilkins.

Kitbachi A, Wall B (1995) Diabetic ketoacidosis. Medical Clinics of North America 79: 9–37.

Kreplick L (2001) Salicylate toxicity. www.emedicine.com/emerg/topic514.htm

Kumar P, Clark M (eds) (1998) Clinical Medicine, 4th edn. Edinburgh: WB Saunders.

Lempert T, Bauer M, Schmidt D (1994) Syncope: a videometric analysis of 56 episodes of transient cerebral hypoxia. Annals of Neurology 36: 233–7.

Lewis R (1999) Diabetic emergencies: Part 1. Hypoglycaemia. Accident & Emergency Nursing 7: 190–6.

Lewis R (2000) Diabetic emergencies: Part 2. Hyperglycaemia. Accident & Emergency Nursing 8: 24–30.

Mandrup-Poulson T (1998) Diabetes – recent advances. British Medical Journal 316: 1221–5.

McDowell J (1991) Prevention is better than coma. Professional Nurse 7(3): 150–4.

Miller J (1999) Management of diabetic ketoacidosis. Journal of Emergency Nursing 25(6): 514–19.

Moller K, Skinhoj P (2000) Guidelines for managing acute bacterial meningitis. British Medical Journal 320: 1290.

Moulton C, Yates D (1999) Lecture Notes on Emergency Medicine, 2nd edn. Oxford: Blackwell Science.

Muir K (2001) Medical management of stroke. Journal of Neurology, Neurosurgery and Psychiatry 70: i 12–16.

National Institute of Neurological Disorders and Stroke (NINDS) rt-PA Stroke Study Group (1995) Tissue plasminogen activator for acute ischemic stroke. New England Journal of Medicine 333:1581–7.

NINDS tPA Stroke Study Group (1997) Generalized efficacy of tPA for acute stroke: subgroup analysis of the NINDS tPA stroke trial. Stroke 28: 2119–25.

Padmore E (1998) Predisposing factors in diabetic emergencies. Accident & Emergency Nursing 6: 160–3.

Paracetamol Information Centre (2001) Paracetamol in overdose. www.pharmweb.net/pwmirror/pwy/paracetamol/pharmwebpic9.html

Shannon B (2000) Poisoning and ingestions. In Jenkins J, Braen G (eds) Manual of Emergency Medicine, 4th edn. Philadelphia: Lippincott/Williams & Wilkins.

Shorvon S (2001) The management of status epilepticus. Journal of Neurology, Neurosurgery and Psychiatry (Suppl II) (70): ii 22–7

Singh R, Perros P, Frier B (1997) Hospital management of diabetic ketoacidosis: are clinical guidelines implemented effectively? Diabetic Medicine 14: 482–6.

Snorgaard O, Eskildsen P, Vadstrup S, Nerup J (1989) Diabetic ketoacidosis in Denmark: epidemiology, incidence rates, precipitating factors and mortality rates. Journal of International Medicine 6: 223–8.

Stephens E (2001) Narcotics toxicity. www.emedicine.com/emerg/topic330.htm

Stroke Unit Trialists' Collaboration (1997) Collaborative systematic review of the randomised trials of organised inpatient (stroke unit) care after stroke. British Medical Journal 314: 1151–9.

Tattersall R, Gale E (1990) Hypoglycaemia. In Diabetes: Clinical Management. Edinburgh: Churchill Livingstone.

van Gijn J, Rinkel G (2001) Subarachnoid haemorrhage: diagnosis, causes and management. Brain 124: 249–78.

van der Wee N, Rinkel G, Hasan D, van Gijn J (1995) Detection of subarachnoid haemorhage on early CT: is lumbar puncture still needed after a negative scan? Journal of Neurology, Neurosurgery and Psychiatry 58: 357–9.

Vermeulen M, van Gijn J (1990) The diagnosis of subarachnoid haemorrhage [Review]. Journal of Neurology, Neurosurgery and Psychiatry 53: 365–72.

West Mercia Guidelines Partnership (2001) Clinical Guidelines: General Adult Medicine. West Mercia: West Mercia Clinical Guidelines Partnership.

CHAPTER 8

Shortness of breath

Susan Hope, Jacqueline Mitchell, Michelle Rhodes, Helen Whitehouse and Ian Wood

Aims

This chapter will:

- describe the initial assessment and management of patients who present with shortness of breath (SOB) to the MAU
- describe the causes (Box 8.1), pathophysiology, investigations and immediate management of the most common causes of SOB seen in the MAU

Box 8.1. Causes of shortness of breath most commonly seen in the MAU

Acute respiratory failure
COPD
Asthma
Pneumothorax
Acute heart failure
Cardiac arrhythmia (see Chapter 5 – Cardiac arrest)
Pulmonary embolism (see Chapter 9 – Chest pain)
Myocardial infarction (see Chapter 9 – Chest pain)

Clinical features

Table 8.1 outlines the clinical features that most commonly accompany SOB.

Table 8.1. Clinical features that commonly accompany shortness of breath (SOB) due to a specific cause

Condition causing SOB	Associated features
Acute respiratory failure	Cyanosis Drowsiness Confusion Tiredness Reduced respiratory rate and effort Loss of consciousness and respiratory arrest
Exacerbation of COPD (British Thoracic Society (BTS) 1997a)	Increased SOB Increased sputum purulence Increased sputum volume Chest tightness Increased wheeze Fluid retention/peripheral oedema Headache Signs associated with significant deterioration: Pyrexia Purulent sputum Severe airways obstruction with audible wheeze Tachypnoea Use of accessory muscles Peripheral oedema Cyanosis Altered consciousness/confusion
Asthma (BTS 1997b)	Acute severe: Peak expiratory flow (PEF) <50% of predicted or best Can't complete sentences in one breath Respirations >25 breaths/min Heart rate >110 beats /min Life-threatening: PEF <33% of predicted or best Silent chest, cyanosis, or feeble respiratory effort Bradycardia or hypotension Exhaustion, confusion or coma
Pneumothorax	Spontaneous pneumothorax: Dyspnoea Pain on inspiration Reduced breath sounds on affected side Tension pneumothorax: Increased respiratory rate and effort Tachycardia Sweating Inability to speak Inequality of chest movement Distended neck veins Cyanosis Tracheal deviation
Acute heart failure	Dyspnoea Tachypnoea Pallor or cyanosis Diaphoresis Anxiety Tachycardia Cool peripheries Possible hypotension Cough Pink, frothy sputum Oliguria

Initial assessment

Assessment of patients presenting with SOB is based on the ABCDE principles outlined in Chapter 2. The following items relate specifically to the assessment of patients who are short of breath.

Airway

Ensure the cause of SOB is not related to an airway obstruction.

Breathing

Record respiratory rate (RR), depth and pattern.
Assess whether chest expansion is equal on both sides of the chest.
Assess the patient's ability to complete sentences.
Listen for wheeze (inspiratory and/or expiratory).
Auscultate for equality of air entry.
Assess use of accessory muscles.
Observe for skin retraction around ribs and clavicles.
Observe the patient's position (e.g. sitting upright to maximise lung capacity).
Observe for signs of fatigue or respiratory distress including mouth opening, pursed lip breathing and flaring of the nostrils.
Feel the position of the patient's trachea (deviation may indicate tension pneumothorax).
Monitor SaO_2 by pulse oximetry (see below for limitations).
Record peak expiratory flow (PEF).
Assess any cough and nature/volume of sputum.
Observe skin colour for central and peripheral cyanosis.

Circulation

Measure capillary refill (normal <2 seconds).
Record heart rate, rhythm and strength of pulse.
Record blood pressure.

Disability

Assess conscious level/changes in consciousness.
Check pupil reactions.
Assess anxiety level.

Assess pain (i.e. on inspiration, expiration, associated with activity, using the PQRST mnemonic).

Exposure

Undress the patient.
Record temperature.
Assess skin temperature and appearance.
Record capillary blood glucose (e.g. BM stix, glucostix).

History taking

Concurrent to the initial ABCDE assessment, gather a history of the patient's presenting complaint and previous medical history (see Chapter 2 – Initial assessment). Information from family and friends can give a valuable insight into the following issues relating to respiratory problems:

- previous admissions
- social history
- smoking habits
- recent changes in respiratory status
- prescribed medications (e.g. nebulisers, theophyllines, long-term oxygen therapy)
- recent changes in medication
- recent exposure to allergens or chemicals
- occupational hazards
- recent illness or injury

Immediate management

Position the patient so that they are in the best possible position to breathe (usually upright, well supported by pillows) in a well-ventilated area. Unless chronic obstructive pulmonary disease (COPD) is suspected, commence 100% oxygen therapy via a non-rebreathing mask and adjust percentage according to SaO_2 measurements. Give patients with COPD oxygen at 24–28% via a Venturi mask. Monitor oxygen saturation and skin colour continuously. Observe for signs of central and peripheral cyanosis. Measure blood gases in patients with COPD before commencing oxygen therapy if possible, and within 30–60 minutes of commencing oxygen. Give nebulised salbutamol 2.5–5 mg or terbutaline 5–10 mg to patients with suspected asthma or COPD. Record a 12-lead ECG if left ventricular failure or a cardiac arrhythmia is suspected and commence continuous cardiac monitoring of heart rate and rhythm. Ensure that intravenous (IV) access is secured.

A. RESPIRATORY FAILURE
(Jacqueline Mitchell)

Introduction

Respiratory failure can be broadly defined as the impairment of pulmonary gas exchange leading to hypoxaemia (low arterial oxygen) and/or hypercapnia (high arterial carbon dioxide) (Singer and Webb 1998).

Causes

The main causes of respiratory failure are listed in Table 8.2, see page 193.

Pathophysiology

In broad terms, respiratory failure is caused by a dysfunction of gas exchange at the alveolus and/or failure of ventilation and perfusion (V/Q mismatch). In practical terms, respiratory failure is said to exist when arterial oxygen (pO_2) is <8.0 kPa and arterial carbon dioxide (pCO_2) is >6.5 kPa. The pathophysiological mechanism of respiratory failure depends on the cause(s) of the underlying condition(s) (Table 8.2). The most common primary lung disorders causing respiratory failure are emphysema (COPD), asthma, chest infection (pneumonia) and adult respiratory distress syndrome (ARDS) (Copstead and Banasik 2000). It is important to remember that a satisfactory cardiac output is required to maintain optimal respiratory function. In addition, an adequate haemoglobin level is needed to deliver cellular oxygen (Field 2000).

Respiratory failure can be categorised into two types, type I and type II.

Type I respiratory failure

Type I failure is essentially acute hypoxaemia (low arterial oxygen) with a normal carbon dioxide level. This type of respiratory failure is usually due to a sudden acute cause (e.g. hypoventilation (RR <10/min), acute pulmonary oedema or pneumonia).

Table 8.2. Causes of respiratory failure

Respiratory	Asthma
	ARDS
	Pneumonia
	COPD/emphysema
	Infection
	Trauma/contusions
	Pneumothorax
	Haemothorax
	Fibrosis
	Aspiration
	Near drowning
	Thoracic surgery
	Sleep apnoea
Central/peripheral nervous system	Cerebrovascular accident
	Raised intracranial pressure
	Drugs (sedatives/opiates)
	Neurological injury
	Guillain–Barré syndrome
	Tetanus
	Failure to reverse anaesthesia
Circulatory	Pulmonary oedema
	Heart failure
	Pulmonary embolus
	Myocardial infarction
Neuromuscular	Motor neurone disease
	Multiple sclerosis
	Myasthenia gravis
Chest wall deformity	Muscular dystrophy
	Kyphoscoliosis
	Chest wall deformity
Other causes	Cardiorespiratory arrest
	Airway obstruction
	Poisons (carbon monoxide/organophosphates)
	Muscle relaxant drugs
	Anaphylaxis
	Fat embolism
	Morbid obesity
	Smoke inhalation
	Status epilepticus

Type II respiratory failure

Type II failure is characterised by hypoxaemia in addition to elevated CO_2 level (usually >7.0 kPa) (Jeffries and Turley 1999). This occurs when alveolar ventilation is insufficient to excrete the volume of CO_2 being produced by tissue metabolism (Field 2000) (Table 8.3).

Table 8.3. Types I and II respiratory failure

Normal values	Type I respiratory failure	Type II respiratory failure
pO_2 10–13.3 kPa	pO_2 <8 kPa	pO_2 <8 kPa
pCO_2 4.8–6.1 kPa	Normal or low pCO_2	pCO_2 of >6.5 kPa
pH 7.35–7.45	Normal or high pH	Low pH <7.35

NB: A stable high pCO_2 can occur in patients with severe stable COPD.

Note: ABG values represent the patient's condition at the time of assessment only, and will change
according to the treatment and/or the underlying condition.

Presenting features

Respiratory failure has presenting features that are common to different causes of respiratory difficulty. Box 8.2 outlines the most important of these.

Box 8.2. Presenting features of respiratory failure

Alteration of breathing pattern
Tachypnoea
Bradypnoea
Cough
Noisy breathing
Pursed lip breathing
Cyanosis
Upright positioning/orthopnoea (i.e. inability to lie flat)
Inability to complete sentences
Use of accessory muscles
Apnoea/periods of apnoea
Drowsiness/confusion/agitation
Headache
Hypertension
Hypotension
Cardiac arrhythmias/tachycardia/bradycardia
Cool, clammy skin
Warm, pink skin
Pyrexia
Pain on breathing

Noisy breathing may be heard on auscultation or often without a stethoscope. Stridor is a high-pitched noise often associated with the presence of a foreign body/obstruction or by presence of laryngeal oedema, often associated with the upper airway. A wheeze is another high pitched sound that can occur during inspiration and/or expiration, associated with air moving through narrowed airways (Field 2000).

Shortness of breath may be characterised by tachypnoea or bradypnoea. Tachypnoea (RR >30/min) indicates increased work of breathing and is usually one of the first indications of respiratory distress (Jevon and Ewens 2001). Bradypnoea (RR <10/min) can indicate hypoventilation or deterioration in condition often due to sedatives, opiates or hypothermia. Patients may be so breathless that they are unable to complete full sentences. Similarly, there may be alteration to the breathing pattern. Respirations may be deep or shallow. Cheyne–Stokes breathing involves a mixture of deep breaths, shallow breaths and periods of apnoea, caused by changes in blood flow to the respiratory centre (Bucher and Melander 1999). In Kussmaul's breathing deep regular breaths are caused by the respiratory system's response to a metabolic imbalance (e.g. diabetic ketoacidosis) in an attempt to excrete CO_2 via the lungs (Bucher and Melander 1999).

Upright positioning may be observed as the patient attempts to relieve dyspnoea. It may also be an indication of long-term respiratory disease. The use of accessory muscles (in the neck, shoulders and abdomen) indicates increased work of breathing due to an increase in oxygen demand (Field 2000). Together these mechanisms are used to increase the capacity of the lungs. Pursed lip breathing and open mouth breathing may be seen together. Open mouth breathing is an attempt to decrease dead space (within the upper respiratory system) and pursed lip breathing occurs on expiration in an attempt to increase lung compliance and increase gas exchange (Field 2000).

Cyanosis may be peripheral (e.g. nail beds) or central (e.g. lips, oral cavity, tongue) The bluish skin colour is caused by the circulation of unoxygenated blood (appearing blue rather than red). Cyanosis is usually a very late sign of respiratory failure.

Cough may be productive or non-productive, and may involve haemoptysis. Pink frothy secretions are associated with pulmonary oedema (Lewis 1999) (see Section E on acute heart failure, below).

Hypertension is an early sign of increased work of breathing. However, hypotension may develop as respiratory distress increases and oxygen demands are not met. As a result, myocardial contractility will be impaired, which can lead to decreased tissue perfusion and signs of shock (Field 2000).

Cardiac arrhythmias, including tachycardia or bradycardia, can occur if hypoxaemia progresses to critical levels (SaO_2 <90%) and the myocardium becomes hypoxic (Woodruff 1999). Increased heart rate, anxiety and pain will increase oxygen demand further. Acid–base imbalances may also exacerbate arrhythmias.

Cool and clammy skin is caused by decreased tissue perfusion. The skin may appear pale as hypoxia (O_2 deficiency in tissues) causes vasoconstriction (Jevon and Ewens 2001). Vasoconstriction reduces the skin temperature, reducing its ability to evaporate sweat. Conversely, the skin may feel warm and look well perfused, as elevated CO_2 levels cause vasodilation of blood vessels resulting in warm peripheries and a bounding pulse.

Drowsiness, confusion and/or agitation may be caused by decreased cerebral oxygenation. Headache may be due to CO_2 retention.

Pyrexia may indicate infection. A raised temperature will increase oxygen demand, which may further exacerbate respiratory failure.

Pain may be due to surgery, trauma, chest infection, pulmonary embolus, cardiac disease and may be exacerbated by exhaustion, anxiety and deep breathing or increased respiratory rate. Pain increases oxygen demand and may worsen respiratory failure.

Periods of apnoea, usually lasting for between 15–20 seconds, may be a result of damage to respiratory centres in the brain (e.g. neurological insult/head injury), airway obstruction or post cardiorespiratory arrest.

Initial assessment

As previously described, initial assessment focuses on the identification and correction of life-threatening and potentially life-threatening conditions using the ABCDE approach.

Immediate management and investigations

Manage the patient's airway according to their level of consciousness. Use of oral/nasal airways or tracheal intubation may be needed if the patient is obtunded. Give high concentration oxygen via a non-rebreathing mask or bag-valve-mask according to the likely underlying cause of respiratory failure. Exercise care if the patient is likely to have COPD. Oxygen is the primary treatment for acute or chronic respiratory failure as it helps correct hypoxaemia and, thereby reduces the work of breathing and decreases myocardial workload (Field 2000). Use a simple facemask or nasal cannulae for patients requiring lower concentrations of oxygen (e.g. those with COPD). Ensure that the length of oxygen tubing is not too long as this can increase dead space and increase the patient's work of breathing. Consider applying humidified oxygen as this reduces the drying of the mucous membranes and will aid expectoration of sputum and secretions.

Nurse the patient in the most appropriate position that will aid their respiration. Fully conscious patients are likely to be sitting upright with backrest support. Those with altered conscious levels will require a position that aids breathing at the same time as ensuring a clear airway. For patients who are unconscious, regular turning not only reduces the incidence of pressure sores but aids the mobilisation of secretions and may improve gas exchange by improving ventilation and perfusion. The supine position reduces the patient's functional residual capacity (Moore 2000) and, therefore, the lateral position may be useful to mobilise secretions. Position patients with unilateral lung disease with their unaffected lung down-most (Thelan et al 1998). It must be remembered that any alteration of position increases oxygen demand. Document positional changes and any effect they may have upon SaO_2, and respiratory rate. Liaise with physiotherapists to enhance respiratory function.

Measure arterial blood gases (ABGs) to monitor the effectiveness of oxygen delivery, CO_2 removal and effects on acid–base balance.

Box 8.3. Limitations of pulse oximetry

Pulse oximetry determines the saturation of oxygen (SaO_2) by reflecting light off haemoglobin. The normal SaO_2 is approximately >95%. Pulse oximetry is an extremely useful assessment tool but it does have limitations. The following limitations should therefore be considered when using pulse oximetry:

- pulse oximetry does not provide an indication of ventilation or lung performance
- an SaO_2 within normal limits does not exclude hypoxaemia or hypoventilation (Lowton 1999)
- altered readings can occur due to poor peripheral perfusion, hypothermia, hypotension, arrhythmias (e.g. atrial fibrillation), vascular disease, peripheral oedema, nail varnish and blood pressure cuff inflation (Moore 2000)
- pulse oximetry does not indicate the presence of carbon monoxide or increasing levels of carbon dioxide (Bourke and Brewis 1998)
- anaemic patients may display a normal SaO_2 even though oxygen-carrying capacity on red blood cells is reduced. A patient with a low haemoglobin may still be 97% saturated with oxygen but their ABG may reveal a low pO_2
- probes can cause skin damage due to pressure and need to be repositioned every few hours (Barker and Shah 1996)
- the effect of motion (e.g. shivering) and excessive light can cause altered readings
- false readings can lead to inappropriate management. Readings can be severely altered as hypoxaemia progresses (Place 2000)

Measure and record the patient's respiratory rate and depth and monitor SaO_2 (Box 8.3). Record the heart rate, blood pressure and feel the pulse volume regularly. Record the patient's temperature and reduce any pyrexia with fan therapy or anti-pyretics. Tepid sponging can cause shivering and increase oxygen demands.

Obtain a portable chest X-ray to assess heart position and size, lung fields and any focus of infection or pathology (e.g. pneumothorax). Take bloods for full blood count (FBC), white cell count (WCC), urea and electrolytes, and glucose.

Observe for presence or development of peripheral oedema. Patients with poor peripheral perfusion due to respiratory failure are already at high risk from pressure sore development.

Drug treatment in respiratory failure

Depending upon the severity of the respiratory failure, measured by ABGs, several approaches can be taken to drug therapy. Nebulised $beta_2$-agonists (e.g. salbutamol) may relieve bronchospasm and aid ventilation. Ipratropium may also be given concurrently with a $beta_2$-agonist. Oral or IV theophyllines relax bronchial smooth muscle (Laurence et al 1997).

Doxapram hydrochloride, given as an IV infusion, is a stimulant used in type II respiratory failure (raised pCO_2 level). It is usually given to rouse the patient, encourage coughing and stimulate respiratory effort in those patients who may be unsuitable for mechanical ventilation (Field 2000). Side effects include twitching, seizures and restlessness and cardiac arrhythmias.

In addition to the medications outlined above, consider the use of steroids (e.g. hydrocortisone) and appropriate antibiotics if infection is identified.

Give appropriate analgesia for pain but exercise care with opiates because of their respiratory depressant effect. Monitor and document the effect of analgesia on respiratory rate and neurological status.

Liaise with respiratory physicians and/or intensivists depending upon the patient's condition. Physiotherapists may have a role to play in the MAU if appropriate.

Mechanical ventilation may be considered if respiratory function continues to deteriorate despite supplemental oxygen and drug therapy, and if ABGs exhibit a worsening acid–base balance. Mechanical ventilation using intermittent positive pressure ventilation (IPPV) may not treat the cause of respiratory failure but will provide support for the respiratory system and enhance oxygenation.

Alternatively, non-invasive ventilation methods may be used to support the patient's existing respiratory effort. Continuous positive airway pressure (CPAP) is a technique used to promote greater ventilation at the alveoli without the need for an endotracheal tube or invasive mechanical ventilation. It is achieved by using a close-fitting, well-sealed nasal or face mask (Brigg 1999). Non-invasive positive pressure ventilation (NiPPV – known as Nippy) allows the patient to be nursed on a ward or high dependency area, thus avoiding admission to an intensive care unit (ICU). In addition, the patient is able to eat, drink and communicate.

B. CHRONIC OBSTRUCTIVE PULMONARY DISEASE (COPD)
(Helen Whitehouse)

Introduction

In England, respiratory disease accounts for 20% of emergency admissions to NHS hospitals (DoH 2001), and in an audit of all medical admissions to a UK health region 25% were due to respiratory disease with over half of those due to COPD (Pearson et al 1994). It is widely acknowledged that COPD is frequently under-diagnosed, as substantial lung damage has usually occurred before clinical symptoms become obvious and it is estimated that most patients experience 50% loss of lung function before they first visit their doctor (Fletcher et al 1976).

Definition of COPD

COPD is the term used to describe a range of clinical features and pathological processes that obstruct airflow. In essence, COPD is a multifaceted disease state that includes chronic bronchitis and/or emphysema, and some cases of chronic asthma (Box 8.4). COPD is characterised by airflow obstruction that is, for the most part, fixed (i.e. not changing for several months or not reversed by bronchodilators) (BTS 1997a). There may, however, be a small degree of reversibility in airway obstruction.

Box 8.4. Definition of diseases associated with COPD

Chronic bronchitis (defined in clinical terms):
'The presence of a chronic cough with sputum production occurring for most days of the week for at least three months in at least two consecutive years when other causes of chronic cough have been excluded (e.g. asthma and bronchiectasis)'
(Medical Research Council 1965)

Emphysema (defined pathologically):
'Abnormal permanent enlargement of the air spaces distal to the terminal bronchioles accompanied by destruction of their walls and without obvious fibrosis'
(Snider et al 1985)

Chronic asthma:
Asthma where 'the inflammation is persistent and can cause permanent structural damage to the airways resulting in irreversible airflow limitation'
(Dagg and Thomson 1996)

Causes of COPD

COPD is associated with a number of risk factors, which can be defined as either definite or probable.

- Definite causes:
  cigarette smoking
  genetic factors (i.e. $alpha_1$-antitrypsin deficiency)
- Probable causes:
  occupational
  environmental
  airway infection
  atopy and airway hyperresponsiveness

Pathophysiology of COPD

The clinical manifestations of COPD, which first become evident on strenuous activity and later occur at rest, include symptoms associated with airway irritation and altered lung mechanics, and vary considerably between patients. For example, patients may have chronic sputum production with no breathlessness whilst other patients may have severe airway obstruction and shortness of breath without any sputum production. The diversity in symptoms serves to highlight the different underlying disease pathologies associated with COPD, which affect the conducting airways (trachea, bronchi and bronchioles), the alveoli, lung parenchyma (tissue) and the pulmonary vasculature. The physiological impact of these changes is described below (Celli et al 1999).

Physiological changes affecting the large or central airways (>2 mm radius), trachea, bronchi and bronchioles

Exposure to irritants (e.g. cigarette smoking) leads to:

- Enlargement of mucus-secreting glands and an increase in the number of goblet cells. This is associated with mucus hypersecretion which leads to sputum production and chronic cough. These changes have minimal effect on airflow limitation.
- Infiltration of the surface epithelium by inflammatory cells, macrophages, T lymphocytes and neutrophils.
- Impaired clearance of mucus due to damaged cilia.

Physiological changes associated with a change in lung mechanics

1. Changes in small or peripheral airways (<2 mm in diameter), bronchioles and terminal bronchioles

- As in the large airways, inflammatory cells, macrophages, T lymphocytes and neutrophils infiltrate the surface epithelium.
- Activated inflammatory cells release a variety of mediators which may damage lung structures and sustain inflammation.
- Chronic inflammation can lead to injury and repair of the airway wall. This may result in structural remodelling of the airway wall with increasing collagen content and scar tissue formation which narrows the lumen.
- Semi-solid mucus plugs may occlude some small bronchi.
- Bronchoconstriction and smooth muscle contraction occur as a result of inflammation. This accounts for a limited amount of airflow limitation in COPD.
- Loss of alveolar attachments due to destructive changes in emphysema leads to airflow limitation. As they contain no cartilage, there is a tendency for bronchioles to collapse when they are compressed.

2. Changes within the alveoli

Emphysema involves the pathological destruction of the alveoli due to irreversible enzymatic destruction of the protein, elastin. Loss of elastin results in disruption of alveolar attachments to the bronchioles, which reduces their ability to maintain patency. This leads to their collapse or narrowing, which in turn limits airflow out of the lungs. Destruction of elastin also causes loss of elastic recoil and damage to alveoli. Damaged alveoli can merge into bullae that are relatively inefficient at gas exchange owing to a loss of surface area.

3. Changes to airway resistance

Resistance from the conducting airways depends predominantly on their radius. A small change in radius results in a significant increase in the resistance. Halving the radius will increase resistance by a factor of 16. Consequently in COPD, narrowing of the airway lumen due to inflammation, remodelling and, to a lesser degree, bronchoconstriction and the tendency of small airways to narrow or collapse, has a huge impact on the airway's resistance to the flow of air. Pushing air through narrowed obstructed airways gets progressively more difficult and exhausts the respiratory muscles. This increased work of breathing results in dyspnoea. The elevated airway resistance seen in COPD causes particular difficulty on exhalation.

When expiratory flow is severely limited, alveolar hyperinflation occurs as a result of slow and incomplete emptying and closure of the small airways. This increase in lung volume supplements elastic recoil and is associated with an increase in end-expiratory alveolar pressure. Consequently, the inadequate supply of fresh air results in alveolar hypoventilation. Hyperinflation also forces the respiratory muscles to work at a length that reduces their contractile strength. This has the effect of flattening the diaphragm and results in a large barrel-shaped chest.

4. Changes to compliance

Lung compliance is a measure of the ease with which the lungs can be inflated and is affected by the elasticity of lung tissue. Both normal and emphysematous lungs distend more easily at lower volumes. This is because at high lung volumes, the distensible components of the alveolar walls have already been stretched out and large increases in pressure only create a small increase in volume. The compliance of the emphysematous lung is increased because, as previously described, the alveolar septae that normally oppose lung expansion have been destroyed. The increased compliance seen in emphysema causes the most over-distended areas (i.e. with a higher lung volume) to receive the least ventilation. Elastic recoil usually helps the lung to return to its normal unstretched volume but in COPD, the decreased elastic recoil of the alveoli leads to a decreased pressure gradient for expiration. Hypoventilation of the alveoli leads to impaired gas exchange because areas are being perfused but not ventilated (i.e. a ventilation–perfusion mismatch).

5. Changes to ventilation and perfusion

Ventilation. In the early stages of COPD, as the lung function declines, the level of oxygen in the circulation falls and the respiratory centre triggers an increase in respiratory effort. This causes the sensation of breathlessness. Accessory muscles, not usually involved in quiet inspiration, help to increase the dimensions of the chest in order to create an adequate pressure gradient. Abdominal muscles, usually passive in quiet breathing, contract and compress the abdominal contents against the relaxed diaphragm, forcing it up in expiration. Respiratory frequency increases, as does the tidal volume. These measures ensure that pO_2 and pCO_2 remain at normal levels in the blood. As lung damage progresses and resistance to airflow increases, these mechanisms prove inadequate, with the respiratory rate continuing to increase, tidal volume decreasing and arterial gases becoming abnormal. Too little O_2 in the blood (hypoxaemia) and too much CO_2 (hypercapnia) affect brain function, leading to headache, insomnia, irritability and confusion. In some patients, the pO_2 falls but CO_2 is still exhaled (type I respiratory failure). In others, the response to low pO_2 is impaired and a dysfunctional respiratory drive develops, whereby pO_2 falls and pCO_2 rises (type II respiratory failure).

Perfusion. Optimal gas exchange occurs when the ratio of lung ventilation (V) to blood flow (Q) is equal (i.e. V/Q ratio = 1). In patients with COPD, the alveoli can become hypoventilated. Initially, the local O_2 supply to the tissues will drop (hypoxia). This results in vasoconstriction and a consequent fall in perfusion to that area. This has the effect of matching blood flow to ventilation. However, worsening airflow limitation results in uneven V/Q with an ensuing reduction in pO_2 (hypoxic hypoxia).

Chronic hypoxia-induced vasoconstriction of the pulmonary capillaries and damage/destruction of many of the small blood vessels in the lungs leads to increased pulmonary vascular resistance. As a result, the heart (particularly the right ventricle) must work harder in order to pump blood through the pulmonary vessels. Over time, this leads to right ventricular hypertrophy and right ventricular failure (i.e. cor pulmonale). Eventually, blood that is unable to empty completely from the right ventricle becomes congested in the venous system. Presence of peripheral oedema associated with this process is indicative of a poor prognosis.

Other physiological changes associated with COPD

Polycythaemia.   Another physiological response to inadequate oxygenation is secondary polycythaemia. Here, an increased production of red blood cells raises the oxygen-carrying capacity of the blood but the associated rise in blood viscosity increases the risk of pulmonary embolus.

Pneumothorax.   Presence of air in the pleural cavity can be caused spontaneously by emphysema. Bullae formed from damaged alveoli may rupture, causing deflation of the affected lung as air enters the pleural space.

Presenting features of an exacerbation of COPD

* Increasing breathlessness
* Cyanosis
* Increased sputum purulence
* Increased sputum volume
* Pyrexia
* Headache
* Chest tightness
* Increased wheeze
* Fluid retention
* Oedema
* Anorexia/weight loss (Anthonisen et al 1987, BTS 1997a)

Initial assessment of the patient with an exacerbation of COPD

The aim of the initial assessment is to determine and record the patient's usual stable respiratory state and the severity of their current respiratory problem. This is achieved by observation, limited verbal questioning (history) and physical examination. Assessment comprises the usual ABCDE framework with the addition of the following specific components.

The assessment of breathing should include:

1. Observation of:
- respiratory rate
- depth and pattern of breathing (shallow, rapid breathing indicates severe ventilatory failure and respiratory fatigue)
- use of accessory (sternomastoid and scalene) muscles on inspiration – these accessory muscles elevate the sternum and help increase the dimensions of the chest
- use of accessory muscles of expiration (prominent abdominal movements)
- pursed lip breathing
- ability to speak in sentences
- skin colour for pallor, cyanosis and/or sweating. Cyanosis is an insensitive physical finding. Although it is useful for alerting and detecting hypoxaemia, absence of peripheral or central cyanosis does not rule out hypoxaemia
- wheeze caused by the sound generated by turbulent airflow through conducting airways. Wheezing may be audible and is particularly common in patients affected by emphysema and over-inflated lungs. The wheeze is usually prominent on expiration
- signs of hypercapnia such as:
  vasodilatation causing warm, flushed skin
  tachycardia with a strong, bounding pulse
  deteriorating level of consciousness (confusion, agitation and drowsiness may all signify hypercapnia)
  flapping tremor
- in addition, use a breathlessness questionnaire (e.g. BORG score (Borg 1982)) or a more detailed questionnaire such as the Baseline and Transition Dyspnoea Index (Mahler et al 1984)

2. History:
- ask about previous mobility distances and whether there has been a reduction
- has the patient's sleep been disturbed (i.e. orthopnoea)? How many pillows are required to sleep?

- use of long-term oxygen therapy (LTOT) which would indicate that pO_2 is continually below 7.3 kPa and forced expiratory volume in 1 second (FEV1) is less than 1.5 litres (both criteria for LTOT)
- headache may indicate hypercapnia
- has there been increased use of inhalers/nebuliser prior to admission?
- was the onset of breathlessness sudden or insidious?
- what was previous lung function or blood gas analysis in a stable state? Access previous reports for comparison.

3. Physical examination:
- lung auscultation
- presence of rhonchi especially on expiration.

The assessment of cough and sputum should consider the following:
- is the cough new or has their usual cough increased?
- how frequent is coughing? Is it constant or intermittent?
- what triggers coughing?
- what type of cough is it? Is it dry/hacking/productive?
- is sputum production new or has volume and/or colour changed?
- what is the colour? (e.g. mucoid, mucopurulent or purulent)
- what is the consistency? (e.g. liquid or semi-solid)
- amount per day (e.g. teaspoon or half eggcupful)
- is the patient pyrexial?
- is haemoptysis present?

Sputum in COPD patients is usually mucoid but becomes yellow or green with exacerbations. Purulence of sputum is due to an increase in degranulating neutrophils and not necessarily bacteria, although many exacerbations may be due to upper respiratory tract viral infections. It is difficult to tell clinically whether an infection is bacterial or viral. If sputum production is continuously purulent, consider bronchiectasis.

The assessment of circulation should include observation for signs of right ventricular failure (e.g. observe the peripheries for signs of oedema). Chest pain should be assessed using the PQRST tool (see Chapter 9 – Chest pain). Pleuritic pain is common and may hinder expectoration of secretions and restrict respiration. Sudden onset may indicate pulmonary embolus (see Chapter 9 – Chest pain).

The assessment of anorexia and/or weight loss should include the following:

- calculation of body mass index (BMI).
- question the patient about any recent weight loss.
- ask about dietary intake.
- is the skin dry (indicating dehydration)?

A diagnosis of COPD is usually suggested by clinical symptoms but can only be truly established by objective measurement (i.e. spirometry). Access to such testing can be limited, so COPD is often diagnosed on the basis of clinical symptoms. Essentially patients with COPD present to the MAU because of an acute exacerbation of their condition. An exacerbation is defined as a new respiratory event or complication superimposed upon their existing COPD. Although the pathophysiology of exacerbations is poorly understood, the new event is often an infection. Many patients with an exacerbation of COPD will be managed at home. However, admission to hospital is indicated if they exhibit one or more of the following features (Barnes 1999):

- unable to cope at home
- live alone
- severe breathlessness
- cyanosis
- worsening peripheral oedema
- acute confusion

Immediate management

Ensure that the patient is sitting as upright as possible and is well supported by a backrest and pillows. Enable them to assume the position most comfortable to them. Constant reassurance and explanations are necessary especially if the patient is confused or agitated. The following three-step approach to the management of COPD is advocated (Brochard 2000).

1. Oxygen therapy and drug treatment.
2. Early use of non-invasive intermittent positive pressure ventilation (NIPPV). In this case, 'early' is defined as when the patient develops moderate acidosis (i.e. pH <7.35) (Plant et al 2000).
3. Transfer to the intensive therapy unit (ITU) if indicated.

Oxygen therapy and drug treatment

Oxygen therapy is the priority in the management of COPD. The aim is to achieve a pO_2 of at least 6.6 kPa without pH falling to below 7.26 (which occurs secondary to a rise in pCO_2). Some patients with COPD will have been in respiratory failure for some time and may have become so accustomed to hypercapnia that their respiratory centre may have lost its normal sensitivity to changes in CO_2 levels. To maintain respiration these patients require low blood oxygen levels (i.e. a 'hypoxic drive'). Giving these patients too much oxygen could reduce the hypoxic drive to breathe.

On arrival in the MAU (following ABGs if possible), give oxygen at between 24 and 28% via a Venturi mask (as these masks deliver the most precise concentration) or nasal cannulae at 2 litres/min (less predictable) until ABGs are known. The suitability of nasal cannulae depends on factors including breathing pattern, nasal or oral breathing, nasal resistance and changing clinical state. They are perhaps best reserved for patients who are clinically more stable. There is no evidence that humidification is necessary with low flow rates. Humidification is only required if flow rate is sustained at >4 litres/min (BTS 1997a).

Check ABGs within 30–60 minutes of starting or altering O_2 therapy. Modify the flow rate according to pO_2 and pH. If the pO_2 is responding and the effect on pH is modest, increase the inspired concentration of O_2 until the pO_2 is above 7.5 kPa. If the pH falls secondary to a rise in pCO_2, consider alternative strategies such as doxapram or non-invasive positive pressure ventilation (NIPPV). A pH of <7.26 indicates a poor prognosis (Jeffrey et al 1992).

Bronchodilators

1. Beta$_2$-agonists. Give salbutamol 2.5–5 mg or terbutaline 5–10 mg via a nebuliser on admission and, thereafter, 4–6-hourly. Both may be given more frequently if required. Nebulised bronchodilators should be continued until the patient's clinical condition improves. Ensure that the fill volume in the nebuliser chamber is at least 4 ml to guarantee correct dose administration. It may be necessary to add 0.9% saline to the medication to make up an adequate fill volume.

2. Anticholinergics. Give nebulised ipratropium bromide 250–500 μg on arrival and at 4–6-hourly intervals thereafter. Ipratropium bromide can lead to pupillary dilation and occasionally glaucoma; these complications are reduced if a mouthpiece is utilised on nebuliser equipment instead of a mask. Studies suggest that ipratropium bromide

is as efficacious as beta$_2$-agonists in treating patients with COPD (Tashkin et al 1994, Combivent Inhalation Aerosol Study Group 1994). Ensure that the nebuliser is driven by compressed air if the pCO$_2$ is raised and/or the pH is low. Continue oxygen therapy via nasal cannulae to prevent hypoxia during administration of the nebuliser.

Methylxanthines

If the patient is not responding to treatment, consider an IV infusion of aminophylline 0.5 mg/kg/h, although there is little evidence to support this treatment (BTS 1997a). Check blood levels daily.

Antibiotics

Commence antibiotics if two or more of the following symptoms are present (Anthonisen et al 1987):

- increased breathlessness
- increased purulence of sputum
- increased sputum volume

Send sputum for culture and sensitivity if infection is suspected. A recent meta-analysis showed a significant but marginal benefit from antibiotics in exacerbations of COPD (Saint et al 1995).

Systemic corticosteroids

There is limited evidence available but systemic corticosteroids are thought to be useful in acute exacerbations of COPD (Thompson et al 1996). Use a 7–10 day course of oral prednisolone 30 mg/day. If already on a maintenance dose, increase the daily dose by 30 mg. If the patient is severely ill and unable to take oral medication, give 100 mg hydro-cortisone 6-hourly as an intravenous (IV) bolus (BTS 1997a).

Relief of chest pain

Avoid medications that cause respiratory depression. Give a non-opiate analgesic 4–6-hourly.

Prophylactic subcutaneous heparin is recommended in patients with acute or chronic respiratory failure due to their higher risk of pulmonary embolism (BTS 1997a).

Treatment of right ventricular failure

Oral diuretics are indicated if there is evidence of peripheral oedema but they must be used carefully to avoid hypotension.

Doxapram

The use of IV doxapram as a respiratory stimulant in COPD is debatable as lung ventilation is limited by mechanical rather than neurophysiological factors. Doxapram may be indicated in the management of an acute exacerbation with hypercapnia and hypoventilation in order to stabilise the patient for 24–36 hours until the underlying cause (e.g. infection) is controlled (BTS 1997a). Careful monitoring is required as doxapram increases the heart rate and blood pressure. It can cause central nervous system stimulation, which may result in confusion and tremor that can become intolerable to the patient. Check ABGs 90 minutes after starting the infusion. If there is no improvement, increase the infusion rate in increments of up to 1 mg/min (max 4 mg/min) and continue to monitor ABGs hourly. Evidence for the use of doxapram is scarce and there is some evidence to suggest that non-invasive positive pressure ventilation is better than doxapram in correcting ABGs in the initial treatment of acute exacerbations (Angus et al 1996).

Non-invasive positive pressure ventilation (NIPPV)

Evidence suggests that NIPPV reduces the need for endotracheal ventilation and can shorten hospital stay (Brochard 2000). In NIPPV, the patient's breathing is assisted by means of positive pressure delivered via a mask and small portable ventilator. It increases tidal volume and supports the patient's own efforts. If successful, NIPPV slowly increases pO_2 over a few hours. If available, NIPPV should be commenced within the MAU.

Transfer to the ITU

If NIPPV is not available, and the patient's condition is deteriorating (i.e. elevated pCO_2, fatigue and/or confusion), consider intubation, intermittent positive pressure ventilation (IPPV) and transfer to the ITU (Box 8.5). The decision to admit the patient to the ITU will be influenced by the patient's existing quality of life, presence of co-existing disease and whether it is their first episode of respiratory failure (BTS 1997a). It should be noted patents with COPD who receive IPPV for respiratory failure do not have a higher mortality rate than patients who receive IPPV for non-COPD causes.

Box 8.5. Indications for positive pressure ventilatory support (BTS 1997a)

- pH <7.26
- pCO$_2$ rising
- Failure to respond to treatment
- Fatigue
- Confusion

The BTS support the use of NIPPV before the patient has deteriorated to this extent

---

Coping and breathing strategies

It is important for MAU nurses to address the psychological factors (i.e. fear and anxiety) that may be exaggerating the patient's sensation and perception of dyspnoea (American Thoracic Society 1999). In addition to the provision of reassurance and explanations about their treatment and investigations, simple relaxation techniques and control strategies can be used within the MAU to help reduce the amount of distress felt by the patient.

- Relaxation techniques include the systematic tensing and relaxing of different parts of the body. Patients with COPD invariably overuse and tense the muscles in the upper body; therefore suggest that they drop their shoulders, whilst gently pressing on them if necessary. Advise the patient to close their eyes and repeat a word such as 'calm'.
- Body positioning – the head down and leaning forward position has been found to reduce dyspnoea. This position is thought to allow the abdominal contents to push up the diaphragm, increasing its resting length and consequently its ability to generate force (Sharp et al 1980). Patients with COPD usually find the best body position to relieve breathlessness themselves.
- Pursed lip breathing – instruct the patient to inhale through the nose and to purse their lips (as if they are going to whistle) and exhale slowly. Pursed lip breathing is often adopted spontaneously and is thought to reduce respiratory rate, which may reduce dynamic hyperinflation and improve V/Q match (Casaburi et al 1997).

Diagnostic investigations

Arterial blood gases (ABGs)

ABGs measure the degree of respiratory failure and should be taken before the initiation of oxygen therapy. However, this is often not possible, as the patient requires oxygen immediately or may have been given oxygen on route to the MAU. Ensure that the percentage of inspired oxygen is recorded at the time that ABGs are taken.

Oxygen saturation (SaO$_2$)

SaO$_2$ (see Section A on respiratory failure) only measures the degree of oxygenation and does not provide any information about the state of ventilation or CO$_2$ retention. Therefore, whilst SaO$_2$ monitoring may reduce the need for painful ABG measurements (providing it is greater than 92% and pH is normal), it should not replace ABG sampling during the initial respiratory assessment or if the patient is deteriorating clinically.

Chest X-ray

A chest X-ray cannot diagnose COPD but can exclude other pathologies including pneumonia, pneumothorax, left ventricular failure, right ventricular failure, pulmonary oedema, lung cancer (of which there is an increased incidence in COPD (Skillrid et al 1986)), pleural effusion and upper respiratory airway obstruction. When cor pulmonale is present, the hilar vasculature may become more prominent and cardiomegaly will be evident on the X-ray.

A plain posterior/anterior chest X-ray may be normal in mild COPD but with progressive disease, hyperinflation will be shown by the presence of increased lung volumes and a low, flat diaphragm.

Blood investigations

Take blood samples for:

- full blood count – to assess for anaemia and raised white cell count
- haematocrit – to assess polycythaemia (haematocrit >47% in women, >52% in men)
- electrolytes – to monitor hypokalaemia and/or hyponatraemia, which may occur in patients treated with diuretics
- blood cultures if sputum is purulent and pyrexia is present

- erythrocyte sedimentation rate (ESR) and C-reactive protein (CRP) should also be obtained if infection is suspected

Peak expiratory flow (PEF)

PEF may be difficult to perform correctly if the exacerbation is severe. In general, a PEF <100 litres/min indicates a severe exacerbation. PEF has limited use in stable COPD as airflow is largely fixed. Comparisons of inpatient recordings may be useful if usual readings in a stable state are known.

Sputum sample collection

Routine culture of non-purulent sputum is unhelpful. Oral antibiotics are only indicated if there are signs of infection (e.g. purulent sputum, increased SOB and/or increase in sputum volume).

ECG

ECG is used to diagnose right ventricular hypertrophy, identify arrhythmias (e.g. atrial fibrillation) or co-existing coronary heart disease.

Preparation for discharge from the MAU

If the patient is to be discharged home, ensure that they have the necessary support. Advise the patient about smoking cessation and refer them for further advice if required. Be certain that the patient understands their treatment and that they are able to use any devices (e.g. nebulisers and inhalers) correctly. Ensure that sufficient medication is provided and inform the patient's GP about their recent treatment in the MAU. It is also wise to recommend the influenza vaccination. If the patient is to be transferred, refer them to a respiratory consultant if possible and try to arrange transfer to a dedicated respiratory ward so that appropriate management and aftercare will be adhered to. Referral to a pulmonary rehabilitation programme, and for lung function testing, LTOT assessment and alpha$_1$-antitrypsin deficiency screening should be considered where appropriate.

Although the primary aim of MAU staff is to deal with the acute situation, it is also within their remit to identify ways that emergency admissions can be prevented. Many hospitals have developed alternative care options in order to reduce emergency admissions and hospital bed days. Such initiatives include:

- hospital at home services (Davies et al 2000)
- acute respiratory assessment services (Gravil et al 1998)
- rapid response nurses
- self-management plans (Watson et al 1997) and symptom diary cards
- specialist COPD nurses
- care pathways
- early discharge from the assessment unit

Reducing COPD admissions and/or length of inpatient stay could have a huge impact on patients themselves and on reducing workload pressures on MAUs and hospital wards alike.

C. ASTHMA
(Susan Hope)

Introduction

The British Thoracic Society (BTS) (1997b) has defined asthma as 'a common and chronic inflammatory condition of the airways whose cause is not completely understood'. Asthma can change over time and can be intermittent, mild, moderate, severe or life-threatening. Patients at any level of severity can have acute severe exacerbations necessitating their referral to the MAU. This section is based on the BTS guidelines for asthma management (1997b), which aim to:

- prevent death
- restore the patient's clinical condition and lung function to their best possible levels as soon as possible
- maintain optimal lung function and prevent early relapse

Types of asthma

- Childhood/young adult asthma: This is allergic or atopic asthma (extrinsic) characterised by an allergic response to identifiable specific triggers. Atopy involves a specific immunoglobulin E mediated reaction and is associated with a genetic predisposition to asthma, hayfever, eczema and urticaria.
- Late onset asthma: Usually older adults, non-atopic (intrinsic) and often with more persistent symptoms.

- Occupational asthma: This is due to exposure to a specific agent or chemical in the workplace, it can be atopic or non-atopic.
- Aspirin-sensitive asthma: A small number of people have symptoms due to aspirin or other non-steroidal anti-inflammatory drugs (NSAIDs).
- Exercise-induced asthma: Only a small number of people have exercise-induced asthma, usually children and young adults.

Pathophysiology

As a result of inflammation, the airways become hyperresponsive and narrow easily in response to a wide range of stimuli. This may result in coughing, wheezing, chest tightness and shortness of breath. These symptoms are often worse at night. Narrowing of the airways is usually reversible but, in some patients with chronic asthma, the inflammation may lead to irreversible airflow obstruction. Characteristic pathological features include the presence in the airway of inflammatory cells, plasma exudation, oedema, smooth muscle hypertrophy, mucous plugging and shedding of epithelium. These changes may be present even in patients with mild asthma when they have few presenting features (BTS 1997b).

Mechanisms of inflammation

One of the most important advances in the management of asthma has been the recognition that asthma is an inflammatory disease rather than a disease characterised by altered smooth muscle function. Although the actual mechanisms causing airway inflammation are still not fully understood, it is thought that there is a genetic predisposition that interacts with the effects of the environment (Holgate 1993).

The inflammatory cells (e.g. activated mast cells, macrophages, eosinophils and T-helper lymphocytes) release multiple inflammatory mediators (including histamine, leukotrienes, prostaglandins and bradykinin). Inflammatory mediators result in brochoconstriction, mucus secretion, exudation of plasma and airway hyperresponsiveness. Multiple intracellular messengers called cytokines (e.g. interleukin-1, interleukin-5) are responsible for co-ordinating, amplifying and perpetuating the inflammatory response and attracting additional inflammatory cells. Structural changes (i.e. airway remodelling) may occur with subepithelial fibrosis (i.e. basement membrane thickening), airway smooth muscle hyperplasia and new vessel formation. These changes may underlie irreversible airflow obstruction (Barnes and Godfrey 2000).

Presenting features

Patients referred to the MAU with asthma may range in the severity of their attack from mild to life-threatening. If not recognised and treated appropriately, acute asthma can be fatal (BTS 1997b). It is, therefore, essential that MAU nurses are able to recognise the presence of acute, severe asthma and identify any life-threatening features (Box 8.6). It is important to note that patients with a severe or life-threatening asthma attack may not be distressed and may not demonstrate all of the symptoms described above. If any of these features are present, seek medical advice immediately.

Initial assessment

In addition to the usual ABCDE assessment, the assessment of patients with suspected asthma focuses specifically on the assessment of respiratory rate and pattern, PEF and pulse rate. Arterial blood gases (ABGs) should be measured if oxygen saturation is less than 92% or if the patient has any life-threatening features.

PEF is the simplest test of lung function and can be measured on simple portable devices in hospital and at home. It is measured as the maximum expiratory flow achieved during forced expiration – usually within the first few milliseconds of the expiratory effort. It is a very effort-dependent but

---

Box 8.6. Presenting features of acute, severe asthma (BTS 1997b)

Features of acute, severe asthma
- Peak expiratory flow (PEF) 33–50% of predicted or best
- Can't complete sentences in one breath
- Respirations >25 breaths/min
- Pulse >110 beats/min

Features of life-threatening asthma
- PEF <33% of predicted or best
- Unable to talk
- Silent chest, cyanosis or feeble respiratory effort
- Bradycardia or hypotension
- Exhaustion, confusion or coma
- ABGs show:
  Normal (5–6 kPa) or high pCO_2 (>6 kPa)
  Severe hypoxaemia: pO_2 <8 kPa (60 mmHg) despite oxygen therapy
  Acidosis (a low pH – <7.35)

reproducible test that reflects mainly large airway obstruction. Measurements are most easily interpreted when expressed as percentages of the predicted normal value (see Figure 8.1) or of the best obtainable value for the individual with optimal treatment. PEF must be interpreted in the light of other features of severity and the patient's history, particularly previous admissions to hospital, attendance at A&E or MAUs and current treatment, especially corticosteroids.

Immediate management and investigations

The immediate management of acute severe asthma is outlined in Figure 8.1.

Administer 40–60% oxygen via a medium concentration mask. Give doses of inhaled beta$_2$ agonists (e.g. salbutamol 5 mg or terbutaline 10 mg) via an oxygen-driven nebuliser and high doses of systemic steroids (e.g. oral prednisolone 30–60 mg or IV hydrocortisone 200 mg), or both if the condition warrants. Ensure that no sedation of any kind is administered as this would depress respiratory function further. Arrange for a chest X-ray to exclude pneumothorax. If life-threatening features are present, add ipratropium bromide (0.5 mg) to the nebulised beta$_2$ agonist (BTS 1997b) and give IV aminophylline (250 mg over 20 minutes) or salbutamol or terbutaline (250 μg over 10 minutes). Do not give bolus aminophylline to patients already taking oral theophyllines. Immediate transfer to the ITU (for mechanical ventilation) is indicated if any of the following features are present:

- deteriorating PEF, worsening or persisting hypoxia (pO$_2$ <8 kPa) despite high flow inspired oxygen or hypercapnia (pCO$_2$ >6 kPa)
- onset of exhaustion, feeble respiration
- altered consciousness (e.g. confusion or drowsiness)
- respiratory arrest (if respiratory arrest occurs, an anaesthetist should ideally perform intubation, as the procedure is very difficult in this type of patient)

Once treatment has begun, monitor the patient continuously to check their response. Monitoring should include the following measures.

- Record PEF 15–30 minutes after starting treatment and chart PEF before and after nebulised beta$_2$ agonists.

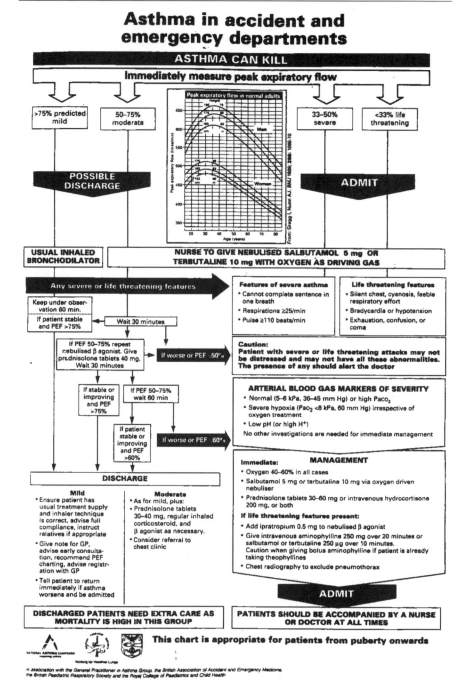

Figure 8.1. Immediate management of acute severe asthma. Reproduced with permission from the British Thoracic Society (1997b) Asthma Management Guidelines. Thorax (52) Supplement 1.

- Record oxygen saturations by pulse oximetry. Continue oxygen therapy, sufficient to maintain saturations above 92%.
- Measure or repeat ABGs within 2 hours of starting treatment if:
  - the initial pO_2 was below 8 kPa (unless the arterial oxygen saturation was above 92%)
  - the initial pCO_2 was normal or raised
  - the patient's condition deteriorates.
- Record the heart rate.
- Measure the serum theophylline concentration if aminophylline is continued for more than 24 hours (aim at a concentration of 55–110 mmol/l).
- Measure serum potassium and blood glucose concentrations.

Treatments that are considered to be unhelpful in the initial stabilisation of asthmatics include:

- any form of sedation
- antibiotics (should only be given if bacterial infection is present)
- percussive physiotherapy

Ongoing management of asthma centres on the use of high concentration oxygen with nebulised beta$_2$ agonists. Continue high dose steroids as above. Ipratropium bromide (0.5 mg) can be added to the nebuliser and consider giving IV salbutamol, subcutaneous terbutaline or an aminophylline infusion (250 mg over 20 minutes) if the patient does not improve or deteriorates. A loading dose of aminophylline is not required unless the patient's condition is deteriorating. Lower doses may be needed for patients with liver disease or heart failure, for those taking cimetidine and most quinolone and macrolide antibiotics. Higher doses are appropriate in smokers.

Preparation for transfer to the ward or discharge home

The majority of patients referred to the MAU will be admitted to hospital. Asthmatics should not be discharged home until their symptoms have cleared and their lung function stabilised or returned to its normal/best level (a PEF >75% of the predicted or best level, or a diurnal variability <25% and no nocturnal symptoms). Careful consideration must be given to patients with certain types of history associated with their asthma (Box 8.7).

Box 8.7. Relative contraindications for discharging a patient with asthma (Moulton and Yates 1999)

Previous ICU admission
Previous severe attacks needing hospitalisation
Already on steroids
Poor social circumstances/referred late at night
Reattendance within 2 weeks
Drug-induced attack (e.g. NSAIDs)

A minority of patients will be discharged home from MAU. These patients are likely to be previously diagnosed asthmatics who are already under the care of their primary care team. As asthma is a chronic disease, the long-term management must focus on prevention of further exacerbations. This necessitates a move towards encouraging patients to take more responsibility for managing their own condition in partnership with health professionals. The use of self-management plans has been demonstrated to be one way of achieving this aim. Self-management plans can range from simple instruction to complex plans including how to adjust treatment according to changes in peak flow or symptoms (Gibson et al 1995, Partridge 1995, Gibson et al 1998, Gibson and Charpin 2000).

Before discharging an asthmatic patient home from MAU, ensure that they have had:

- their inhaler technique checked, corrected if necessary and recorded
- a PEF of 75% of predicted or best level
- advice regarding compliance with usual medication
- a discharge letter for their GP and practice nurse
- a PEF meter and PEF/symptom diary
- a written management plan of what to do if their asthma deteriorates
- a written plan of their current treatment including oral and inhaled steroids
- the reasons for their exacerbation and referral identified

D. SPONTANEOUS PNEUMOTHORAX
(Ian Wood)

A pneumothorax is a condition in which air enters the space between the visceral and parietal pleurae.

Pathophysiology

In normal respiration, as the chest expands the negative pressure in the potential space between the visceral pleura (attached to the lung surface) and parietal pleura (attached to the inside of the chest wall) ensures that the lung expands. As the lung expands, the negative pressure inside draws air into the lung for gaseous exchange. When the visceral pleura loses its integrity (often as a result of a ruptured bulla), air is able to leak from the lung into the space between the pleurae. In so doing, the negative pressure between the two layers is lost and the lung does not inflate as the chest expands. Consequently, the affected lung collapses and is unable to function effectively. If the air leak stops, a simple pneumothorax develops. If, however, the leak continues, air will leak into the pleural space increasing the pressure within it. This pressure can continue to build until it is sufficient to compress the mediastinal contents, thereby making expansion of the unaffected lung more difficult, and impairing venous return and cardiac function. This condition is known as a tension pneumothorax. If untreated, the increasing pressure within the chest will cause cardiac arrest (see Chapter 5 – Cardiac arrest).

Presenting features

Pneumothorax usually occurs in two groups of patient (Moulton and Yates 1999):

• young adults, usually male, who are previously fit and healthy
• older patients with emphysema

Features may be difficult to detect if the pneumothorax is small or when emphysema is present (Box 8.8).

Box 8.8. Features of spontaneous pneumothorax

Dyspnoea (degree depends on size of pneumothorax)
Pain on inspiration
Reduced breath sounds on the affected side
Reduced chest expansion on the affected side
Resonance on percussion of the affected side

Tension pneumothorax is an immediately life-threatening condition that requires immediate management (Box 8.9).

Box 8.9. Features of tension pneumothorax (Moulton and Yates 1999, ALSG 2001)

Signs of increasing respiratory distress
Increased respiratory rate and effort
Tachycardia
Sweating
Inability to speak
Reduced breath sounds on the affected side on auscultation
Inequality of chest movement/expansion
Hyperresonance of the chest on percussion
Distended neck veins
Cyanosis (late sign)
Tracheal deviation (late sign)

Initial assessment

Assessment centres on the ABCDE approach already described. Patients who are younger and previously healthy will tolerate a relatively large pneumothorax whereas an older patient with emphysema is likely to be symptomatic with a relatively small air leak. It is important to assess accurately the patient's breathing at regular intervals for signs of a developing tension pneumothorax.

Immediate management and investigations

A simple pneumothorax is usually confirmed on chest X-ray (anterior/posterior and lateral films will be needed). The results of the X-ray will guide the treatment required (ALSG 2001). Patients who exhibit signs of developing a tension pneumothorax should *not* be X-rayed but should have a needle chest decompression (thoracocentesis) performed immediately after securing IV access. The latter is necessary because pneumothoraces can involve haemothorax if vessels have been damaged by the air leak from the lung. After needle decompression, an underwater seal chest drain should be inserted as definitive treatment. Chest X-ray is performed once the chest drain has been inserted.

Simple pneumothoraces in asymptomatic patients can be treated with analgesia (e.g. NSAIDs), observation and reassurance (Moulton and Yates 1999). Patients with larger pneumothoraces will require treatment with a chest drain and admission to hospital.

E. ACUTE HEART FAILURE (LVF)
(Michelle Rhodes)

Introduction

Acute heart failure is caused by failure of the left ventricle or the right ventricle. Acute left ventricular failure (LVF) is typically caused by acute myocardial infarction (AMI), cardiac arrhythmia or acute dysfunction of the aortic or mitral valve. Right ventricular failure (RVF) is usually a result of pulmonary embolism or right ventricular MI (Timmis et al 1997). Both give rise to the typical symptoms listed in Table 8.4. RVF has been considered in other chapters (Chapters 5 and 9); this section will therefore focus on the assessment and treatment of the patient with LVF.

Table 8.4. Presenting features of acute heart failure

Acute LVF	Acute RVF
Increasing dyspnoea	Signs of low cardiac output:
Cough	Cool skin
Frothy sputum, which may be pink	Hypotension
Unable to tolerate recumbent position	Peripheral cyanosis
Anxiety and agitation	Elevated jugular venous pressure
Weakness and fatigue	
Tachycardia	
Cool peripheries	
Pallor	
Central cyanosis	
Hypotension* (systolic blood pressure <90 mmHg)	
Dizziness and confusion*	
Oliguria*	
Low cardiac output*	

*Indication of cardiogenic shock.

Causes of LVF

LVF can be attributed to three main causes:

* volume overload
* pressure overload
* myocardial dysfunction

Volume overload occurs when the ventricle is expected to pump more blood than normal (e.g. in conditions such as mitral regurgitation and aortic regurgitation). Pressure overload occurs when the ventricle pumps the blood against greater resistance (e.g. in hypertension or aortic stenosis). Myocardial dysfunction, usually as a result of AMI, reduces the contractility of the left ventricle and is the commonest cause of acute LVF (Julian et al 1998).

Pathophysiology of acute LVF

When the heart starts to fail, the volume of blood in the left ventricle rises, cardiac output falls and a number of compensatory mechanisms are stimulated in an attempt to maintain an adequate circulation. Unfortunately, many of these mechanisms actually make the condition worse. In response to the increased volume of blood in the ventricle, the left ventricle dilates. As the size of the ventricle increases, more tension is required to expel blood. This process increases ventricular oxygen requirements and further impairs contractility, which contributes to additional deterioration in the function of the left ventricle (Julian et al 1998). Components of the neuroendocrine system are also stimulated in acute LVF. Activation of the sympathetic nervous system increases heart rate and contractility and causes vasoconstriction of arteries and veins. These responses help to maintain blood pressure but also increase the workload of the heart. Stimulation of the renin–angiotensin– aldosterone system causes vasoconstriction, which increases vascular resistance of blood within the left ventricle. It also triggers the secretion of aldosterone, which causes sodium and water retention, thus increasing blood volume and escalating congestion of blood within the left ventricle. (Julian et al 1998).

As congestion in the left side of the heart increases, pressure in the left ventricle, left atrium, pulmonary veins and capillaries rises. When the pressure within the pulmonary capillaries exceeds the osmotic pressure exerted by plasma proteins, fluid leaks into the interstitial tissues (interstitial oedema). If the capillary and interstitial pressure exceed the intra-alveolar air pressure, fluid leaks into the alveoli (alveolar pulmonary oedema) (Kumar 1997). This fluid reduces the compliance of the lungs, making breathing more difficult and interfering with oxygen and carbon dioxide exchange.

Presenting features of LVF

The features of LVF result from pulmonary congestion and reduced cardiac output (see Table 8.4). The reduced lung compliance that accompanies interstitial oedema causes dyspnoea, particularly on exertion, orthopnoea and an inability to tolerate lying in a recumbent position. On auscultation, crackles will be heard in the dependent parts of the lung. Alveolar pulmonary oedema causes the patient to expectorate frothy, pink sputum as the fluid invades the large airways (Laurent-Bopp 2000). Mucus production is increased, leading to a cough and wheeze (Jowett and Thompson 1996). Impaired gas exchange leads to tachypnoea and cyanosis due to hypoxaemia. Reduced cardiac output causes the heart rate to rise. Pulsus alternans (an alternating pulse strength) may be present and indicates altered left ventricular function (Laurent-Bopp 2000). In very severe cases, hypotension will develop, signifying the onset of cardiogenic shock (see Chapter 6 – Shock).

Initial assessment

Acute LVF is a medical emergency requiring immediate assessment and management. The aim of the assessment is to recognise life-threatening features promptly and to identify the underlying cause, so that appropriate treatment can be commenced. The assessment should follow the ABCDE principles outlined in Chapter 2.

Position the patient close to resuscitation equipment and ensure that they are continuously observed. Obtain medical assistance immediately so that appropriate medications can be administered without delay. Continuously monitor SaO_2, respiratory rate, pattern of breathing and skin colour to identify the severity of respiratory distress and pulmonary oedema. Monitor haemodynamic status for signs of cardiogenic shock. Check blood pressure and pulse at least every 15 minutes, and with any change in condition. Commence continuous cardiac monitoring of heart rate and rhythm to detect arrhythmias and record a 12-lead ECG to identify any underlying cause (e.g. AMI). In very severe cases, it will be necessary to insert a urinary catheter so that a precise, hourly record of urine output can be maintained. Secure IV access and obtain blood for full blood count, urea and electrolytes to assess renal function and cardiac markers to identify or eliminate AMI as a cause.

Immediate management and investigations

The aims of initial management within the MAU are to:

1. Improve tissue oxygenation.
2. Relieve pulmonary congestion.
3. Improve the haemodynamic status.
4. Treat the underlying cause (Millane et al 2000).

Initial measures to improve tissue oxygenation

Sit the patient upright and help them to maintain as comfortable a position as possible. Administer 100% oxygen and monitor SaO_2 continuously. Measure ABGs to accurately assess oxygenation and acid–base balance. Arrange an urgent chest X-ray to assess the extent of pulmonary oedema. Constant reassurance is essential as the patient will be frightened and may be agitated due to hypoxia. Maintain constant contact with the patient and provide reassurance and explanation regarding all treatment and investigations.

Initial measures to relieve pulmonary congestion

Give an IV diuretic (e.g. furosemide (frusemide)). Furosemide (frusemide) causes venodilation, thereby reducing the amount of blood returning to the heart (preload) and reducing venous congestion before its diuretic effect takes effect (Millane et al 2000). As a diuretic, furosemide (frusemide) quickly promotes a large diuresis, thus reducing circulating blood volume, reducing preload and relieving venous congestion (Julian et al 1998). Furosemide (frusemide) may also cause potassium depletion; therefore, monitor the serum potassium level closely. Administer IV diamorphine 2.5–5 mg to reduce anxiety and promote venodilation (reduce preload). Diamorphine also helps to reduce myocardial oxygen demand. Finally, administer a nitrate such as glyceryl trinitrate (GTN), either IV or by the buccal or sublingual routes. GTN causes venous and coronary artery dilation, helping to improve blood supply to the myocardium and reducing preload on the failing ventricle. As nitrates cause hypotension, they can only be administered if the systolic blood pressure is greater than 90 mmHg.

Initial measures to improve the haemodynamic status

The therapies described above should positively influence haemodynamic status, by reducing venous congestion. If, however, cardiac output is low, IV inotropes (e.g. dobutamine and/or dopamine) may be commenced. Dobutamine increases myocardial contractility, whereas low dose dopamine improves renal perfusion and helps to maintain a diuresis (Millane et al 2000).

Initial measures to treat the underlying cause

The investigations performed in the initial assessment will reveal the cause of the patient's sudden deterioration. In most cases, the cause will be attributed to AMI. Cardiac echocardiography can be performed as an emergency within the MAU as this is a useful means of evaluating cardiac function. If the ECG indicates AMI, treatment should not be delayed (see Chapter 9 – Chest pain). Similarly, if a mechanical complication is suspected, urgent referral to a cardiologist is necessary.

The patient's response to treatment should be prompt but if this is not the case, respiratory function may deteriorate and respiratory arrest may occur. In some cases, endotracheal intubation and intermittent positive pressure ventilation will be necessary. In these cases, MAU nurses have an important role to play in the safe transfer of the patient to the intensive care unit.

Summary

This chapter has provided a comprehensive guide to the assessment and initial management of patients who present with the most common causes of SOB to the MAU. A vast number of disorders can cause the patient to experience SOB; some less common causes are listed in Box 8.10. The detailed description of the causes, pathophysiology, presenting features, immediate management and investigations for each of the most common disorders provides the reader with an understanding of how the breathless patient should be managed in the MAU. The reader is directed to the sources of further reading listed at the end of the chapter for information on the continuing management of the patient with SOB.

Box 8.10. Less common causes of shortness of breath

- Diabetic ketoacidosis (see Chapter 7 – Altered consciousness)
- Anaphylaxis (see Chapter 6 – Shock)
- Anxiety, hyperventilation
- Anaemia
- Renal failure
- Fractured ribs/chest trauma
- Pleural effusion
- Lung cancer
- Smoke inhalation

References

Advanced Life Support Group (ALSG) (2001) Acute Medical Emergencies: The Practical Approach. London: BMJ Books.

American Thoracic Society (1999) Dyspnea: mechanisms, assessment, and management: a consensus statement. American Journal of Respiratory Critical Care Medicine 159: 321–40.

Angus R, Ahmed A, Fenwick L (1996) Comparison of the acute effects of gas exchange of nasal ventilation and doxapram in exacerbations of chronic obstructive pulmonary disease. Thorax 51: 1048–50.

Anthonisen N, Manfreda J, Warren C et al (1987) Antibiotic therapy in exacerbations of chronic obstructive pulmonary disease. Annals of Internal Medicine 106: 96–204.

Barker S, Shah N (1996) Effects of motion on the performance of pulse oximeters in volunteers. Anaesthesiology 85(4): 1774–81.

Barnes P (1999) Managing Chronic Obstructive Pulmonary Disease. London: Science Press.

Barnes P, Godfrey S (2000) Asthma, 2nd edn. London: Martin Dunitz.

Borg A (1982) Psychophysical bases of perceived exertion. Medicine and Science in Sport and Exercise 14(5): 377–81.

Bourke SJ, Brewis RAL (1998) Respiratory Medicine, 5th edn. Oxford: Blackwell Science.

Brigg C (1999) The benefits of non-invasive ventilation and CPAP therapy. British Journal of Nursing 8(20): 1355–61.

British Thoracic Society (1997a) Guidelines for the management of chronic obstructive pulmonary disease. Thorax 52 (Supplement 5).

British Thoracic Society (1997b) Asthma management guidelines. Thorax 52 (Supplement 1).

Brochard L (2000) Non-invasive ventilation for acute exacerbations of COPD: a new standard of care. Thorax 55: 817–18.

Bucher L, Melander S (1999) Critical Care Nursing. Philadelphia: WB Saunders.

Casaburi R, Porzasz J, Buens R et al (1997) Physiological benefits of exercise training in rehabilitation of patients with severe COPD. American Journal of Respiratory and Critical Care Medicine 155: 1541–51.

Celli B, Benditt J, Albert R (1999) Chronic obstructive pulmonary disease. In Albert R, Spiro S, Jett J (eds) Comprehensive Respiratory Medicine. London: Mosby.

Combivent Inhalation Aerosol Study Group (1994) In chronic obstructive pulmonary disease, combination of ipratropium and albuterol is more effective than either agent alone. Chest 105: 1411–19.

Copstead L-E, Banasik J (2000) Pathophysiology: Biological and Behavioral Perspectives. Philadelphia: WB Saunders.

Dagg K, Thomson N (1996) Asthma in adults. Respiratory Medicine Update October: 252–9.

Davies L, Wilkinson M, Bonner S et al (2000) 'Hospital at home' versus hospital care in patients with exacerbations of chronic obstructive pulmonary disease: prospective randomised controlled trial. British Medical Journal 321: 1265–8.

DoH (2001) Hospital Episode Statistics 1998/99: Table 3 Primary Diagnosis. http://www.doh.gov.uk/hes/site

Field D (2000) Respiratory care. In Sheppard M, Wright M (eds) Principles and Practice of High Dependency Nursing. Edinburgh: Baillière Tindall/RCN.

Fletcher CM, Peto R, Tinker C et al (1976) The Natural History of Chronic Bronchitis and Emphysema: An Eight Year Study of Early Chronic Obstructive Lung Disease in Working Men in London. London: Oxford University Press.

Gibson P, Charpin D (2000) Educating adolescents about asthma. Chest 118: 1514–15.

Gibson P, Coughlan J, Wilson A (1998) Review: Limited asthma education reduces the number of visits to emergency departments but does not improve patient outcomes. Evidence-Based Medicine July/August: 121.

Gibson P, Talbot P, Toneguzzi R (1995) Self-management autonomy, and quality of life in asthma. Chest 107: 1003–8.

Gravil J, Al-Rawas, Cotton O et al (1998) Home treatment of exacerbations of chronic obstructive pulmonary disease by an acute respiratory assessment service. Lancet 351: 1853–5.

Holgate S (1993) Asthma: past, present and future. The 1992 Cournand Lecture. European Respiratory Journal 6: 1507–20.

Jeffrey A, Warren P, Flenley D (1992) Acute hypercapnic respiratory failure in patients with chronic obstructive pulmonary disease: risk factors and use of guidelines in management. Thorax 47: 34–40.

Jeffries A, Turley A (1999) Mosby's Crash Course Respiratory System. London: Mosby.

Jevon P, Ewens B (2001) Assessment of a breathless patient. Nursing Standard 15(16): 48-53.

Jowett N, Thompson D (1996) Comprehensive Coronary Care, 2nd edn. London: Baillière Tindall.

Julian D, Cowan J, McClenachan J (1998) Cardiology, 7th edn. London: WB Saunders.

Kumar A (1997) Chest X-ray. In Thompson P (ed) Coronary Care Manual. London: Churchill Livingstone.

Laurence DR, Bennett PN, Brown MJ (1997) Clinical Pharmacology. New York: Churchill Livingstone.

Laurent-Bopp D (2000) Heart failure. In Woods S, Froelicher E, Motzer S (eds) Cardiac Nursing, 4th edn. Philadelphia: Lippincott.

Lewis A (1999) Respiratory emergency! Nursing 99: 62–4.

Lowton K (1999) Pulse oximeters for the detection of hypoxaemia. Professional Nurse 14(5): 343–50.

Mahler D, Weinberg D, Wells C et al (1984) The measurement of dyspnoea: contents, interobserver agreement and physiological correlates of two new clinical indices. Chest 85: 751–8.

Medical Research Council (1965) Definition and classification of chronic bronchitis, clinical and epidemiological purposes; a report to the Medical Research Council by their committee on the etiology of chronic bronchitis. Lancet i: 775–80.

Millane T, Jackson G, Gibbs C, Lip G (2000) ABC of heart failure: acute and chronic management strategies. British Medical Journal 320: 559–62.

Moore T (2000) Supporting respiration. In Bassett C, Makin L (eds) Caring for the Seriously Ill Patient. London: Arnold.

Moulton C, Yates D (1999) Lecture Notes on Emergency Medicine, 2nd edn. Oxford: Blackwell Science.

Partridge M (1995) Asthma: lessons from patient education. Patient Education and Counselling 26: 81–86.

Pearson M, Littler J, Davies P (1994) An analysis of medical workload by speciality and diagnosis in Mersey: evidence of a specialist mismatch. Journal of the Royal College of Physicians 28: 230–4.

Place B (2000) Pulse oximetry: benefits and limitations. Nursing Times 96(26): 42–4.

Plant P, Owen J, Elliott M (2000) A multicentre randomised controlled trial of the early use of non-invasive ventilation for acute exacerbations of chronic obstructive pulmonary disease on general respiratory wards. Lancet 355: 1931–5.

Saint S, Bent S, Vittinghoff E et al (1995) Antibiotics in chronic obstructive pulmonary disease exacerbations: a meta-analysis. Journal of the American Medical Association 273: 957–60

Sharp JT, Drutz S, Moisan T et al (1980) Postural relief of dyspnea in severe chronic obstructive pulmonary disease. American Review of Respiratory Disease 122: 201–11.

Singer M, Webb AR (1998) Oxford Handbook of Critical Care. Oxford: Oxford University Press.

Skillrid D, Offord K, Miller R (1986) Higher risk of lung cancer in chronic pulmonary disease. A prospective matched case-controlled study. Annals of International Medicine 105: 503–7.

Snider G, Kleinerman J, Thurlbeck W et al (1985) The definition of emphysema: a report of the National Heart and Blood Institute, Division of Lung Diseases Workshop. American Review of Respiratory Disease 132:182–5.

Tashkin D, Detels R, Simmons M et al (1994) The UCLA population studies of chronic obstructive respiratory disease 6. Impact of air pollution and smoking on annual change in forced expiratory volume in one second. American Journal of Respiratory and Critical Care Medicine 149: 1209–17.

Thelan L, Urden L, Lough M, Stacy K (1998) Critical Care Nursing Diagnosis and Management, 3rd edn. St Louis: Mosby.

Thompson W, Nielson C, Carvalho P (1996) Controlled trial of oral prednisolone on outpatients with acute COPD exacerbations. American Journal of Respiratory and Critical Care Medicine 154: 407–12.

Timmis A, Nathan A, Sullivan I (1997) Essential Cardiology, 3rd edn. Oxford: Blackwell.

Watson P, Town G, Holbrook N et al (1997) Evaluation of a self-management plan for chronic obstructive pulmonary disease. European Respiratory Journal 10: 1267–71.

Woodruff DW (1999) How to ward off complications of mechanical ventilation. Nursing 99 29(11): 35-9.

Further reading

Barnes P, Godfrey S (2000) Asthma, 2nd edn. London: Martin Dunitz.

Barnes P, Grunstein M, Leff A (1997) Asthma: Philadelphia: Lippincott.

Bassett C, Makin L (2000) Caring for the Seriously Ill Patient. London: Arnold.

Bateman N, Leach R (1998) Acute oxygen therapy. British Medical Journal 317: 798–801.

Bourke S, Brewis R (1998) Lecture Notes on Respiratory Medicine. Oxford: Blackwell Science.

Brewis R, Corrin B, Geddes D, Gibson G (1995) Respiratory Medicine. London: Harcourt.

BTS (1997) The British guidelines on asthma management: 1995 review and position statement. Thorax 52 (Supplement 1).

BTS (1997) Current best practice for nebuliser therapy. Thorax 52 (Supplement 2).

BTS (1997) Guidelines on the management of COPD. Thorax 52 (Supplement 5).

BTS and the association of Respiratory Technicians and Physiologists (1994) Guidelines for the measurement of respiratory function. Respiratory Medicine 88: 165–94.

Cox C, McGrath A (1999) Respiratory assessment in critical care units. Intensive and Critical Care Nursing 15: 226–34.

Dean B (1997) Evidence based suction management in Accident & Emergency: a vital component of airway care. Accident and Emergency Nursing 5: 92–7.

Gibbs R (2000) ABC of Heart Failure. London: BMJ Books.

Hinchliff SM, Montague SE, Watson R (1996) Physiology for Nursing Practice, 2nd edn. London: Baillière Tindall.

Pauwels R (2000) National and International Guidelines for COPD: the need for evidence. Chest 117 (Supplement): S20–2.

Peate I, Lancaster J (2000) Safe use of medical gases in the clinical setting: practical tips. British Journal of Nursing 9(4): 231–6.

Sheppard M, Davis S (2000) Oxygen therapy – 1. Nursing Times 96(29): 43–4.

Sheppard M, Wright M (2000) Principles and Practice of High Dependency Nursing. London: Baillière Tindall.

Stockley R (1999) Alpha 1 antitrypsin deficiency – uncharted territory. Respiratory Disease in Practice 16: 21–3.

Waugh A, Grant A (2001) Ross and Wilson Anatomy and Physiology in Health and Illness, 9th edn. London: Churchill Livingstone.

For further information on any lung disorders:
British Lung Foundation
78 Hatton Garden
London
EC1N 8LD
Tel 020 7831 5831
Website http://www.blf@britishlungfoundation.com

CHAPTER 9

Chest pain

MICHELLE RHODES

Aims

This chapter will:

- describe a systematic approach to the initial assessment and management of patients with chest pain
- describe the presenting features, pathophysiology, investigations and management of patients who present with the most common causes of chest pain

Introduction

Between 20 and 30% of emergency medical admissions comprise patients with acute, central chest pain, although less than half of these patients will have a final diagnosis of acute myocardial infarction (AMI) or unstable angina (Blatchford and Capewell 1999). A number of potentially life-threatening and non-life-threatening conditions may cause the patient to experience chest pain (Table 9.1) and may give rise to specific presenting features (Table 9.2).

Initial assessment of patients with chest pain

The initial assessment of patients with chest pain uses the ABCDE principles (see Chapter 2 – Initial assessment). The priority is the identification of high-risk patients with life-threatening conditions who require immediate treatment.

Table 9.1. The causes of chest pain

	Cardiac	**Pulmonary**	**Gastro-intestinal**	**Musculo-skeletal/other**
Most common causes of chest pain:				
Life-threatening causes	Acute coronary syndrome: AMI or unstable angina	Pulmonary embolism		
Non-life-threatening causes	Stable angina		Oesophagitis Gastro-oesophageal reflux Hiatus hernia	Costochondritis
Less common causes of chest pain:				
Life-threatening causes	Dissecting thoracic aortic aneurysm Pericarditis Arrhythmia Aortic valve stenosis	Pneumothorax Severe chest infection	Peptic ulcer	
Non-life-threatening causes		Pleurisy		Rib fractures Osteoarthritis Cervical spondylosis Anxiety/depression

Airway

Is the patient's airway clear?

Breathing

Is the respiratory rate elevated or depressed?

Is the patient having difficulty breathing?

Is chest expansion equal?

Is there peripheral or central cyanosis (indicating shock)?

Is there a cough? Is sputum being produced? Is the sputum frothy and/or blood-stained (indicating pulmonary oedema)?

Is the patient's trachea central? Deviation may indicate tension pneumothorax.

Has the patient received an opioid analgesic, which may be causing respiratory depression? If so, administer naloxone 400 μg intravenously (IV) (British Medical Association and the Royal Pharmaceutical Society of Great Britain (BMA and RPSGB) 2000).

Table 9.2. Symptoms commonly associated with chest pain due to a specific cause

Condition causing chest pain	Associated symptoms
Cardiac ischaemia: acute myocardial infarction unstable angina stable angina	Pallor Diaphoresis Dyspnoea Pink frothy sputum Nausea and vomiting
Cardiac arrhythmia **Aortic valve stenosis**	Weakness Dizziness Palpitations Indigestion Syncope Shock
Dissecting thoracic aortic aneurysm	Tearing chest pain, typically in interscapular area, but may radiate to throat and/or both arms Pain more severe at onset Paralysis of limbs Unequal BP and pulse on each arm History of untreated hypertension Shock
Pericarditis	Pleuritic pain, worse on inspiration and relieved by sitting forwards
Pulmonary: pulmonary embolism pneumothorax chest infection	Collapse Signs of deep vein thrombosis Tachypnoea Dyspnoea Cough with/without haemoptysis Cyanosis Desaturation Shock Pleuritic chest pain
Gastrointestinal: oesophageal spasm gastro-oesophageal reflux peptic ulcer hiatus hernia	Vomiting Dyspepsia Dysphasia Regurgitation Bloating History of poor diet
Musculoskeletal: costochondritis rib fracture osteoarthritis cervical spondylosis	Limb numbness and weakness Limb tingling History of recent strenuous activity Precipitated by abrupt movement Pleuritic chest pain

Psychogenic:
anxiety
depression
	Hyperventilation
	   panic attacks, numbness, tingling
	   dizziness
	   light-headedness
	   palpitation

Circulation

Measure the heart rate (HR).

Is the peripheral pulse strong, or thready and weak (indicating shock)?

Is the HR regular or irregular (indicating an arrhythmia)?

If the patient is on a cardiac monitor, what is the heart rhythm?

What is the blood pressure (BP)? Is the systolic BP <90 mmHg (hypotension) or >140 mmHg (hypertension)?

Is the patient's skin warm and dry (normal perfusion) or cool, clammy and wet (indicating shock)?

Disability

Assess the patient's conscious level according to the AVPU scale (Alert, responds to Voice, responds to Pain or Unresponsive). Have they received an opioid analgesic? If so and they are P or U on the scale, administer naloxone as above.

Assess the patient's pain. Use the PQRST mnemonic to assess the pain (see Chapter 2 – Initial assessment) and to differentiate between the chest pain caused by specific conditions (Table 9.2).

Does the patient have any relevant prior history (e.g. myocardial infarction, angina, pulmonary embolism or aortic aneurysm)?

Look for any other clinical signs or symptoms accompanying the pain (Table 9.2).

Exposure

Undress the patient's chest initially and attach cardiac monitoring electrodes.

Record the temperature.

Check the capillary blood sugar (e.g. BM stix, glucostix). This is especially important in diabetic patients (see Chapter 7 – Altered consciousness).

Undress the patient fully.

Observe for peripheral oedema/signs of deep vein thrombosis (DVT).

Initial management of the patient with chest pain

- Secure IV access.
- Commence continuous cardiac monitoring of heart rate and rhythm.
- Record a 12-lead ECG.
- Administer 100% oxygen via a non-rebreathing mask unless the patient has COPD.
- Give 300 mg aspirin to chew, if acute coronary syndrome suspected.
- Pain relief (sublingual glyceryl trinitrate (GTN) and/or IV diamorphine 2.5–5 mg).
- Consider administering an anti-emetic (e.g. metoclopramide 10 mg IV).

- Access to immediate basic life support (BLS) and advanced life support (ALS) in case of cardiac arrest.

Acute coronary syndromes

Coronary heart disease (CHD) is the commonest cause of premature death (in people under 75 years of age) in the UK (British Heart Foundation (BHF) 2000). The BHF has estimated that 1.5 million people in the UK have angina, and that each year 270 000 experience a myocardial infarction, of whom about 135 000 die (BHF 2000). Most patients who die from AMI do so in the first hour after the onset of symptoms as the result of a fatal cardiac arrhythmia (Ryan et al 1999).

The term 'acute coronary syndrome' (ACS) is now widely used to define the acute manifestations of CHD, namely AMI (Q-wave MI), non-Q wave MI (minimal myocardial injury) and unstable angina (Fox 2000). All three arise as a result of the same pathophysiological processes. However, the manifestation depends on a number of factors, including the severity of the coronary artery obstruction, the presence or absence of a collateral blood supply to the myocardium and the myocardial oxygen requirements within the area affected by the obstruction (Fox 2000). Only AMI is treated with immediate reperfusion and therefore requires prompt recognition and distinction from the other coronary syndromes.

Pathophysiology

Atherosclerosis, the underlying condition that gives rise to the symptoms of AMI or angina, begins as an accumulation of lipid-laden cells within the intima of the coronary arteries. A plaque develops as deposits of cholesterol, lipid, smooth muscle cells, inflammatory cells, fibrous tissue, fibrin and blood are deposited and covered by a fibrous cap. Such plaques are present in a large proportion of the adult population but do not necessarily cause symptoms (Weissberg 2000). Symptoms may develop if the plaque becomes so large that it restricts blood flow to an area of myocardium with resultant angina on exertion. If, however, the plaque ruptures, platelets rapidly accumulate at the site of rupture, leading to fibrin deposition, the formation of a thrombus with possible occlusion of the coronary artery and the symptoms of AMI or unstable angina (Weissberg 2000). When the blood supply to myocardial cells is critically reduced or ceases completely, severe myocardial ischaemia occurs. In the absence of a collateral blood supply, myocardial cells will die if the ischaemia lasts for more than 30–45 minutes. The area of necrosis starts at the centre of the ischaemic zone and spreads outwards from the sub-endocardium (inner wall of the heart) towards the epicardium (outer wall of the heart). Unless reperfusion occurs in time to limit the necrosis, the area of infarction will involve the entire ischaemic zone and will become transmural (Fletcher 1997). Since all of the cells within the area of infarction are irreversibly damaged, the pumping function of the heart or the conduction of electrical impulses may be compromised, leading to acute heart failure and/or cardiac arrhythmias (see later).

In response to AMI, the autonomic nervous system is stimulated, so that in addition to the typical chest pain that is experienced, several other symptoms arise including nausea, vomiting, burping, sweating and clamminess (Fletcher 1997). Different types of myocardial infarction lead to different types of autonomic nervous system response. With anterior MI, tachycardia and vasoconstriction lead to an increase in BP that may also be a consequence of left ventricular dysfunction. In an inferior MI reflex bradycardia and vasodilation lead to a reduction in BP, and ischaemia of the sino-atrial and atrioventricular nodes may cause bradyarrhythmias (Fletcher 1997).

Presenting features of ACS

Table 9.3. Presenting features frequently associated with cardiac chest pain (Fletcher 1997, Del Bene and Vaughan 2000)

Presenting features	Mechanism of action
Nausea and vomiting Sweating Shortness of breath Pale Anxious and distressed Indigestion Weakness Light-headed Hypertension	Occur as a result of increased sympathetic nervous system activity and pain
Cough – producing pink, frothy or blood-stained sputum	Indicating acute left ventricular failure and pulmonary oedema
Hypotension, pallor and confusion	Indicating cardiogenic shock or arrhythmia
Dyspnoea and tachypnoea	Suggesting significant left ventricular dysfunction or arrhythmia
Loss of consciousness	Indicating hypotension due to arrhythmia or shock

It is important to remember that although 75–80% of all patients who present with AMI experience some chest discomfort, a small percentage of patients experience no chest symptoms (Del Bene and Vaughan 2000). It is known that certain groups of people commonly present with atypical symptoms of AMI. These groups include women, people with diabetes mellitus, older people and people from ethnic minorities (DoH 2000). All patients who present with chest discomfort require very careful, detailed assessment of their symptoms to differentiate between the symptoms of ACS and other conditions that can mimic ACS (e.g. pulmonary embolism and aortic dissection) (Table 9.3).

Initial assessment of ACS

The aim of the initial assessment within the MAU is to detect patients with an acute coronary syndrome and to categorise them into one of two groups (Ryan et al 1999):

- definite AMI requiring immediate reperfusion
- patients with a non-diagnostic ECG (included in this group are patients with suspected or confirmed unstable angina or non-Q wave MI, patients with non-cardiac chest pain and patients at low risk, with conditions like stable angina)

Patients with definite AMI must be identified quickly so that the appropriate reperfusion therapy can be commenced. Such an approach will reduce the patient's risk of disability or death both during and after hospitalisation (DoH 2000). The MAU nurse, therefore, has a fundamental role in the rapid assessment and identification of patients with AMI.

The diagnosis of AMI is based on the presence of at least two of the following three criteria (Norris 2000):

1. Clinical history of cardiac-type chest pain or discomfort.
2. Sequential ECG changes.
3. Rise in cardiac markers to at least twice the upper limit of normal.

Within the MAU, the primary screening of all patients who present with chest pain will involve recording a 12-lead ECG and evaluating the patient's symptoms (Ryan et al 1999). Bedside blood tests for cardiac markers (which identify myocardial necrosis) are now available in some hospitals. Where this is not the case, blood should be taken and sent to the laboratory to permit the later detection of AMI in patients who present with a non-diagnostic ECG. Assessment of the patient's clinical symptoms will permit the detection of complications (e.g. acute left ventricular failure, cardiogenic shock or arrhythmia).

1. Evaluation of chest pain

When evaluating the patient's pain, reassurance and explanations will help to allay the patient's anxiety. Calm questioning and the use of a chest pain evaluation tool (such as the PQRST tool suggested here, Table 9.4) will permit the rapid and detailed assessment of the patient's pain. At the same time, take a brief, targeted history; obtain information about the patient's personal and family risk factors for coronary heart disease and information about any contraindications to thrombolytic therapy. The emphasis should be on obtaining accurate information, with the minimum of delay and avoidance of repetition. This requires good teamwork and collaboration between ambulance, medical and nursing staff. In many MAUs, chest pain assessment proformas have been developed to aid this process.

Table 9.4. Assessment of cardiac chest pain (Thompson 1997a, Del Bene and Vaughan 2000)

Characteristics of cardiac chest pain		
P	Provokes	Chest discomfort occurs at rest, or with less physical exertion than usual angina. Not relieved by GTN or rest.
Q	Quality	Aching, burning sensation. Gripping, tightening, crushing, constricting, oppressive. Typically described like a heavy weight on the chest.
R	Radiation	Left arm to the elbow, both arms. Neck, lower jaw, upper jaw. Epigastrium. Interscapular area.
S	Site and severity	Central chest. Retrosternal. Severe – the worst pain possible. Highest score on a chest pain evaluation tool. Associated with apprehension.
T	Time	Prolonged, lasting more than 15 minutes.
Atypical features of chest discomfort associated with AMI: Pain presenting as isolated lower jaw pain or epigastric pain. Pain isolated to interscapular area, shoulders or ante-cubital fossa.		

Chest pain is often accompanied by a number of other symptoms (Table 9.3), which may arise simply as a result of the pain itself or as a result of the compromising effects of the AMI on the cardiovascular system.

2. ECG changes associated with AMI

The 12-lead ECG is central to the diagnosis of AMI and other acute coronary syndromes. ST-segment elevation and/or abnormal Q waves or left bundle branch block (LBBB) indicate the presence of myocardial infarction and identify those patients who will benefit from reperfusion with thrombolytic therapy or primary angioplasty (Ryan et al 1999). As Q waves can take up to 12 hours to develop (Thompson and Ilton 1997), diagnosis of AMI within the MAU will usually rely on the detection of ST elevation or LBBB. Only half of the patients who present to the MAU with AMI will have such unequivocal ECG changes; the remainder will display other less specific and undiagnostic ECG changes (Gibler et al 1990). These patients will require more detailed evaluation by a cardiologist.

A 12-lead ECG should be recorded within 10 minutes of the patient's arrival in MAU. Accurate and immediate interpretation of the ECG is essential and should be carried out by appropriately trained MAU nurses. The aim is to differentiate between those patients with a diagnostic ECG who require immediate evaluation regarding their suitability for reperfusion therapy and those patients whose ECG is undiagnostic. The first stage of ECG interpretation involves identifying any changes indicating AMI or other acute coronary syndrome (Table 9.5).

Once the presence of ST elevation and/or Q waves in two or more leads has been confirmed, the next stage of the interpretation involves classifying the AMI according to its location within the heart (Table 9.6). AMI usually involves the walls of the left ventricle and is classified as being anterior, posterior or lateral (Del Bene and Vaughan 2000). AMI may also involve the right ventricle. Significant right ventricular infarctions almost always occur in the presence of an inferior MI (Anderson et al 1987). Therefore, evidence of right ventricular infarction (ST elevation of 1 mm or more in V4R, which may resolve within 10 hours of symptom onset) (Robalino et al 1989) should be sought in all patients with acute inferior MI (Figure 9.1).

The location of the MI can have a significant impact on the patient's prognosis. Infarcts involving the anterior wall of the left ventricle (Figure 9.2) may severely affect the function of the left ventricle, resulting in complications such as acute left ventricular failure and cardiogenic shock (Del Bene and Vaughan 2000) (see Chapter 6 – Shock and Chapter 8 – Shortness of breath). Anterior infarcts may cause extensive damage to the interventricular septum and the bundle branch system, leading to conduction disturbances (e.g. bundle branch block) and/or rhythm disturbances (e.g. heart block). These may require temporary and, sometimes, permanent cardiac pacing (Thompson 1997b) (see Chapter 5 – Cardiac arrest). In the majority of cases, anterior MI is accompanied by sinus tachycardia due to sympathetic nervous system stimulation (Del Bene and Vaughan 2000).

Table 9.5. ECG changes indicating presence of AMI (Thompson and Ilton 1997, Ryan et al 1999)

ECG change diagnostic of AMI	Pathophysiology
ST-segment elevation In 2 or more contiguous leads: >1 mm in limb leads: II, III, AVF, I AVL >2 mm in chest leads: V1–V6 >1 mm in II, III, AVF and V4R Localised to area of infarction Typically accompanied by peaking of T waves, followed by T wave flattening and T wave inversion ST elevation gradually lowers as the T wave inverts	Occurs within 1–2 minutes of coronary occlusion. Indicates the early phase of myocardial injury. May be reversed by early reperfusion. The number of leads involved indicates the extent of the injury. The height of ST elevation tends to reflect the amount of injury.
Tall peaked T waves Localised to the area of infarction	Represents the hyperacute phase of infarction and can occur before ST elevation.
Deep T wave inversion Localised to the area of infarction	Part of the sequence of changes indicating AMI. Occurs in both Q wave and non-Q wave MI. Usually resolves after weeks/months.
Development of abnormal Q waves Q waves >0.04 seconds in duration (1 small square) and more than 25% of the height of the R wave In 2 or more contiguous leads: limb leads: II, III, AVF, I AVL chest leads: V1–V6	Indicates myocardial cell death and Q wave myocardial infarction. Begins to develop 2–12 hours after the onset of symptoms. Usually persists but can occasionally return to normal after 3 years.
New or presumed new left bundle branch block (LBBB) NB. In the presence of right bundle branch block (RBBB) the diagnosis of AMI is still possible	Diagnosis of AMI in the setting of LBBB is very difficult, as the presence of ST elevation, Q waves and T wave inversion is obscured. Therefore, presume LBBB is a result of AMI.
Other ECG changes	
ST-segment depression Flat, horizontal or down sloping of the junction of the ST segment with the QRS (ST depression confined to V1–V4 without ST elevation indicates posterior wall MI)	When present in 2 or more leads without ST elevation – represents myocardial ischaemia. When present alongside ST elevation may represent a reciprocal change.

Table 9.6. Classification of acute myocardial infarction (Thompson and Ilton 1997, Ryan et al 1999)

Site of infarct	ECG leads involved
Inferior wall of left ventricle	II, III, AVF
Right ventricle	V4R (V4 lead placed on the right side of the chest, in the 5th intercostal space on the mid-clavicular line)
Anterior wall of left ventricle	V2, V3, V4
Lateral wall of left ventricle	I, AVL, V5, V6
Antero-lateral walls of left ventricle	I, AVL, V2–V6
Posterior wall of left ventricle	Tall R wave and ST depression in V1 ST depression V1–V4

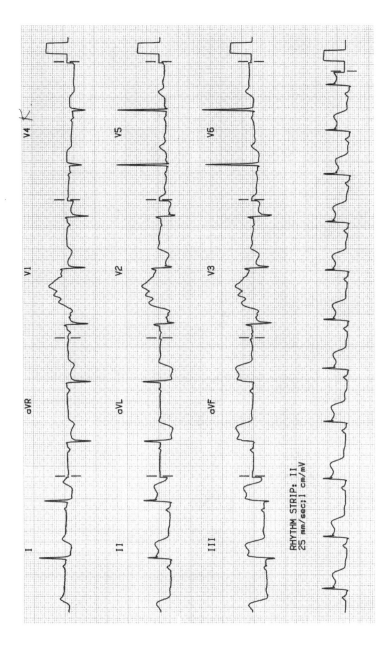

Figure 9.1. Inferior MI and right ventricular MI.

Note: ST-segment elevation >1 mm in leads II, III, AVF indicating acute inferior MI. Abnormal Q wave in lead III. ST-segment elevation >1 mm in V4R indicating acute right ventricular MI. ST-segment depression in I, AVL, V1–V3 indicating a reciprocal change.

N.B. V4R replaces usual V4 lead.

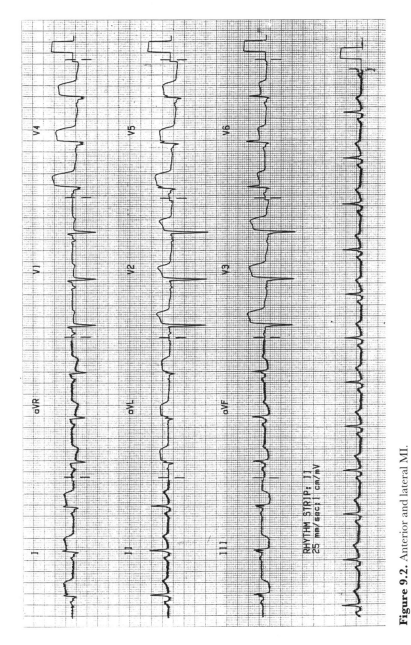

Figure 9.2. Anterior and lateral MI.

Note: ST-segment elevation >1 mm in leads I, AVL, and >2 mm in leads V2–V6 indicating acute antero-lateral MI. ST-segment depression in leads III, AVF indicating a reciprocal change. Loss of R wave and appearance of Q wave in leads V2–V5. Abnormal Q wave in leads I, AVL.

Patients with inferior MI (Figure 9.1) often develop cardiac rhythm disturbances due to ischaemia or necrosis of the atrioventricular node. This may lead to heart block, which may require temporary cardiac pacing if the patient becomes symptomatic (Thompson 1997b) (See Chapter 5 – Cardiac Arrest). Inferior MI is often accompanied by sinus bradycardia and hypotension due to activation of the parasympathetic nervous system (Del Bene and Vaughan 2000). Up to 50% of all patients with inferior MI will also have ECG evidence of right ventricular involvement, although only 10–15% will develop significant right ventricular infarction leading to haemodynamic abnormalities (Ryan et al 1999) (see Chapter 6 – Shock). When right ventricular MI does accompany inferior MI, mortality is significantly higher than for inferior MI alone (Zehender et al 1993). It is, therefore, essential that, as part of the continuing assessment, the MAU nurse maintains continuous close observation of the patient's heart rate and rhythm, circulatory and respiratory function for signs of shock.

Following this assessment, the patient can now be categorised into one of the two groups identified in Table 9.7.

Table 9.7. Categorisation of patients according to ECG changes (Ryan et al 1999)

Group 1	Patients with ST-segment elevation or left bundle branch block indicating a diagnosis of AMI and the need for immediate reperfusion (the so-called 'barn door MI')
Group 2	Patients with a non-diagnostic ECG. This group will comprise patients with non-cardiac pain or cardiac pain due to: • unstable angina • small MI • posterior MI • multiple coronary artery disease with left ventricular dysfunction This group of patients will require more detailed assessment (see later). NB. Patients with AMI without ST elevation are more likely to have multiple coronary artery disease and to have had a prior AMI than patients with ST elevation (group 1). They are also more likely to be elderly, diabetic, hypertensive and to have co-existing heart failure and/or peripheral vascular disease than patients with ST elevation.

At this point, contact the relevant doctor or specialist nurse to perform a brief physical examination, confirm the diagnosis and begin the appropriate treatment. In most MAUs, the initial management strategy will be outlined within the individual unit's policies and procedures. This should follow the algorithm presented in Figure 9.3.

For patients with a definite AMI, the initial assessment, physical examination and ECG should be completed within 20 minutes of their arrival in the unit (Del Bene and Vaughan 2000). This will help to ensure

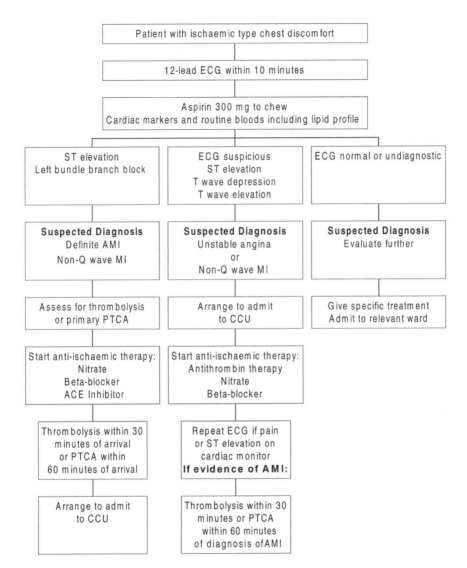

Figure 9.3. Algorithm for the initial management of patients with suspected acute coronary syndromes in the MAU. (Adapted from Ryan T et al (1999) on behalf of the Committee on Management of Acute Myocardial Infarction (1999) 1999 update: American College of Cardiology/American Heart Association guidelines for the management of patients with acute myocardial infarction. Journal of the American College of Cardiology 34: 890–911.)

the administration of thrombolysis to eligible patients within 20 minutes of their arrival at hospital, as currently recommended (DoH 2000). Thrombolysis should be commenced within the MAU before transferring the patient to the coronary care unit (CCU) for continuing management (DoH 2000). This will help to avoid any unnecessary delays.

3. Serum cardiac markers of AMI

Cardiac markers are released into the bloodstream by damaged myocardium and are an indication of myocardial cell necrosis. Traditional markers include the cardiac enzymes creatine kinase (CK), lactic dehydrogenase (LDH) and aspartate aminotransferase (AST). The newer markers include the troponins (troponin I and T) (Ryan et al 1999).

For patients who present to the MAU with an obvious AMI, cardiac markers have little impact on the initial treatment decisions made. However, where the diagnosis is less clear, cardiac markers have an important role in the detection of patients with unstable angina or AMI without ST elevation or Q waves (Fox 2000). They may also permit the later evaluation of the success of thrombolytic therapy (Ryan et al 1999). For these reasons, blood should be taken for cardiac markers, along with other routine haematological and biochemical tests (e.g. full blood count, urea and electrolytes, glucose, and lipid profile) as soon as the patient has been stabilised in the MAU. The specific markers measured, the methods of analysis used and the length of time taken to receive results will vary according to local hospital policy They should include total creatine kinase (total CK), its isoenzyme CK-MB and troponin I and/or T.

Creatine kinase and CK-MB. Total CK lacks specificity for myocardial necrosis, as it is present in tissues other than the myocardium. CK-MB is a cardiac-specific component of total CK and is much more widely used to diagnose AMI. CK-MB is usually measured as a ratio of CK-MB to total CK. In addition, serial measurements should be obtained during the first 72 hours following symptom onset to allow its rise and fall to be evaluated (Wooding Baker 2000). In AMI, total CK and CK-MB rise within 4–6 hours after symptom onset. They peak within 12–24 hours to more than six times their normal value and return to normal within 2–4 days. A CK-MB >5% of the total CK is indicative of AMI (Wooding Baker 2000).

CK-MB isoforms have recently been identified as new and potentially very early (within 1–4 hours of infarction) markers of myocardial necrosis (Ryan et al 1999). They are, therefore, especially useful for the early diagnosis of AMI and for detecting recurrent myocardial infarction (as their early return to normal levels permits their re-evaluation).

Troponins. Troponin I and troponin T are extremely sensitive, specific markers of myocardial necrosis (Hillis and Fox 1999). As they are not normally found in the blood of healthy people, their presence has been linked directly to an increased risk of AMI (Hillis and Fox 1999). Troponin I and T are not found in the blood until 6 hours after the onset of symptoms and they peak at between 12 and 24 hours. Troponin I remains elevated for up to 7 days and troponin T for 10–14 days (Ryan et al 1999). For these reasons, admission values of troponins may be most beneficial for the diagnosis of patients with a non-diagnostic ECG. Table 9.8 represents the ECG and enzyme marker features associated with the acute coronary syndromes.

Many patients who present to the MAU with a history suggesting AMI have no diagnostic clinical or ECG findings when they arrive (Hillis and Fox 1999). In these patients continuing assessment is necessary by checking serum troponin and repeating the ECG (especially during any further episodes of chest pain) (Fox 2000). This permits the identification of patients who have sustained a small myocardial infarction (non-Q wave MI) and patients with unstable angina (Fox 2000) (Table 9.8). There is no evidence to support the administration of thrombolytic therapy to these patients; indeed it may increase mortality. It has been found that patients who present with abnormalities in their QRS who do not develop a Q wave MI are at high risk of death (Ryan et al 1999) and, therefore, require very early assessment by a cardiologist.

In cases where non-Q wave MI or unstable angina are suspected, arrange admission to the CCU for continuing evaluation and diagnosis. Continue monitoring the heart rate and rhythm, and repeat the ECG if the patient experiences any further chest pain. Treatment to relieve the pain should include GTN, which may be given IV or sublingually. Additional anti-ischaemic therapy will include anti-thrombin agents and beta-blockers (Ryan et al 1999).

Immediate management of the patient with ACS

The immediate management of patients with ACS in the MAU involves:

1. Relief of pain and anxiety.
2. Treatment of potentially life-threatening ventricular arrhythmias.

Table 9.8. Diagnosis of acute coronary syndromes

Clinical syndrome	ECG features	Pathophysiology	Enzyme marker features	Indication for reperfusion
Acute myocardial infarction (AMI) Q wave MI	ST elevation New bundle branch block ECG changes of posterior MI Evolution of Q waves	Abrupt occlusion of coronary artery by thrombus, leading to acute ischaemia and infarction usually resulting in Q wave MI	> 2 times upper limit of CK-MB, CK Troponin T > 0.2 ng/dl Troponin I* > 1.0–1.5 ng/dl	Requires immediate reperfusion
Non-Q wave MI (Minimal myocardial injury)	Aborted ST elevation MI Transient ST elevation ST depression T inversion Minor non-specific ECG changes	Partial coronary artery obstruction with distal ischaemia and, therefore, minor enzyme rise usually resulting in non-Q wave MI	< 2 times elevation CK-MB, CK Troponin T 0.01–0.2 ng/dl Troponin I* 0.1 or 0.4 to 1.0–1.5 ng/dl	No indication for immediate reperfusion
Unstable angina	Transient ST elevation ST depression T inversion Minor non-specific ECG changes Normal ECG	Non-occlusive coronary thrombus without enzyme rise	CK-MB, CK < upper limit of normal Troponin T < 0.01 ng/dl Troponin I* < 0.1 or 0.4 ng/dl	No indication for immediate reperfusion

*Troponin I cut-off values depend upon assay system.

Adapted from Fox KAA (2000) Acute coronary syndromes: presentation – clinical spectrum and management. Heart 84: 93–100.

3. Reduction of the size of the infarct and reperfusion of the affected coronary artery.
4. Early detection/prevention of complications.

1. Relief of pain and anxiety

Once the patient has undergone initial assessment, they should be given pain relief as soon as possible. Pain increases myocardial oxygen demand by increasing the heart rate and blood pressure. It can, therefore, increase the area of infarction (Ryan et al 1999).

Commence 100% oxygen via a non-rebreathing mask (unless the patient also has severe COPD) in all patients suspected of having an AMI. Monitor and maintain oxygen saturation at >95–98%. Giving supplemental oxygen may reduce the amount of myocardial ischaemia (Maroko et al 1975) and reduce the amount of ST elevation (Madias and Hood 1976). Observe the patient for signs of hypoxaemia (e.g. shortness of breath or cyanosis). This may indicate the presence of a complication (e.g. left ventricular failure and pulmonary oedema), which will require immediate medical intervention, and, in some cases, mechanical ventilation (Ryan et al 1999). In uncomplicated cases, oxygen can be discontinued after 3 hours (Ryan et al 1999).

Gain IV access or, if already in situ, ensure the patency of the cannula before commencing any drug therapy. Check which drugs (if any) the patient has already received. To relieve chest pain and reduce the patient's anxiety, give an opioid analgesic. Diamorphine is usually the drug of choice. Diamorphine should be administered by a slow (1 mg/minute) IV injection of 5 mg, followed by further doses of 2.5–5 mg until the chest pain is relieved. In frail or elderly patients, reduce the dose by half (BMA and RPSGB 2000). As opiates can cause respiratory depression and hypotension, monitor BP and respiratory rate continuously. If the respiratory rate drops significantly, administer naloxone $400\,\mu g$ IV to reverse the effects, and repeat every 3 minutes to a maximum of three doses if necessary (Ryan et al 1999). Remember that once reversed by naloxone, the analgesic effects of diamorphine will be lost. To combat any pre-existing or concomitant nausea and vomiting, administer an anti-emetic such as metoclopramide 10 mg IV over 1–2 minutes or cyclizine 50 mg IV (if no left ventricular dysfunction).

In cases where the ECG is non-diagnostic, sublingual GTN may be given. GTN is known to relieve cardiac ischaemic pain by dilating the coronary arteries and is, therefore, effective in patients with unstable angina. Nitrates, such as GTN, also dilate peripheral arteries and large veins, which may benefit the patient. They can, however, cause bradycardia or significant hypotension with reflex tachycardia (Ryan et al 1999). Therefore, monitor the patient's BP and heart rate closely during and after nitrate therapy. Do not give nitrates to patients with a systolic BP less than 90 mmHg, a bradycardia less than 50 bpm, a tachycardia or a suspected right ventricular MI (Ryan et al 1999).

2. Prevention and treatment of potentially life-threatening ventricular arrhythmias (VF or VT)

Patients with AMI are at high risk of sudden death, especially during the first hour, due to potentially fatal cardiac arrhythmias such as VF or VT (Ryan et al 1999).

Ensure that the patient is monitored continuously via a cardiac monitor connected to a central monitoring station. Resuscitation equipment should be easily accessible. MAU nurses should be trained in advanced life support so that when VF or pulseless VT is recognised and loss of consciousness confirmed, defibrillation can be performed within 15 seconds (Thompson and Morgan 1997) (see Chapter 5 – Cardiac arrest).

Primary VF may occur within the first 48 hours of AMI, though the risk is highest in the first 4 hours (Campbell et al 1981). Primary VF is not associated with heart failure or cardiogenic shock (Volpi et al 1990). A number of factors may precipitate VF and these include increased sympathetic nervous system activity (e.g. during pain), hypokalaemia, hypomagnesaemia, acidosis and reperfusion of the ischaemic myocardium (Campbell 1994, Norderhaug and von der Lippe 1983, Higham et al 1993). For this reason, check the serum electrolyte levels whilst the patient is in the MAU and maintain the serum potassium at >4.0 mmol/l. The use of prophylactic anti-arrhythmic agents is not recommended in the routine management of AMI, or for the treatment of non-sustained VT, ventricular ectopic beats or accelerated idioventricular rhythm (Ryan et al 1999).

Secondary VF or VT that occurs 48 hours after AMI requires careful evaluation regarding the cause. VF or VT that occurs in association with heart failure or cardiogenic shock has a poor prognosis (Ryan et al 1999).

3. Reperfusion of coronary arteries and reduction of infarct size

The following approaches can be adopted to aid reperfusion of the affected coronary arteries and reduce the size of the infarcted area:

Anti-platelet therapy:	Aspirin
Reperfusion:	Thrombolytic therapy
	Percutaneous transluminal
	coronary angioplasty (PTCA)
Anti-ischaemic therapy:	Beta-blockers
	ACE inhibitors

Anti-platelet therapy. Aspirin has been shown to have a positive effect on reducing mortality from AMI (ISIS-2 Collaborative Group 1988). If aspirin has not already been administered, and providing there are no contraindications (e.g. aspirin hypersensitivity, asthma, bleeding peptic ulcer or bleeding disorders), give 300 mg as soon as possible (BMA and RPSGB 2000). This initial dose of aspirin should be chewed to promote its rapid absorption (Ryan et al 1999). Aspirin causes an anti-thrombotic effect by inhibiting platelet aggregation and is important in reducing coronary reocclusion and ischaemia after thrombolytic therapy (Roux et al 1992). The main side effects of aspirin are dose related and include gastrointestinal bleeding. Clopidogrel may be used as a substitute when aspirin is contraindicated because of hypersensitivity (Ryan et al 1999).

Reperfusion therapy – thrombolytic therapy. The primary goal of reperfusion therapy is the restoration of normal blood flow through the affected coronary artery (Robinson and Timmis 2000). The most widely used and best-tested method of reperfusion is the administration of thrombolytic therapy. As the benefits of thrombolytic therapy are time related, the earlier treatment is begun, the better the outcome for the patient in terms of mortality and morbidity reduction. Whilst benefit is greatest when treatment is started within the first 3 hours of symptom onset, patients still benefit when treatment is given up to 12 hours from onset (FTT Collaborative Group 1994). As many patients suffering an AMI find it difficult to identify the precise time that their symptoms started, it is important for MAU nurses to obtain a detailed history regarding their symptoms. The time of symptom onset should be taken as 'the beginning of the continuous, persistent discomfort that brought the patient to hospital' (Ryan et al 1999). The indications for thrombolytic therapy are listed in Table 9.9.

Thrombolytic agents currently used in the UK include streptokinase, which is administered as an IV infusion over 60 minutes, t-PA (Actilyse), which is given as an accelerated infusion over 90 minutes, and r-PA (Reteplase), which is given as two IV bolus doses 30 minutes apart. A new

Table 9.9. Indications for thrombolytic therapy

ECG	ST ↑ >1 mm in 2 or more contiguous limb leads ST ↑ >2 mm in 2 or more contiguous chest leads
	ST ↓ confined to V1–V4 (suggesting posterior wall infarction due to occlusion of circumflex artery)
	Hyperacute T waves before ST elevation indicates early sign of injury; therefore repeat ECG every 15 minutes
	Left bundle branch block – new or presumed new
Chest pain	Typical cardiac pain and accompanying symptoms
	<12 hours since onset of symptoms
	>12 hours since onset if ongoing cardiac chest pain and accompanied by extensive ST elevation

Adapted from Ryan T et al (1999) 1999 update: American College of Cardiology/American Heart Association guidelines for the management of patients with acute myocardial infarction. Journal of the American College of Cardiology 34: 890–911.

agent (TNK) is a single bolus injection, which has recently been licensed for use in the UK (BMA and RPSGB 2000). All the current thrombolytic agents act as plasminogen activators by enzymatically converting plasminogen to plasmin, which degrades the fibrin within the blood clot and causes the thrombus to break up (Ryan et al 1999, BMA and RPSGB 2000).

The choice of thrombolytic agent depends very much on the individual hospital's policy. Whilst accelerated t-PA and r-PA have produced the most favourable results in terms of restoring early coronary reperfusion, they both require the concomitant infusion of IV heparin. Both produce slightly higher rates of intracranial haemorrhage (ICH) (a potentially fatal complication of all the agents) when compared to streptokinase (Ryan et al 1999). Consequently, both these agents should be reserved for younger patients (with a lower risk of ICH) who present early after symptom onset with larger infarcts (anterior MI), or patients in whom streptokinase is contraindicated because of previous administration or allergic reaction (Ryan et al 1999).

Administration of streptokinase causes a non-specific fibrinolytic state, resulting in the systemic breakdown of the coagulation system. As a result, there is little need for concomitant anticoagulation therapy, whereas t-PA and the related agents r-PA and TNK are more fibrin specific, leading to a variable effect on the coagulation system with very little breakdown of fibrinogen. For this reason, t-PA and r-PA should be accompanied by an intravenous infusion of heparin for 48 hours in most patients, to increase their effectiveness (Ryan et al 1999). For those patients with a high risk of sustaining an embolic stroke (large anterior MI, left ventricular thrombus, history of previous embolus or atrial fibrillation) IV heparin should be given after thrombolysis, regardless of the thrombolytic agent used (Ryan et al 1999).

The benefits of thrombolytic therapy occur regardless of the patient's gender or age, although elderly patients (over 75 years of age) are at higher risk of death anyway. Most benefit is achieved when thrombolytic therapy is given to patients with large anterior MIs, people with diabetes mellitus, low blood pressure (systolic <100 mmHg) and/or a tachycardia (heart rate >100 bpm) and people with a previous history of AMI. Patients with inferior MI tend to obtain less benefit, apart from when it is associated with a right ventricular or posterior MI (Ryan et al 1999).

The complications associated with thrombolytic therapy relate largely to bleeding problems, and in particular to haemorrhagic stroke, allergic reactions (with streptokinase) and cardiac arrhythmias. Because of the large number of risks, and in order to reduce the likelihood of complications, there are a large number of contraindications to thrombolytic therapy, against which the patient must be assessed before a decision regarding their suitability for therapy can be made (Table 9.10). In most hospitals, proformas (which include indications for thrombolytic therapy, contraindications and cautions) have been developed to assist MAU nurses and doctors to obtain relevant information and to hasten the assessment process. The aim is to ensure that thrombolytic therapy is commenced within 30 minutes of the patient's arrival at hospital (door-to-needle time). By April 2003, the door-to-needle time target will be reduced to 20 minutes (DoH 2000).

Table 9.10. Contraindications and cautions for immediate thrombolytic therapy (Ryan et al 1999)

Contraindications	Previous stroke within one year, or any previous haemorrhagic stroke
	Known intracranial pathology
	Any active internal bleeding (does not include menstruation)
Cautions or relative contraindications	Hypertension (>180/110 mmHg) on admission or history of severe hypertension
	Previous stroke > one year
	Current use of anticoagulants or known bleeding disorder
	Prolonged cardiopulmonary resuscitation >10 minutes, surgery, trauma or head injury in previous 3 weeks
	Non-compressible puncture
	Recent internal bleeding (2–4 weeks)
	Active peptic ulcer
	Pregnancy

Reperfusion therapy – primary percutaneous transluminal coronary angioplasty (primary PTCA).   Thrombolytic therapy restores blood flow in 60–80% of cases (GUSTO Angiographic Investigators 1993, Cannon et al 1994), although normal blood flow only returns in 30–55% of cases, and in 5–10% reocclusion of the artery occurs. An alternative, and more successful, method of reperfusion is primary PTCA, which leads to a return of normal blood flow in 90–93% of cases (Grines et al 1999), results in greater reductions in mortality from AMI (Zijlstra et al 1999) and reduces risk of ICH (Zijlstra 2001). When PTCA is followed by the implantation of an intracoronary stent, the benefits may be even greater (Grines et al 1999); therefore, primary PTCA and stent may be the optimum reperfusion strategy (Robinson and Timmis 2000).

Only a small number of hospitals in the UK have the facilities to offer a 24-hour PTCA service. If primary PTCA is indicated, the patient may need to be transferred to another hospital before reperfusion therapy can be commenced. This delay may offset some of the benefits of this therapy (Zijlstra 2001). It has been suggested, therefore, that primary PTCA should be reserved for the patients who are at greatest risk, including those with large AMI, diabetes, tachycardia and/or hypotension and patients in whom thrombolytic therapy is contraindicated (Oneil et al 1998). MAU nurses should be aware of the indications for primary PTCA and procedures for transferring patients for this urgent procedure.

Anti-ischaemic therapy.   *Beta-blockers* should be given to all patients who present with AMI to reduce morbidity and mortality (Dana and Walker 1999). They are, however, contraindicated by the presence of asthma, pulmonary oedema, hypotension, bradycardia or heart block. When given early (within 12 hours of the AMI), beta-blockers reduce the workload of the heart by reducing contractility and heart rate. They have an important role in reducing the size of the AMI, the incidence of ischaemic chest pain and ventricular arrhythmias (Ryan et al 1999), and should be continued for at least one year post AMI (DoH 2000).

Angiotensin converting enzyme (ACE) inhibitors should be given to all patients with anterior MI or heart failure (without hypotension) within the first 24 hours of the AMI (Ryan et al 1999), unless contraindicated by the presence of hypotension, renal failure or previous complications with ACE inhibitors (Dana and Walker 1999). ACE inhibitors reduce the incidence of ischaemia and left ventricular dysfunction. Treatment should be reviewed after 4–6 weeks, but may continue indefinitely in patients with symptomatic heart failure (DoH 2000).

4. Early detection/prevention of complications

Patients who are admitted to the MAU with AMI are at risk from a number of life-threatening complications. The MAU nurse must therefore be aware of these complications, and ensure that patients are monitored continuously whilst in the unit, so that any deterioration in the patient's condition can be detected promptly.

Recurrent chest pain (ischaemia or pericarditis). The patient may experience recurrent chest pain, which in the first 12 hours is often related to the original infarction (Ryan et al 1999). Chest pain after 12 hours is usually due to either ischaemia or pericarditis. If the patient experiences additional pain, record an ECG and look for signs of pericarditis (concave upward ST elevation in most leads) or ischaemia (ST elevation or ST depression, inverted T waves becoming upright) (Ryan et al 1999). Assess the patient's chest pain and symptoms. The chest pain of pericarditis is usually pleuritic in nature, made worse by lying down, radiates to the left shoulder and is often accompanied by a pericardial friction rub. Pericarditis is usually successfully treated with a non-steroidal anti-inflammatory drug (NSAID). If the chest pain is similar to the initial pain experienced by the patient and occurs at rest, or on minimal exertion, suspect reinfarction (Ryan et al 1999). Cardiac markers should be repeated and immediate referral made to a cardiologist for urgent coronary angiography.

Cardiac rupture. Rupture of the left ventricular free wall is usually preceded by chest pain, ST and T wave changes on the ECG. It may occur within 24 hours of symptom onset or between 4 and 7 days after AMI and leads rapidly to shock, cardiac tamponade and pulseless electrical activity on the ECG (for treatment see Chapter 5 – Cardiac arrest). Cardiac rupture occurs most commonly in patients with anterior MI, the elderly, women and people who have received late thrombolytic therapy (>14 hours after symptom onset) or NSAIDs (Ryan et al 1999).

Left ventricular failure (LVF) in AMI. The development of LVF after AMI represents a poor prognosis for the patient and usually occurs when a large area of left ventricle has infarcted. If more than 40% of the left ventricle has been damaged, cardiogenic shock may develop. This is associated with a very poor prognosis (see Chapter 6 – Shock). In LVF, reduction in the contractility of the left ventricle causes pressure within the ventricle to rise, and stroke volume and cardiac output to fall. The increased pressure is transmitted to the left atrium and pulmonary veins, leading to the development of pulmonary oedema (Fletcher 1997) (see Chapter 8 – Shortness of breath). Continuous monitoring of BP is essential, as hypotension (systolic BP <90 mmHg) indicates a low cardiac output and cardiogenic shock (see Chapter 6 – Shock). LVF requires treatment with IV furosemide (frusemide) to reduce the amount of blood returning to the heart (preload). IV nitrates (e.g. GTN) promote venodilation and reduce preload. They also promote coronary vasodilation and thus reduce coronary ischaemia. The use of an ACE inhibitor to promote vasodilation (reduce afterload) prevents worsening of left ventricular function, providing there is no evidence of renal dysfunction or hypotension (Ryan et al 1999).

Acute LVF may also occur as a result of mechanical complications such as ventricular septal defect, mitral valve regurgitation, papillary muscle rupture or left ventricular aneurysm. All of these lead to sudden or progressive deterioration in the patient's condition. If the patient is hypotensive and/or pulmonary oedema develops post AMI, urgent referral to a cardiologist is required so that the cause can be identified and appropriate treatment commenced (Ryan et al 1999).

AMI of the right ventricle may lead to right ventricular dysfunction and cardiogenic shock (see Chapter 6 – Shock). Therefore, patients with inferior MI accompanied by hypotension, clear lung fields and raised jugular venous pressure should be treated with 0.5–1.0 litres of 0.9% saline IV to resolve hypotension. If BP does not return to normal, inotropic support with IV dobutamine is required. Drugs that reduce preload and BP (e.g. nitrates and diuretics) must be avoided (Ryan et al 1999).

Cardiac arrhythmias. Disturbances in the cardiac rhythm are very common after AMI and only require treatment if they are life-threatening, cause symptoms or increase the workload of the heart (Thompson 1997b). MAU nurses should be skilled in the recognition and management of the following arrhythmias that commonly accompany AMI.

1. *Atrial fibrillation (AF)*: AF usually occurs in the first 24 hours after AMI and is often a temporary arrhythmia. It is associated with large (anterior) infarcts, acute heart failure and pericarditis and may be exacerbated by factors such as hypokalaemia, hypomagnesaemia and hypoxia (Ryan et al 1999). Patients who develop AF may become symptomatic because of a rapid ventricular rate or because of the loss of atrial contraction. Signs of haemodynamic compromise (e.g.

hypotension, shortness of breath, chest pain) indicate the need for rapid treatment (see Chapter 5 – Cardiac arrest).

2. *Bradycardia*: Sinus bradycardia often accompanies inferior MI and requires treatment with 500 μg atropine IV if the patient develops symptoms such as a heart rate less than 50 bpm, hypotension, chest pain, ventricular escape (late) beats or ventricular ectopic (early) beats (Ryan et al 1999). Profound bradycardia due to a significant pause in electrical activity may occur following successful reperfusion of the right coronary artery (Ryan et al 1999) (see Chapter 5 – Cardiac arrest).

3. *Atrioventricular (AV) block*: This comprises first degree AV block, second degree AV block (Mobitz type I and type II) and third degree AV block (complete heart block or CHB). AV block is associated with a higher mortality as it often occurs as a result of extensive myocardial damage (anterior MI). When AV block occurs following inferior MI, it is usually due to localised AV node ischaemia and often does not require treatment with a temporary pacemaker. AV block accompanying anterior MI is associated with a much poorer prognosis and requires treatment with a temporary pacemaker. In some cases this will need to be followed by a permanent pacemaker (Thompson 1997b) (see Chapter 5 – Cardiac arrest).

Ongoing assessment

The ongoing assessment of the patient with AMI focuses on the need to reduce the workload of the heart and to ensure the effective detection and relief of pain. Whilst in the MAU, ensure that the patient is kept under constant observation. Continuous cardiac monitoring (preferably through a centralised monitoring system) will permit the rapid identification of any change in heart rate or rhythm, and also prompt the recording of a repeat 12-lead ECG if changes in QRS, ST segment and/or T waves are noted. Ensure that the patient has complete bed rest for at least 12 hours. During this time continuously observe the patient for any complications following reperfusion therapy (e.g. bleeding or ICH), life-threatening arrhythmias (e.g. VF/VT, profound bradycardia or AV block), mechanical complications and/or acute heart failure. Be alert to the greater risks associated with certain patient groups such as diabetics, the elderly and those with large or previous infarcts. Assess for signs of haemodynamic compromise by regular BP recording (the frequency depends on the individual patient's condition) and oxygen saturation monitoring. Be aware of the particular needs of the patient's family and ensure that they are included in the plan of care. Arrange for the patient to be transferred to the CCU (or local equivalent) as soon as possible.

Pulmonary embolism (PE)

Causes

In more than 70% of patients, PE is caused by a thrombus, which travels from its site of origin, usually a DVT (British Thoracic Society (BTS) 1997), to the pulmonary vasculature, where it obstructs pulmonary blood flow (Timmis et al 1997). Alternatively the thrombus may originate within the right atrium or may be the result of IV drug misuse or an infected vascular access site (Lea and Zierler 2000). PE may also occur as a result of air, amniotic fluid or fat embolism (Timmis et al 1997), although such causes are rare.

A number of risk factors for the development of DVT and PE have been identified in Chapter 11 (Extremity pain and swelling). Those that indicate the greatest risk of developing PE are listed in Box 9.1. Between 80 and 90% of patients with PE are found to possess one or more risk factors (BTS 1997).

Box 9.1. Major risk factors for the development of PE (BTS 1997)

>7 days immobilisation
History of previous venous thromboembolism
Recent surgery or fractures (especially lower limbs)
Age >40 years
Presence of multiple risk factors
Non-surgical factors:
  cardiorespiratory disease
  lower limb immobility
  malignancy

Pathophysiology

The severity of PE depends upon the degree of the obstruction to pulmonary blood flow. A massive PE occurs when more than 50% of the pulmonary blood flow is obstructed. A minor PE occurs when less than 50% of the pulmonary blood flow is obstructed (Timmis et al 1997). As a result of the obstruction, vasoconstriction and bronchoconstriction occur which lead to a ventilation–perfusion (V/Q) mismatch (see Chapter 8 – Shortness of breath). For adequate gas exchange to occur, ventilation and perfusion must be equal. The reduction in lung perfusion that accompanies PE leads to a reduction in the pO_2 (hypoxaemia) (Lea and Zierler 2000). In order to increase arterial oxygen levels, the respiratory rate increases. This increase causes too much carbon dioxide to be exhaled with the result that pCO_2 falls. The low pCO_2 then stimulates further bronchoconstriction and vasoconstriction, which exacerbates the V/Q mismatch (Lea and Zierler 2000).

A number of haemodynamic changes also occur in massive PE, due to the reduced pulmonary blood flow. Pulmonary artery pressure and right ventricular pressure increase because of the increased work required to overcome the obstruction within the pulmonary vasculature. This will eventually lead to dilatation of the right ventricle followed by right ventricular failure. The reduction in blood flow to the left side of the heart (lowered left ventricular preload) causes cardiac output and, eventually, blood pressure to drop (Lea and Zierler 2000). Minor PE (<50%) does not usually compromise the circulation in this way (Timmis et al 1997).

Presenting features

The features of PE vary considerably. The most common symptoms are listed in Box 9.2. Dyspnoea and tachypnoea occur in almost all cases and are usually accompanied by pleuritic chest pain (BTS 1997).

Box 9.2 Presenting features of PE (BTS 1997)

Dyspnoea
Tachypnoea
Pleuritic pain
Apprehension
Tachycardia
Cough
Haemoptysis
Leg pain
Deep vein thrombosis

Massive PE is a medical emergency and is associated with a high mortality (Riedel 2001a). Early recognition of massive PE (Box 9.3) is essential so that the appropriate management can be commenced promptly (Riedel 2001a).

Patients with PE usually present in one of three ways (BTS 1997) (Box 9.4).

Box 9.3. Symptoms associated with massive PE

Hypotension
Tachycardia
Shock
Chest pain (not usually pleuritic)
Sudden onset of dyspnoea
Tachypnoea
Cyanosis

Box 9.4. Typical presentations of PE

1. **Circulatory collapse (usually due to extensive vascular obstruction):**
    Hypotension and/or loss of consciousness
    Faintness on sitting up
    Central chest tightness
    Signs of right ventricular failure (elevated jugular venous pressure)
    ECG changes (of right ventricular strain)
    Chest X-ray may be normal
    ABGs show marked hypoxaemia and hypocapnia (due to hyperventilation)
2. **Pulmonary haemorrhage (usually due to peripheral pulmonary emboli):**
    Pleuritic pain and/or haemoptysis
    Chest X-ray may show changes at the site of pleuritic pain which resolve rapidly
    ECG often normal
    ABGs may be normal
3. **Isolated dyspnoea (usually due to a central embolus):**
    Acute shortness of breath with no other symptoms
    ABGs show hypoxaemia
    Risk factor(s) for thromboembolism

Initial assessment

The aim of the initial assessment is to identify any features indicative of a massive PE (Box 9.3) and to make a distinction between PE and other medical disorders (e.g. AMI, LVF, pericarditis, dissecting thoracic aortic aneurysm, pneumothorax and pneumonia) (BTS 1997). Assessment should follow the ABCDE framework (Chapter 2 – Initial assessment).

Immediate management and investigations

The immediate management of patients with PE in the MAU involves:

*   effective relief of pain and anxiety
*   provision of supplemental oxygen

- monitoring and maintenance of haemodynamic function
- dissolution of the blood clot (in acute massive PE)
- commencement of anticoagulation
- rapid transfer for appropriate investigations

Position the patient appropriately. If normotensive, help the patient to sit upright to assist breathing. If they are hypotensive (systolic <90 mmHg), the semi-recumbent or recumbent position is preferred. Record the respiratory rate (>20/minute indicates tachypnoea). Observe skin colour for cyanosis and administer 100% oxygen. Monitor oxygen saturation continuously. Obtain ABGs to monitor hypoxaemia and hypocapnia (which occurs due to hyperventilation). Give appropriate IV opiate analgesia to relieve chest pain. As this can cause hypotension and respiratory depression, monitor blood pressure and respiratory rate closely. Given the risk of cardiac arrest associated with massive PE, the patient should be nursed in an area where they can be continuously observed with resuscitation equipment close by.

Continuous cardiac monitoring of heart rate and rhythm is essential. In patients with hypotension, a central venous line should be inserted to monitor right atrial pressure and to allow the administration of IV drugs (Riedel 2001b). A right atrial pressure of 15 mmHg is desirable. This can be maintained by the cautious infusion of 0.9% saline or 5% dextrose so that right ventricular output is maintained (Riedel 2001b). Avoid drugs that cause vasodilation (Riedel 2001b) and would reduce cardiac output further. Small IV doses of noradrenaline may be administered (providing blood pressure, heart rate and rhythm are monitored continuously) to increase blood pressure by inducing vasoconstriction (Riedel 2001b). Take blood to establish the pre-treatment clotting screen including activated partial thromboplastin time (aPTT), prothrombin time, fibrinogen and platelets. Full blood count, urea and electrolytes should be routinely obtained in the critically ill patient.

The patient and their family will be extremely anxious given the presenting features of PE. Ensure that detailed explanations about the nature and purpose of any investigations and treatment are given and that questions are answered openly and honestly.

An algorithm for the treatment of suspected PE is given in Figure 9.4. As previously stated, massive PE is a life-threatening condition with mortality up to 30% in untreated cases (Riedel 2001a). Whilst it is probable that such patients will be transferred to either the intensive care unit (if mechanical ventilation is required) or coronary care unit for invasive monitoring and

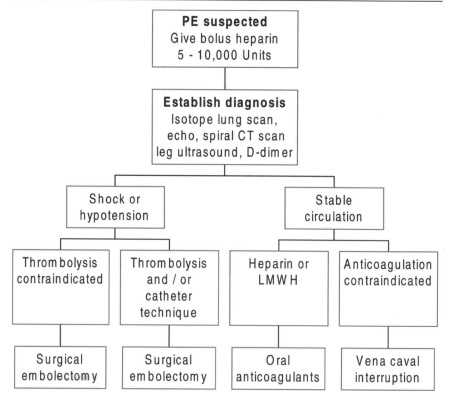

Figure 9.4. Algorithm for the treatment of PE. (Adapted from Riedel M (2001a) Acute pulmonary embolism 2: treatment. Heart 85: 351–60.)

intervention, MAU nurses have an important role in the initial stabilisation and management of these patients.

The exact nature of the investigations performed will depend upon the individual hospital. However, the recommendations of the BTS (1997) should be followed wherever possible and are detailed below.

If massive PE is obvious, contact senior medical staff urgently. Initially, an urgent echocardiogram (echo) may be used to confirm the diagnosis or to exclude other causes. If the echo does not confirm PE, immediate (within one hour) angiography or spiral CT scan is required (BTS 1997). Stable patients should have an isotope lung scan (V/Q) within 24 hours. Such scans are widely available, give an indication of the probability of PE, and should be interpreted in conjunction with clinical symptoms. In addition, plasma D-dimer and leg ultrasound are also recommended to identify the existence of proximal DVT (see Chapter 11 – Extremity pain and swelling).

Other investigations include ABGs, chest X-ray and ECG. The chest X-ray is particularly useful for excluding other possible diagnoses. A normal chest X-ray in an acutely breathless and hypoxic patient is highly indicative of PE (BTS 1997). The 12-lead ECG is important for excluding AMI and pericarditis and should be recorded soon after admission. ECG abnormalities are common with a massive PE due to right-sided heart strain (BTS 1997). Look for non-specific changes in the ST segment and T wave, such as an S wave in lead I, Q wave in lead III and inverted T wave in lead III (Timmis et al 1997). ABGs reveal the degree of hypoxaemia and hypocapnia. Hypoxaemia usually correlates with the degree of obstruction to pulmonary blood flow (BTS 1997).

Drug treatment

The British Thoracic Society guidelines for drug treatment of PE are shown in Table 9.11.

Thrombolytic therapy

Thrombolytic therapy, given either IV or directly into the pulmonary artery, is indicated in patients who have evidence of PE with haemodynamic compromise (hypotension, oliguria or severe hypoxaemia) or PE with a large proximal DVT (Riedel 2001b). Thrombolytic agents including streptokinase, t-PA and urokinase work by actively dissolving blood clots and are effective when given up to 10–14 days after the onset of symptoms of PE (Riedel 2001b). No single drug has yet demonstrated superiority and the choice of drug will depend upon local policy. Heparin should be discontinued before thrombolytic therapy is commenced. Once the obstruction has been removed, pressure on the right ventricle will be reduced and right ventricular failure will resolve. As a result, cardiac output and blood pressure will both increase and the patient's condition will begin to stabilise. As in the treatment of AMI, thrombolytic therapy is contraindicated in patients with active internal bleeding, intracranial haemorrhage, recent surgery or trauma and uncontrolled severe hypertension. The main complication is bleeding, with the risk of major haemorrhage occurring in 10% and cerebral haemorrhage in 0.5–1.5% of patients (Riedel 2001b).

Because of the risk of bleeding after thrombolytic therapy, closely observe blood pressure and heart rate during and after the infusion and also check any venous or arterial puncture sites. Anticoagulation with heparin should be commenced as soon as possible after the completion of

Table 9.11. Drug treatment for PE

Intravenous thrombolysis

	Initial treatment	Further treatment
rt-PA	100 mg in 2 hours	
Streptokinase*	250 000 units in 20 min	100 000 units/hour for 24 hours
Urokinase	4400 IU/kg in 10 min	4400 IU/kg/hour for 12 hours

Before treatment, stop heparin; after treatment, use maintenance dose as below.

Intravenous heparin

	Initial dose	Maintenance dose
Standard	5000–10 000 IU	1300 IU/hour
Weight-adjusted	80 IU/kg	18 IU/kg/hour

Adjust infusion rate until aPTT is 1.5–2.5 × control (45–75 seconds)

aPTT monitoring	After initial bolus	4–6 hours later
	After any dose change	6–10 hours later
	aPTT in therapeutic range	Daily

Discontinue heparin 5 days after starting warfarin if INR at least 2.0.

Warfarin

Initial doses	5–10 mg daily for 2 days
Subsequent treatment	1–10 mg daily

Adjust dose to INR = 2–3 × control, initial measured every 1–2 days

*Plus hydrocortisone to prevent further circulatory instability.
Reproduced with permission from the British Thoracic Society Standards of Care
Committee (1997). Suspected acute pulmonary embolism – a practical approach Thorax 52:
Supplement 4.

thrombolytic therapy. Measurement of fibrinogen and aPTT will dictate the point at which heparin can be started safely. This is usually when aPTT is greater than twice the upper limit of normal or fibrinogen <1 g/l. Measurements should be repeated every 4 hours until this point is reached (Riedel 2001b).

Heparin

Unfractionated heparin is the standard treatment for all cases of PE and should be continued after thrombolytic therapy. Heparin, which should be given IV for at least 7 days in cases of major PE, has been shown to reduce mortality and morbidity from PE by preventing the redevelopment of the thrombus, the development of new thrombi and subsequent recurrence of PE (Riedel 2001b). To be effective, heparin must be maintained at a therapeutic level (aPTT 1.5–2.5 times the patient's pre-treatment level or the laboratory control level).

Unfractionated heparin is best given via continuous IV infusion so that fluctuations in plasma heparin concentration are avoided and therapeutic levels are maintained in the optimum range. Measure aPTT 4–6 hours after commencing heparin and 6 hours after any change in heparin dosage. In most MAUs, a heparin regime will specify the amount required for any given aPTT. If the aPTT is not maintained within the desired range, the patient will be at risk of further thromboembolism (Riedel 2001b). Heparin is associated with complications (e.g. haemorrhage and thrombocytopenia) although the former is more likely to occur in patients with a pre-existing bleeding disorder or risk factor (Riedel 2001b).

Low molecular weight heparin (LMWH) may become an alternative to unfractionated heparin in the treatment of PE. At the present time, there is insufficient evidence to recommend its routine use, especially in the case of massive PE (Riedel 2001b).

Oral anticoagulation

Warfarin should be started in conjunction with heparin therapy, and the two treatments should be given together for at least 5 days before heparin is discontinued. It is essential that a therapeutic dose of warfarin is administered. This is determined by the international normalised ratio (INR), which is a measure of the prothrombin time. The aim should be to maintain the INR within the range 2.0–3.0.

Other treatment

Surgical pulmonary embolectomy is indicated when other treatments have failed and where death is almost certain. It may also be indicated in patients with acute massive PE where thrombolytic therapy is contraindicated or has not worked effectively (Riedel 2001b).

Catheter embolectomy is an alternative to surgical embolectomy in patients with massive PE who are able to maintain a BP (Riedel 2001b).

Venous interruption procedures, such as the implantation of a filter within the inferior vena cava to prevent emboli getting to the pulmonary vasculature, have been used in patients in whom anticoagulation has failed or is contraindicated (Riedel 2001b).

Other common causes of non-cardiac chest pain

For the majority of patients who are admitted to the MAU with chest pain, the cause will be non-cardiac, often due to a non-life threatening respiratory, gastrointestinal, musculoskeletal or anxiety-related cause (Chambers et al 1999). MAU nurses need to be able to distinguish between different causes of chest pain, in a patient group that will include people with co-existing CHD and people with more than one non-cardiac cause for their pain (Chambers et al 1999). This assessment is particularly difficult in patients who are very anxious, patients who are perceived to be at high risk of CHD or patients with an abnormal ECG (Dowling 1997). Patients with chest pain should have a thorough assessment of their pain and symptoms utilising the PQRST principles. The assessment of all patients who present with chest pain should comprise an assessment of risk factors for CHD so that patients at risk can be identified and referred to appropriate personnel for further evaluation. The most common causes of non-cardiac chest pain are detailed in Table 9.12.

Summary

This chapter has considered in detail the initial assessment and management of patients who present to the MAU with chest pain. Chest pain is a common complaint, which usually arises because of a disorder of the cardiac, respiratory, musculoskeletal or gastrointestinal systems or may be related to a psychological disorder. MAU nurses require skill in differentiating between the different life-threatening causes of chest pain and this chapter has provided a detailed guide to that assessment. The management of patients with the most common, life-threatening disorders has been discussed in detail and the reader is encouraged to refer to the recommended further reading at the end of the chapter for information on the continuing management of such patients (beyond their first 24 hours in hospital).

Table 9.12. Evaluation of non-cardiac chest pain in the MAU (Becker 2000, Chambers et al 1999, Dowling 1997)

Source of chest pain	Assessment of chest pain	Associated features	Assessment and investigations	Initial treatment for chest pain
Respiratory: Pneumonia	Pleuritic chest pain, worse on deep inspiration Induced by coughing	Fever, sputum, dyspnoea, cough	Temperature, pulse, respiratory rate Chest X-ray Sputum culture	Simple oral analgesia Steam inhalation
Pneumothorax	Pleuritic chest pain	Sudden onset of dyspnoea Signs of tension pneumothorax (see Chapter 5 – Cardiac arrest)	Chest X-ray and examination ABGs	Simple oral analgesia
Musculoskeletal:	Brief duration (<1 minute) to constant pain lasting days Precipitated by abrupt movement or application of pressure to the chest wall Induced by exercise and subsides slowly	History of recent strenuous activity	Physical examination History	Simple oral analgesia Non-steroidal anti-inflammatory drug (NSAID) Heat
Costochondritis	Sharp, pleuritic pain localised to costochondral or costosternal junctions	Localised swelling		
Cervical and upper thoracic osteoarthritis	Chest pain worse when bending or moving, coughing or sneezing. Pain can be traced to an initiating event	Numbness, tingling, weakness, stiffness, vertigo, paraesthesia		
Gastrointestinal: Oesophageal	Chest pain typically described as heartburn, warmth, fullness, pressure, gnawing Provoked by food, especially hot or cold food, large meals or eating after moving from a recumbent position Pain usually substernal, may extend to the left or right of the chest and the jaw Pain lasts for hours, disturbs sleep and is precipitated by swallowing, exercise and/or emotion Often relieved by GTN (though not quickly)	Dysphagia, oesophageal reflux, belching, regurgitation of stomach contents, epigastric pain	History Endoscopy	Antacid H2 antagonist Proton pump inhibitor
Psychological causes: Anxiety	Pain in infra-mammary region, near to the apex of the heart Pain dull and aching or sharp and stabbing Pain lasts seconds to hours Not caused by exertion Related to emotional strain	Numbness, dizziness, light-headedness, weakness, headache, palpitations, depression, fatigue Hyperventilation, shortness of breath Panic attack	Ask about panic attacks History of unexplained medical symptoms History of recent upsetting events	Investigation Reassurance Provide positive explanation about cause of pain

References

Anderson H, Falk E, Nielsen D (1987) Right ventricular infarction: frequency, size and topography in coronary heart disease: a prospective study comprising 107 consecutive autopsies from a coronary care unit. Journal of the American College of Cardiology 10: 1223–32.

Becker R (2000) Chest Pain. Boston: Butterworth Heinemann.

Blatchford O, Capewell S (1999) Emergency medical admissions in Glasgow: general practices vary despite adjustments for age, sex and deprivation. British Journal of General Practice 49: 551–4.

British Heart Foundation (BHF) (2000) Coronary Heart Disease Statistics. London: BHF.

British Medical Association and the Royal Pharmaceutical Society of Great Britain (2000) British National Formulary. London: BMJ Books and Pharmaceutical Press.

British Thoracic Society (1997) Suspected acute pulmonary embolism: a practical approach. Thorax 52 (Supplement 4).

Campbell R (1994) Arrhythmias. In Julian D, Braunwald E (eds) Management of Acute Myocardial Infarction. London: WB Saunders.

Campbell R, Murray A, Julian D (1981) Ventricular arrhythmias in first 12 hours of acute myocardial infarction: natural history study. British Heart Journal 46: 351–7.

Cannon C, McCabe C, Diver D et al (1994) Comparison of front-loaded recombinant tissue-type plasminogen activator, anistreplase and combination thrombolytic therapy for acute myocardial infarction: results of the TIMI 4 trial. Journal of the American College of Cardiology 24: 1602–10.

Chambers J, Bass C, Mayou R (1999) Non-cardiac chest pain: assessment and management. Heart 82: 656–7.

Dana A, Walker M (1999) Acute myocardial infarction: extended review. Journal of the Royal College of Physicians of London 33(2): 131–40.

Del Bene S, Vaughan A (2000) Diagnosis and management of myocardial infarction. In Woods S, Froelicher E, Motzer S (eds) Cardiac Nursing, 4th edn. Philadelphia: Lippincott.

Department of Health (2000) National Service Framework for Coronary Heart Disease. London: DoH.

Dowling J (1997) Other causes of chest pain. In Thompson P (ed) Coronary Care Manual. London: Churchill Livingstone.

Fibrinolytic Therapy Trialists (FTT) Collaborative Group (1994) Indications for fibrinolytic therapy in suspected acute myocardial infarction: collaborative overview of early mortality and major morbidity results from all randomised trials of more than 1000 patients. Lancet 343: 311–22.

Fletcher P (1997) Pathophysiology of myocardial infarction. In Thompson P (ed) Coronary Care Manual. London: Churchill Livingstone.

Fox K (2000) Acute coronary syndromes: presentation – clinical spectrum and management. Heart 84: 93–100.

Gibler W, Lewis L, Erb R et al (1990) Early detection of acute myocardial infarction in patients presenting with chest pain and nondiagnostic ECGs: serial CKMB sampling in the emergency department. Annals of Emergency Medicine 19: 1359–66.

Grines C, Cox D, Stone G et al (1999) Coronary angioplasty with or without stent implantation for acute myocardial infarction. New England Journal of Medicine 341:1949–56.

GUSTO Angiographic Investigators (1993) The comparative effects of tissue plasminogen activator, streptokinase, or both on coronary artery patency, ventricular function and survival after acute myocardial infarction. New England Journal of Medicine 329: 1615–22.

Higham P, Adams P, Murray A et al (1993) Plasma potassium, serum magnesium and ventricular fibrillation: a prospective study. Quarterly Journal of Medicine 86: 609–17.

Hillis G, Fox K (1999) Cardiac troponins in chest pain. British Medical Journal 319: 1451–2.

ISIS-2 (Second International Study of Infarct Survival) Collaborative Group (1988) Randomised trial of intravenous streptokinase, oral aspirin, both, or neither among 17,187 cases of suspected acute myocardial infarction. Lancet ii: 349–60.

Lea H, Zierler B (2000) Hematopoiesis and coagulation. In Woods S, Froelicher E, Motzer S (eds) Cardiac Nursing, 4th edn. Philadelphia: Lippincott.

Madias J, Hood W Jr (1976) Reduction of precordial ST-segment elevation in patients with anterior myocardial infarction by oxygen breathing. Circulation 53 (Supplement 1): 198–200.

Maroko P, Radvany P, Braunwald E et al (1975) Reduction of infarct size by oxygen inhalation following acute coronary occlusion. Circulation 52: 360–8.

Norderhaug J, von der Lippe G (1983) Hypokalaemia and ventricular fibrillation in acute myocardial infarction. British Heart Journal 50: 525–9.

Norris R (2000) The natural history of acute myocardial infarction. Heart 83: 726–30.

Oneil W, de Boer M, Gibbons R et al (1998) Lessons from the pooled outcome of the Pami, Zwolle and Mayo clinic randomised trials of primary angioplasty vs thrombolytic therapy of acute myocardial infarction. Journal of Invasive Cardiology 10: 4A–10A.

Riedel M (2001a) Acute pulmonary embolism 2: treatment. Heart 85: 351–60.

Riedel M (2001b) Emergency diagnosis of pulmonary embolism Heart 85: 607–9.

Robalino B, Whitlow P, Underwood D et al (1989) Electrocardiographic manifestations of right ventricular infarction. American Heart Journal 118: 138–44.

Robinson N, Timmis A (2000) Reperfusion in acute myocardial infarction. British Medical Journal 320: 1354–5.

Roux S, Christeller S, Ludin E (1992) Effects of aspirin on coronary reocclusion and recurrent ischaemia after thrombolysis: a meta-analysis. Journal of the American College of Cardiology 19: 671–7.

Ryan T et al on behalf of the Committee on Management of Acute Myocardial Infarction (1999) 1999 update: American College of Cardiology/American Heart Association guidelines for the management of patients with acute myocardial infarction. Journal of the American College of Cardiology 34: 890–911.

Thompson P (1997a) Patient history. In Thompson P (ed) Coronary Care Manual. London: Churchill Livingstone.

Thompson P (1997b) AMI: management of cardiac arrhythmias. In Thompson P (ed) Coronary Care Manual. London: Churchill Livingstone.

Thompson P, Ilton M (1997) Electrocardiography. In Thompson P (ed) Coronary Care Manual. London: Churchill Livingstone.

Thompson P, Morgan J (1997) AMI: emergency department care. In Thompson P (ed) Coronary Care Manual. London: Churchill Livingstone.

Timmis A, Nathan A, Sullivan I (1997) Essential Cardiology, 3rd edn. Oxford: Blackwell.

Volpi A, Cavalli A, Santoro E et al (1990) Incidence and prognosis of secondary ventricular fibrillation in acute myocardial infarction: evidence for a protective effect of thrombolytic therapy. Circulation 82: 1279–88.

Weissberg P (2000) Atherogenesis: current understanding of the causes of atheroma. Heart 83: 247–52.

Wooding Baker M (2000) Laboratory tests using blood. In Woods S, Froelicher E, Motzer S (eds) Cardiac Nursing, 4th edn. Philadelphia: Lippincott.

Zehender M, Kasper W, Kauder E et al (1993) Right ventricular infarction as an independent predictor of prognosis after acute inferior myocardial infarction. New England Journal of Medicine 328: 981–8.

Zijlstra F (2001) Acute myocardial infarction: primary angioplasty. Heart 85: 705–9.

Zijlstra F, Hoorntje C, de Boer M et al (1999) Long-term benefit of primary angioplasty as compared with thrombolytic therapy for acute myocardial infarction. New England Journal of Medicine 341: 1413–19.

Further reading

Becker R (2000) Chest Pain. Boston: Butterworth Heinemann.

British Thoracic Society (1997) Suspected acute pulmonary embolism: a practical approach Thorax 52 (Supplement 4).

Department of Health (2000) National Service Framework for Coronary Heart Disease. London: DoH.

Ryan T et al on behalf of the Committee on Management of Acute Myocardial Infarction (1999) 1999 update: American College of Cardiology/American Heart Association guidelines for the management of patients with acute myocardial infarction. Journal of the American College of Cardiology 34: 890–911.

Thompson P (ed) (1997) Coronary Care Manual. London: Churchill Livingstone.

Woods S, Froelicher E, Motzer S (eds) (2000) Cardiac Nursing, 4th edn. Philadelphia: Lippincott.

CHAPTER 10

Abdominal pain and upper gastrointestinal bleeding

RUTH HARRIS AND TERRY WARDLE

Aims

This chapter will:

- provide a framework for the accurate assessment of the acutely ill medical patient with abdominal pain and/or upper gastrointestinal (GI) bleeding
- describe the investigations and initial management associated with these patients in the MAU
- describe the specific management of three of the most common conditions (acute upper GI bleeding, acute gastroenteritis and inflammatory bowel disease)
- provide brief details of the less common conditions referred to the MAU

Clinical features

Patients referred to an MAU with abdominal pain and/or upper GI bleeding may present with a variety of clinical features (Box 10.1). Some of these features are specific to GI disorders whilst others are common to a range of conditions. It is important for the MAU nurse to recognise this and for an effective assessment to be conducted to exclude underlying conditions.

Initial assessment

The initial assessment of the patient referred to MAU with abdominal pain and/or upper GI bleeding can be divided into primary and secondary

---

**Box 10.1. Common presenting features associated with abdominal pain
and/or gastrointestinal bleeding**

Haematemesis
Melaena
Vomiting
Tachypnoea
Tachycardia
Diarrhoea
Hypotension
Constipation
Weight loss
Anorexia
Dysphagia
Dysuria/frequency
Pyrexia

---

assessments. In the primary assessment life-threatening conditions are identified and treated whilst in the secondary assessment, a detailed history and thorough examination is completed. During these assessments, investigations may be requested and necessary treatment instigated. Following completion of the secondary assessment, further investigations can be arranged and additional treatment established.

MAU nursing priorities in respect of these patients mirror the priorities set out above. In addition, MAU nurses have an important role in giving psychological support to the patient and their family. In this respect, it is important to preserve the patient's dignity given that they may exhibit repeated vomiting and/or require frequent use of toileting facilities. In high activity settings such as MAUs, it is easy to forget the simple necessities required by patients such as hand-washing facilities and oral hygiene.

Primary assessment

The aim of the primary assessment is to identify and treat the patient presenting with a life-threatening cause of acute abdominal pain or upper GI haemorrhage.

Box 10.2 lists the life-threatening conditions that may be present in the patient with abdominal pain.

The components of the primary ABCDE assessment are outlined in Chapter 2 (Initial assessment). However, the following issues pertinent to abdominal pain and upper GI bleeding should be emphasised.

Box 10.2. Life-threatening conditions associated with abdominal pain

Acute pancreatitis
Gastrointestinal haemorrhage
Septicaemia (e.g. following perforation of colon) (see Chapter 6 – Shock)
Leaking abdominal aortic aneurysm
Acute myocardial infarction (see Chapter 9 – Chest pain)
Diabetic ketoacidosis (see Chapter 7 – Altered consciousness)
Small bowel infarction (mesenteric artery occlusion)
Ectopic pregnancy
Splenic rupture (may occur weeks after trauma)

Airway

The airway is at risk in any patient who has haematemesis or vomiting. This risk is increased in those who have a reduced level of consciousness. Endotracheal intubation should be considered in all patients with a reduced level of consciousness who are unable to protect their own airway (Glasgow Coma Score ($\leq 8/15$). Pass a large bore nasogastric tube to drain fluid and air from the stomach and to reduce the risk of aspiration in patients suspected of having gastric outflow obstruction or small bowel obstruction.

Breathing

A patient with severe abdominal pain may exhibit dyspnoea because of splinting of chest movement. Likewise, pain can cause tachypnoea from activation of the sympathetic nervous system. Cardiorespiratory conditions in which dyspnoea is common may present with abdominal pain (e.g. acute myocardial infarction, pneumonia) or may co-exist (e.g. chronic obstructive pulmonary disease). Kussmaul's respiration (i.e. deep sighing breathing) occurs in metabolic acidosis (e.g. diabetic ketoacidosis which can present with abdominal pain).

Circulation

Circulatory assessment in patients with abdominal pain and, in particular, where there is evidence of upper GI bleeding, is important in order to establish or exclude signs of hypovolaemia. In patients presenting with abdominal pain, circulatory collapse (shock) may occur as a result of a critical reduction in cardiac preload or afterload or both:

- preload reduction occurs in hypovolaemia. The cause of hypovolaemia may be overt (e.g. haematemesis, diarrhoea) or covert (e.g. intra-abdominal haemorrhage from a leaking aortic aneurysm).
- afterload reduction occurs with vasodilatation (e.g. in sepsis).

The treatment of shock needs to be tailored to the most likely cause. However, if the cause is not clear, treat both preload and afterload. The treatment of shock is outlined in Chapter 6 but, in addition, consider the following measures for patients with abdominal pain and/or upper GI bleeding. Through a 14G cannula, before commencing fluids, take blood for:

- full blood count (FBC) – a raised white cell count is commonly found in this group of patients but does not necessarily mean an infective cause of the abdominal pain (e.g. patients with diabetic ketoacidosis often complain of abdominal pain and have a neutrophil leucocytosis in the absence of infection)
- urea, electrolytes and creatinine – electrolyte disturbance and renal failure may occur secondary to diarrhoea and/or vomiting
- glucose – hypoglycaemia can mimic shock. If not already done, do a rapid stick test (e.g. BM stix) in addition to sending a sample to the laboratory
- amylase – a normal amylase does not exclude acute pancreatitis and a raised amylase may occur in a variety of other conditions including cholecystitis, perforated peptic ulcer and diabetic ketoacidosis
- blood group +/– cross-match
- clotting studies if the patient is taking anticoagulants, if coagulopathy is suspected or if liver disease is suspected
- liver function tests (LFTs) – in all patients who are jaundiced or if liver/biliary disease is suspected
- calcium – symptoms of hypercalcaemia include abdominal pain, vomiting and constipation
- blood cultures – if patient is pyrexial or sepsis is suspected
- a sickle cell screen for patients of Afro-Caribbean descent

Although the results of some of these investigations may not affect immediate management, it saves time to obtain all the blood investigations together.

Hypovolaemia resulting from bleeding (e.g. from the GI tract or from an aneurysm) requires replacement with blood. Whilst waiting for blood, 2 litres of warm crystalloid can be given intravenously (IV). If there is no improvement in haemodynamic status following this, 'O' negative blood should be given until cross-matched blood is available. The aim of fluid resuscitation is to maintain a systolic blood pressure of approximately 100 mmHg (i.e. 'controlled hypotension'). Blood pressure at higher levels may encourage continued bleeding by disturbing clots that have formed in conditions such as bleeding oesophageal varices or leaking aortic aneurysm.

If septic shock is suspected, consider:

- a broad-spectrum antibiotic initially (e.g. cefotaxime 1 g twice daily (up to 12 g daily in 3–4 divided doses)) and alter appropriately when the results of cultures are known
- IV fluids
- inotropes. In sepsis, peripheral vasodilatation results in reduced systemic vascular resistance and, if hypotension remains despite adequate fluid replacement, a vasoconstrictor such as noradrenaline (norepinephrine) may be required. This is given by IV infusion via a central venous catheter and the dose adjusted according to response. Side effects include hypertension, arrhythmias and peripheral ischaemia.

Consider calling the surgical team. Indications for referral to the surgical team include, but are not limited to, suspected:

- peritonitis (generalised or local)
- bowel obstruction
- pancreatitis
- leaking abdominal aortic aneurysm
- bowel infarction or ischaemia
- upper GI bleeding in a high-risk patient (Box 10.3)
- lower GI bleeding

In the majority of medical patients presenting with abdominal pain and/or upper GI bleeding, it is likely that the primary assessment will be completed within minutes.

Box 10.4 lists some of the many conditions that can present with abdominal pain. As soon as any immediately life-threatening conditions

---

Box 10.3. High-risk patients with upper GI bleeding (from Travis et al 1998)

High-risk patients are patients with three or more of the following criteria:

- Age >60 years
- Fresh haematemesis with melaena – twice the mortality of either alone
- Non-steroidal anti-inflammatory drug (NSAID) intake
- Continued bleeding, or a rebleed in hospital
- Heart failure
- Chronic airflow limitation
- Chronic liver disease
- Onset of bleeding in a patient already in hospital for another reason
- Pulse >100 bpm – suggests the need for transfusion
- Systolic BP <100 mmHg – but it may be preserved until very late in young patients
- Postural drop in systolic BP >15 mmHg on sitting up
- Endoscopic stigmata present. These are:
  active arterial bleeding (80% risk of rebleed)
  visible vessel in the ulcer bare (50% risk of rebleed)
  fresh adherent clot or oozing (30% risk of rebleed) or
  black dots on the ulcer base (5% risk of rebleed)
- Endoscopic evidence of oesophageal varices or portal hypertensive gastropathy

---

have been treated or excluded and the patient's vital signs stabilised, a relevant history should be obtained and an appropriate examination completed.

Secondary assessment

The aim of the secondary assessment is to identify all conditions not detected in the primary assessment. This is achieved by seeking corroborative evidence for a provisional diagnosis through the history of the presenting complaint and physical examination. Following the secondary assessment, further investigations may be requested and an appropriate initial management plan established.

History

Obtaining a clear history, particularly of the presenting problem, is extremely important. If the patient is not able to give this, gather a collaborative history from relatives or carers, the patient's general practitioner and/or ambulance personnel. In addition to the elements of history taking outlined in Chapter 2, the following approach can be used. Box 10.5 indicates the elements of a medical history.

Box 10.4. Conditions that can present with acute abdominal pain and/or upper GI bleeding that are not necessarily immediately life-threatening

Intra-abdominal conditions:
Gastroenteritis
Acute appendicitis
Acute cholecystitis, gall bladder and biliary tract disease
Peptic ulcer disease
Intestinal obstruction
Pseudo-obstruction
Acute pancreatitis
Perforated viscus
Neoplastic disease
Diverticular disease
Infarction of bowel or spleen
Inflammatory bowel disease
Primary infective peritonitis

Urological conditions:
Lower urinary tract infection/pyelonephritis
Ureteric/renal colic
Acute urinary retention
Testicular torsion

Gynaecological and obstetric conditions:
Miscarriage
Pelvic inflammatory disease
Ovarian disease: ovarian torsion, haemorrhage into an ovarian cyst
Ectopic pregnancy
Retained products of conception
Labour
Abruption of placenta

Toxins/poisoning:
Certain foods
Alcohol
Iron
Lead
Aspirin

Cardiorespiratory conditions:
Myocardial infarction
Basal pneumonia
Pulmonary embolus

Other conditions:
Diabetic ketoacidosis
Sickle cell crisis
Addisonian crisis
Hypercalcaemia
Herpes zoster

Non-specific abdominal pain

Box 10.5. Essential elements of a medical history

Pain assessment
Presenting features
Past medical and surgical history
Medications/drugs
Allergies
Family history
Social history
Review of body systems

It is important with this group of presenting complaints to assess the patient's pain effectively. In this respect, the PQRST mnemonic can be used to collect the following information regarding the patient's pain. Other pain measurement tools can be used to supplement this assessment.

Pain assessment

Provoking/relieving factors

A patient with peritonitis will find movement, coughing and deep inspiration painful. Vomiting may provide transient relief of pain in small intestinal obstruction.

Quality (duration and character)

Pain can be constant and steady (e.g. in bowel infarction) or intermittent (e.g. gastroenteritis). An obstructed viscus usually results in colicky pain (present all the time but with fluctuating intensity). Patients often find it difficult to describe the character of pain and different terms can mean different things to different people. However, sharp pain usually indicates somatic pain. Visceral pain is more likely to be described as a dull ache.

Radiation

Abdominal pain may radiate to the patient's back (e.g. pain from a leaking abdominal aortic aneurysm). Upper abdominal pain radiating to the back is suggestive of pancreatitis. Hypogastric pain radiating to the patient's back and thighs suggests large bowel pathology.

Site and severity (Figure 10.1)

An ill-defined site suggests visceral pain early in a disease process or a metabolic, toxic or psychological cause. Migration of pain is characteristic of an inflamed viscus. Examples of this would be migration from the peri-umbilical region to the right iliac fossa in acute appendicitis or from the epigastrium to the right hypochondrium in cholecystitis.

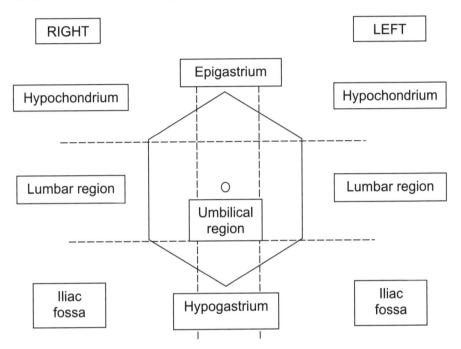

Figure 10.1. Areas of the abdomen.

Time and treatment

Sudden onset of severe pain is characteristic of a vascular problem (e.g. leaking abdominal aortic aneurysm). Pain from pancreatitis may develop relatively rapidly, but over minutes rather than seconds. Diverticulitis or appendicitis tend to progress more slowly over hours or days.

In addition to assessment of abdominal pain, it is important to gather information regarding other associated clinical features.

Presenting features

Haematemesis (vomiting of blood)

Haematemesis is a feature of peptic ulcer disease. Vomiting a small amount of bright red blood after repeated retching is suggestive of a Mallory–Weiss tear. Copious amounts of haematemesis often occur in oesophageal variceal haemorrhage, which is the cause of upper GI haemorrhage in <5% of cases (Travis et al 1998). A brown fluid ('coffee ground') vomit without any other symptoms or signs is unlikely to be due to a significant GI bleed.

Melaena (passage of black, tarry stool per rectum)

Melaena is altered blood and this implies bleeding proximal to the splenic flexure of the colon. Ingestion of iron supplements, which may have been obtained 'over the counter', often results in black stool.

Vomiting

Faeculent vomiting indicates intestinal obstruction.

Diarrhoea

Blood-stained or mucus-stained diarrhoea can occur in inflammatory bowel disease, ischaemic bowel, malignancy or certain infections (e.g. *Campylobacter, Shigella, Salmonella, E. coli* and amoebiasis) (Hope et al 1998).

Constipation

Absolute constipation with abdominal pain and vomiting is indicative of intestinal obstruction.

Weight loss with anorexia

This commonly occurs in the presence of malignant disease.

Dysphagia

Preceding dysphagia may indicate an underlying oesophageal malignancy.

Trauma

Splenic rupture characterised by shock, left shoulder tip pain with abdominal tenderness and distension may occur weeks after blunt abdominal trauma.

Past medical and surgical history

Ask the patient if they have had any episodes similar to their present problem. In addition, ask about the results of investigations undertaken, treatment prescribed and their outcome. Collect details of any previous abdominal surgery and other conditions such as:

* diabetes mellitus
* cardiovascular disease
* cerebrovascular disease
* respiratory conditions
* infections (e.g. tuberculosis)
* psychiatric illness

Medications

Record details of all the patient's medications, including the dose and dosing schedule. Ask about and record the patient's use of 'over the counter' medications.

The use of NSAIDs (including aspirin) and warfarin should be specifically asked about in patients presenting with upper GI bleeding. Previous treatment with glucocorticoids is particularly important to note as the clinical and laboratory responses to inflammation or perforation of an abdominal viscus may be masked. Also, patients who have been taking long-term glucocorticoids may have adrenal suppression and, on admission, the dose of glucocorticoids should be at least doubled, to mimic the usual stress response to acute illness.

Allergies

Note any adverse reactions/allergies to medications, topical antiseptics and cleansing agents (e.g. iodine) or wound dressings.

Family history

Ask the patient if any of their family have GI disorders (e.g. inflammatory bowel disease, carcinoma) or any relevant inherited conditions (e.g. sickle cell disease, acute intermittent porphyria).

Social history

Social history in respect of abdominal pain should specifically include details of smoking habits, detailed alcohol history and contact with other people with similar symptoms.

Review of body systems

Particular attention should be paid to the following systems.

Respiratory system

A recent cough productive of purulent sputum could indicate a basal pneumonia that might be presenting as abdominal pain. Any history of haemoptysis needs further investigation in its own right. However, the combination of upper abdominal pain and haemoptysis might occur in a pulmonary embolus.

Cardiovascular system

Preceding chest pain on exertion could suggest that the patient's upper abdominal pain is resulting from an inferior myocardial infarction.

Urinary system

Dysuria and frequency of micturition may suggest a urological cause for the abdominal pain, but remember that an inflamed appendix or a colonic diverticulum abutting the ureter or bladder can cause urinary symptoms.

From women, obtain a gynaecological history including details of menstrual pattern and contraception.

Physical examination

Medical colleagues will usually conduct a physical examination of patients presenting with abdominal pain and/or upper GI bleeding. However, in the future, consultant nurses and advanced practitioners may undertake some of these roles. The physical examination comprises general observation, inspection, palpation, percussion and auscultation.

General observation

Patients with visceral pain (e.g. ureteric colic) tend to roll around in the bed whilst patients with generalised peritonitis tend to lie still and have rapid, shallow respiration. Whilst looking at the patient's face, ask the patient to cough. An observation of abdominal pain, flinching or a protective movement of hands towards the abdomen suggests peritonitis.

Inspection

Asking the patient to take a deep breath may reveal organomegaly or masses in the abdomen. Inspect the mouth for telangiectasia (permanent dilatation of groups of superficial blood vessels), peri-oral pigmentation and pigmentation on the buccal mucosa (Addison's disease). Inspect the sclera for signs of jaundice and the conjunctiva of the lower eyelid for pallor that may indicate anaemia. Box 10.6 gives details of the characteristic signs of chronic liver disease.

Box 10.6. Characteristic features of chronic liver disease

- Palmar erythema
- Dupuytren's contracture
- Leuconychia (white finger nails)
- Clubbing of the finger nails
- Spider naevi
- Abnormal veins around the umbilicus (in portal hypertension the direction of flow of these veins below the umbilicus is down, dilated veins can also occur around the umbilicus in inferior vena caval obstruction where the direction of flow below the umbilicus is upwards)
- Loss of body hair
- Gynaecomastia
- Testicular atrophy
- Ascites
- Signs of encephalopathy (e.g. flapping tremor, apparent when hands dorsiflexed on outstretched arms)

The clinical features outlined in Box 10.7 may also be observed in relation to their respective disorders.

Palpation

It is important that the examiner's hands should be warm for the patient's comfort. Furthermore, cold hands might cause the patient to flinch or grimace and thereby make it difficult to assess areas for tenderness.

Box 10.7. Presenting features associated with their respective disorders

- Pigmentation of Addison's disease may also be seen in scars and the creases of the palm
- Visible pulsation of an abdominal aortic aneurysm may be seen
- Visible peristalsis implies bowel obstruction
- An everted umbilicus occurs with gross ascites
- Bluish discoloration around the umbilicus (Cullen's sign) can occur when blood is in the peritoneal cavity (e.g. in acute pancreatitis or ruptured ectopic pregnancy)
- Discoloration in the flanks (Grey Turner's sign) is occasionally seen in haemorrhagic pancreatitis and in other causes of retroperitoneal haemorrhage (e.g. leaking abdominal aortic aneurysm)
- Erythema nodosum (painful, red nodular lesions on the anterior shins, thighs or forearms) is associated with inflammatory bowel disease
- Hernial orifices should be carefully examined. A small, incarcerated femoral hernia can be missed easily
- Look for lymphadenopathy. Virchow's node is an enlarged left supraclavicular lymph node associated with cancer of the stomach. Troisier's sign describes enlargement of left supraclavicular nodes due to carcinomatous deposits from carcinoma of stomach or lung

---

To examine the patient's abdomen, the examiner should either kneel or sit. In either of these positions, the examining hand is more relaxed and in more contact with the patient than if the examiner is standing. Therefore, more information can be obtained. Examination should start in an area away from pain.

Palpate each area sequentially whilst looking at patient's face for any evidence of pain, tenderness or guarding (tensing of abdominal muscles because of pain or fear of it). Localised tenderness suggests an inflammatory source of the patient's pain. Rebound tenderness (pain is greater when removing hand pressure) is a sign of local peritoneal inflammation, but if this becomes generalised, rigidity will occur.

Feel for organomegaly and masses. A central, pulsatile mass is likely to be an aortic aneurysm, but this will not be felt if the aneurysm has ruptured. Dry skin with reduced skin turgor implies chronic dehydration due to extracellular fluid loss, which can occur in gastroenteritis or intestinal obstruction.

Percussion

Shifting dullness and a fluid thrill imply the presence of ascites.

Auscultation

Bowel sounds are high-pitched in obstruction and absent when there is a perforated viscus with peritonitis. It is important to realise that bowel sounds may be normal even in cases of serious intra-abdominal pathology.

Concluding the physical examination

The physical examination is usually concluded by the doctor performing a digital rectal examination. This is mandatory for patients who present with abdominal pain and/or GI bleeding. Any peri-anal disease (which may indicate Crohn's disease), the colour of the stool and presence of blood and/or mucus should be noted. The finding of melaena on digital rectal examination confirms a GI bleed proximal to the splenic flexure.

Elderly patients

In comparison with younger patients, fever, tachycardia and leucocytosis are less common in inflammatory conditions such as appendicitis. Pain tends to be less predominant and delayed presentation is more common. The presence of co-existent conditions is likely to lead to a variety of symptoms and signs.

Immediate management and investigations

In the initial management of acutely ill medical patients presenting with abdominal pain and/or upper GI bleeding, the following should be considered:

- analgesia
- control of vomiting
- fluid resuscitation
- antibiotics

Analgesia

Adequate analgesia is paramount in any patient presenting with acute abdominal pain. Opioid analgesia is often required and should be given by slow IV injection and titrated against the patient's pain (e.g. diamorphine, initially 2.5–5 mg, given at a rate of 1 mg/minute, with further doses as required).

Control of vomiting

An anti-emetic (e.g. metoclopramide) should be prescribed if the patient is/has been vomiting OR if opioid analgesia has been administered. A large bore nasogastric tube should be passed if any of the following are suspected:

* gastric outflow obstruction
* small bowel obstruction
* pancreatitis
* persistent vomiting despite the use of anti-emetic medication

Fluid resuscitation

During the primary assessment, patients with circulatory failure will have been identified and appropriate IV fluid resuscitation will have been commenced. Careful fluid balance is mandatory in any patient who is seriously ill and involves co-operation and communication between the medical and nursing staff. Fluid and electrolytes need to be replaced with an appropriate crystalloid. This is particularly important for patients who might need urgent surgery. For elderly patients (or those with cardiac disease) who are at risk of the complications of fluid overload, consider central venous pressure monitoring.

Antibiotics

Antibiotics should be used when there is evidence or high clinical suspicion of infection. Blood cultures and other appropriate cultures should be taken before giving an antibiotic. Antibiotic choice should be tailored to the most likely organism/s causing the sepsis. Consult local hospital guidelines for the prescription of antibiotics.

Investigations

During the primary and secondary assessments, a range of investigations may be considered depending upon findings. Appropriate investigations may include:

* blood tests
* urine tests
* electrocardiogram (ECG)
* radiological investigations

Blood tests

In addition to the blood investigations outlined above, arterial blood gases should be taken in patients with pancreatitis, shock or co-existent respiratory disease.

Urine tests

Perform a urinalysis (dipstick) on all patients presenting with abdominal pain. The following results give an indication of underlying pathology:

- urobilinogen/bilirubin – indicative of liver or biliary tract disease
- blood – may suggest a renal or urological cause of the pain (e.g. urinary tact infection or renal stone)
- ketones and glucose – indicate diabetic ketoacidosis

A urine pregnancy test should be requested in all women of childbearing age presenting with abdominal pain. The results of such tests are confidential to the patient.

ECG

Consider recording a 12-lead ECG in all patients as an acute myocardial infarction can present with abdominal pain.

Radiological investigations

An erect chest X-ray is required if a perforated viscus is suspected and should be considered in patients with co-existent chest pathology. The patient should be sitting up for at least 5 minutes before the X-ray is taken. If the patient is unable to sit or stand, an abdominal lateral decubitus film might show extraluminal gas.

A supine abdominal X-ray can be helpful if either intestinal obstruction or toxic megacolon is suspected. If either ureteric or renal colic is the differential diagnosis, a KUB (kidneys, ureter and bladder) film should be requested. An erect abdominal X-ray is rarely helpful and should not be requested 'routinely'.

Subsequent investigations may include:

- Ultrasound scan. If a leaking abdominal aortic aneurysm is suspected, an ultrasound scan is required urgently. Suspected biliary tract or urinary tract obstruction is also an indication for urgent ultrasound scanning.

- Intravenous urography (IVU). An IVU is often required in patients presenting with ureteric colic to illustrate a calculus and assess the extent of any obstruction of the ureter and kidney.
- CT scan. This is likely to provide more information than an ultrasound scan in the investigation of pancreatic abnormalities. It might be the preferred investigation for a patient presenting with an abdominal mass. It is prudent to discuss the appropriate radiological investigation in the acute setting with a radiologist.
- Angiography. Mesenteric angiography may be used to establish the bleeding point in GI haemorrhage. It has the advantage over a labelled red cell scan that therapeutic embolisation can be achieved at the time of angiography. A labelled red cell, however, is more sensitive in detecting the area of bleeding. Mesenteric angiography is also useful if mesenteric ischaemia is suspected.
- Unprepared contrast enema. This might be required urgently to establish the cause of a suspected large bowel obstruction and to exclude a pseudo-obstruction.

Indications for referral

During the primary assessment, the patient might have been referred to the surgical team. Having completed the secondary assessment, it is worth reconsidering the indications for referral to the surgical team. These include, but are not limited to, suspected:

- peritonitis, generalised or local
- bowel obstruction
- pancreatitis
- leaking abdominal aortic aneurysm
- bowel infarction or ischaemia
- upper GI bleeding in a high-risk patient (see Box 10.3)
- lower GI bleeding

Patients with ureteric colic should be referred to the urology team or general surgeons depending on local arrangements.

Gynaecological assessment is required if any of the following conditions are suspected:

- ectopic pregnancy
- miscarriage
- pelvic inflammatory disease
- complications of an ovarian cyst

Causes of abdominal pain and upper GI bleeding

Thirteen per cent of patients presenting with a medical emergency have an acute GI condition (Advanced Life Support Group 2001). There are many causes of abdominal pain and upper GI bleeding (Box 10.4), with no specific diagnosis being made in a third of patients presenting with acute abdominal pain (Travis et al 1998).

In the following sections, the pathophysiology, assessment and management of three of the more common conditions will be discussed:

- acute upper GI bleeding
- acute gastroenteritis
- inflammatory bowel disease

Features of some of the less common, but still important, conditions will be highlighted.

Acute upper GI bleeding

Causes

Upper GI bleeding is a common cause for acute medical admission and, overall, has a mortality of 14% (Rockall et al 1995). Many conditions can cause acute upper GI bleeding. Although, in approximately 20% of cases no lesion is detected, the following conditions are most often found (in order of frequency):

- duodenal ulcer
- gastric ulcer
- gastric erosions
- Mallory–Weiss tear

Less common causes of upper GI bleeding include:

- duodenitis
- oesophageal varices

- oesophagitis
- tumours

Pathophysiology

Duodenal ulcer

Ninety-five per cent of duodenal ulcers are associated with the presence of *Helicobacter pylori* (McDonald et al 1999), which causes an antritis, hypergastrinaemia and increased gastric acid secretion resulting in ulceration in the duodenal cap. Ingestion of NSAIDs can precipitate or exacerbate bleeding from a duodenal ulcer.

Gastric ulcer

More than eighty per cent of gastric ulcers are associated with *Helicobacter pylori* (McDonald et al 1999), which is characterised, in this situation, by a chronic inflammation of the body of the stomach. Use of NSAIDs increases the risk of developing a gastric ulcer by 80% (Hope et al 1998). Chronic, benign ulceration is associated with smoking. Additional proposed mechanisms include impairment of the mucus–bicarbonate barrier, acid–pepsin damage, deficient gastric mucosal blood flow and duodenogastric reflux. Benign gastric ulcers tend to occur on the lesser curve of the stomach. Ulcers on the greater curve, fundus and in the antrum are more commonly malignant.

Gastric erosions

Gastric erosions are small, shallow lesions, usually <5 mm in diameter, which heal with no sign of scarring. They are commonly seen in an acute gastropathy associated with ingestion of NSAIDs or alcohol. Gastritis is a term that should be reserved for a histological diagnosis.

Mallory–Weiss tear

This is a mucosal tear at the oesophago-gastric junction caused by forceful vomiting.

Presenting features

Haematemesis and/or melaena are often, but not always, present. A patient who has had an upper GI bleed may present with shock and few other clinical features. There may be a previous history of weight loss or dysphagia, which may be suggestive of underlying malignancy. Establish whether there is a history of GI bleeding and, if so, its cause. Make a note of medications, particularly NSAIDs and warfarin, alcohol, liver disease and any other co-morbidity. Determine if the patient has had an aortic graft as, in these cases, an aortoenteric fistula can form which leads to upper GI bleeding (Travis et al 1998).

On presentation, if the patient shows signs of shock, initiate treatment as outlined in the primary assessment. During the examination in the secondary assessment, note the presence or absence of signs of chronic liver disease. If abdominal scars are present, establish their history. The presence or absence of melaena must be confirmed by a digital rectal examination.

Numerical scoring systems can be used after acute upper GI haemorrhage (e.g. Rockall et al 1996). These may be used to identify patients who are at low risk of rebleeding and can be considered for early discharge or outpatient treatment.

Immediate management and investigations

The aims of managing patients presenting with acute upper GI bleeding are to:

- resuscitate/stabilise the patient
- stop active bleeding
- prevent recurrent bleeding

The immediate management of a shocked patient has been described earlier in this chapter (and in Chapter 6 – Shock). Endoscopic therapy has an important role in stopping active bleeding and should be arranged as soon as possible. The surgical team should be involved before an operation is necessary rather than when it is inevitable. Ideally, the patient should be admitted to a designated high-dependency unit.

Initial investigations include full blood count, coagulation studies (when liver disease is present or suspected), urea, electrolytes, creatinine and arterial blood gases (in those with respiratory disease). An upper GI endoscopy should be undertaken as soon as possible. In addition to confirming the diagnosis, therapeutic intervention can be performed in situations that include active bleeding from peptic ulcer or oesophageal varices. The exact timing and place of endoscopy will depend on local arrangements, but should take place within 24 hours. Remember that measured haemoglobin is a poor indicator of transfusion requirement. Haemodynamic status is a better guide.

Ongoing assessment

The ongoing assessment in a patient who has had an upper GI bleed is very important. Initially, monitor vital signs every 15 minutes. A rising pulse rate, rising diastolic blood pressure with reduction in pulse pressure, falling systolic blood pressure or decreasing urine output suggest continued bleeding or a rebleed. The insertion of a central venous line to monitor the central venous pressure is appropriate in elderly patients and those with a history of cardiac disease or poor peripheral venous access.

Acute gastroenteritis

Causes

Acute gastroenteritis is usually caused by the ingestion of bacteria, viruses and toxins (bacterial and chemical) from contaminated food or water. It can also have an airborne source (e.g. Norwalk virus).

Pathophysiology

There are three different pathophysiological mechanisms: inflammatory diarrhoea, secretory (non-inflammatory) diarrhoea and systemic infection.

Inflammatory diarrhoea

Bacterial invasion of the mucosa of the distal small bowel and colon results in both impairment of the absorptive function of the intestine together with loss of blood protein and mucus leading to blood- and mucus-stained diarrhoea. Typical organisms causing this include *Salmonella enteritidis*, *Shigella*, *Campylobacter jejuni* and *Entamoeba histolytica*. *Clostridium difficile* and verotoxin-producing *Escherichia coli* (e.g. *E. coli* 0157) produce cytopathic toxins.

Secretory (non-inflammatory) diarrhoea

A toxin blocks the *passive* absorption of sodium (and water) and stimulates active sodium (and water) excretion in the small bowel, resulting in large amounts of isotonic fluid being secreted into the bowel lumen. This situation exceeds the absorptive capacity of the intestine with resulting profuse watery diarrhoea. *Active* sodium absorption by a glucose-dependent mechanism is not generally affected; therefore rehydration can be achieved by oral glucose solutions which contain both sodium and carbohydrate. Classically, the enterotoxin of *Vibrio cholera* causes secretory diarrhoea, but *Giardia lamblia*, *Cryptosporidium*, *Bacillus cereus* (found in rice), enterotoxogenic *Escherichia coli* and rotavirus, among others, can do so.

Systemic infection

This occurs when infection penetrates the mucosa of the distal small bowel, invades lymphatic structure and causes a bacteraemia. Such invasive organisms include *Salmonella typhi*, *Salmonella paratyphi* and *Yersinia enterocolitica*.

Presenting features

Diarrhoea, abdominal pain, fever, nausea and/or vomiting can occur in various combinations with varying severity.

The presence of blood and pus in diarrhoea is indicative of an inflammatory origin. Inflammatory diarrhoea characteristically contains faecal leucocytes on microscopy. Severity varies from short-lived episodes of diarrhoea with spontaneous resolution to severe colitis complicated by toxic megacolon, perforation, septicaemia and death.

In cases of secretory (non-inflammatory) diarrhoea, there is profuse watery diarrhoea with vomiting. This can cause severe dehydration, leading to hypovolaemic shock and death.

With a systemic infection, about 50% of patients with typhoid fever develop constipation that precedes the diarrhoea and fever. Other features include malaise, headache, cough, relative bradycardia with high fever, myalgia, abdominal pain and splenomegaly. Complications include small bowel ulceration and occasionally perforation.

A history of overseas travel, or of similar symptoms in family members or other contacts might be considered. Preceding antibiotic use or hospital admission might suggest *C. difficile* colitis.

Immediate management and investigations

Fluid replacement with monitoring of fluid balance and oral rehydration may be sufficient in most cases. Antibiotics are rarely required but should be considered in the following cases:

- cholera
- typhoid

- *Clostridium difficile* toxin related diarrhoea
- severe *Salmonella* or *Campylobacter* infections, particularly in those who are immune compromised or who have co-existent medical problems
- parasitic infections

These cases should be discussed with colleagues at the local Public Health Laboratory. Anti-diarrhoeal agents should be avoided but analgesia and anti-emetics can be given as required. Remember that the Consultant in Communicable Disease Control (CCDC) must be notified regarding the following diseases:

- cholera
- dysentery (amoebic, typhoid/paratyphoid)
- food poisoning (any)

A stool specimen for microscopy (leucocytes, red blood cells, ova, cysts and parasites), culture (*Salmonella, Shigella, Campylobacter* and *E. coli* 0157) and toxin detection (*C. difficile*) should be sent as soon as possible. If appropriate, a hot stool should be sent for examination for trophozoites of *Amoeba*. Relevant blood tests are likely to include full blood count, urea, creatinine, electrolytes and blood cultures.

Ongoing assessment

In the continuing assessment of patients with acute gastroenteritis, it is important to look for dehydration, shock and abdominal symptoms and signs of perforation.

Inflammatory bowel diseases (ulcerative colitis and Crohn's disease)

Cause

The cause of the inflammatory bowel diseases is not known. Ulcerative colitis is a recurrent inflammatory disease of the large bowel and virtually always involves the rectum and spreads in continuity proximally to involve a variable amount of the colon. Crohn's disease can affect any part of the gastrointestinal tract from the mouth to the anus with unaffected areas between the transmural inflammation. However, Crohn's disease usually affects the terminal ileum and ileo-caecal region.

Presenting features

Abdominal pain tends to be a more prominent feature in Crohn's disease than in ulcerative colitis. Patients with Crohn's disease may present with abdominal pain associated with vomiting, diarrhoea and weight loss. The site of the disease influences presentation. Crohn's disease involving the colon may present like ulcerative colitis. In ulcerative colitis, the principal symptoms are diarrhoea with rectal bleeding. Patients with ulcerative colitis often complain of abdominal discomfort with cramps but severe, persistent pain suggests a complication or different diagnosis.

In those with severe ulcerative colitis, or less frequently, Crohn's colitis and other forms of colitis, toxic dilatation of the colon can occur. Features associated with toxic dilatation include fever, tachycardia, hypotension and abdominal tenderness.

It is important to remember that patients who have a previous history of inflammatory bowel disease can, and do, develop other conditions. For example, a patient, with a previous history of Crohn's disease, who presents with right hypochondrial pain may have acute cholecystitis, not an exacerbation of Crohn's disease.

Immediate management and investigations

The immediate management of patients with inflammatory bowel disease will depend on the type, site, extent and severity of the disease. Attention should be given to analgesia, fluid balance, nutrition and the administration of steroids with or without antibiotics. The patient should be reassessed regularly. Involvement of the surgical team should be considered early.

Remember that the clinical appearance can be deceptive if a patient is taking steroids. Despite impending perforation in toxic dilatation, the patient may have few symptom and signs.

The initial investigations in patients who are admitted with inflammatory bowel disease, or suspected inflammatory bowel disease, include blood tests (FBC, urea, electrolytes, creatinine, glucose, albumin, inflammatory markers and blood cultures) and radiological investigations (abdominal X-ray ± an erect chest X-ray). In severe colitis, consider performing an abdominal X-ray on a daily basis to look for colonic dilatation. Stool should be sent for microscopy and culture, with examination for *Clostridium difficile* toxin.

Serological investigation for *Yersinia* antibodies and titre is indicated when terminal ileal disease is diagnosed in the absence of a proven diagnosis of Crohn's disease. *Yersinia enterocolitica* is a Gram-negative bacillus and, in some countries is a common cause of gastroenteritis (Cash et al 2001). Subsequent investigations may include lower GI endoscopy (with limited or no preparation) and contrast radiological examination.

Ongoing assessment

Patients with toxic dilatation of the colon, and those who are at risk of developing it, need close, regular assessment. Symptoms, including the severity of abdominal pain and frequency of defaecation, need to be recorded. Temperature, pulse and blood pressure should be monitored at least 2-hourly in those with severe colitis.

Other causes of abdominal pain and upper GI bleeding

A variety of other conditions can cause abdominal pain and/or upper GI bleeding (Box 10.4). There are too many to discuss in detail in this chapter but features of some important, albeit sometimes rare, conditions are highlighted here.

Diabetic ketoacidosis

Severe abdominal pain occurs in approximately 10% of patients presenting with diabetic ketoacidosis (Travis et al 1998) (see Chapter 7 – Altered consciousness). Acute pancreatitis must be excluded in these patients, but remember that a mildly elevated serum amylase can occur in diabetic ketoacidosis without associated acute pancreatitis.

Hypercalcaemia

Causes of hypercalcaemia include malignant disease (myeloma, bone metastases, production of parathyroid hormone related peptide (PTHrP)) and primary hyperparathyroidism. Symptoms include abdominal pain, vomiting, constipation, confusion and renal failure. Rehydration with IV fluids is very important in the immediate management of hypercalcaemia.

Adrenal insufficiency

Patients with adrenal insufficiency can occasionally present with abdominal pain. Other symptoms include weight loss, myalgia and confusion. In acute adrenal insufficiency (Addisonian crisis) the patient may present with shock. Usually, the patient will be known to have Addison's disease but, alternatively, the patient may have been taking steroids long-term and suddenly stopped them. Hyperpigmentation may be seen on examination. Blood tests are likely to show hyponatraemia, hyperkalaemia and an elevated urea.

Yersinia infection

Yersinia infection can cause a variety of clinical syndromes. These include acute mesenteric adenitis and terminal ileitis. A mistaken diagnosis of appendicitis or Crohn's disease may be made initially. A serological test for antibodies (and titre) will confirm the diagnosis.

Acute intermittent porphyria

Abdominal pain, vomiting and constipation are features of acute intermittent porphyria. Usually, but not always, there is a family history of porphyria. Drugs such as phenobarbital, sulphonamides and oestrogens (DeLoughery 2001) and alcohol can precipitate attacks. Urine porphobilinogen is raised during attacks and often between them.

Lead poisoning

'Lead colic' was described first by Hippocrates. Severe lead poisoning causes abdominal pain (which is usually diffuse), constipation, vomiting and encephalopathy. The 'classic' sign of a fine blue line on the gums is rarely seen. Basophilic stippling of red blood cells occurs and may be observed on microscopy. The blood lead level can be measured.

Joint management

In some hospitals, conditions such as pancreatitis and GI haemorrhage are managed jointly by the medical and surgical units, on specialist units. In these cases, it is important that communication and referral arrangements are in place to ensure effective continuity of care for the patient and their family.

Summary

MAU nurses have an important role in providing physical and psychological support for patients referred with abdominal pain and upper GI bleeding. This chapter has described how to assess these patients accurately, and three of the most common conditions (acute GI bleeding, acute gastroenteritis and inflammatory bowel disease) have been described with reference to cause, pathophysiology, presenting features, immediate management, diagnostic tests/investigations and ongoing assessment. Several other conditions which are not as common, but nevertheless important, have been discussed briefly.

References

Advanced Life Support Group (2001) Acute Medical Emergencies: The Practical Approach. London: BMJ Publishing Group.

Cash B, Johnston M, Martin G (2001) Yersinia enterocolitica. eMedicine Journal 2(5): 21 May (www.emedicine.com/med/topic2434.htm).

DeLoughery T (2001) Porphyria, acute intermittent. eMedicine Journal 2(6): 26 June (www.emedicine.com/med/topic1880.htm).

Hope R, Longmore J, McManus S, Wood-Allum A (1998) Oxford Handbook of Clinical Medicine, 4th edn. Oxford: Oxford University Press.

McDonald J, Burroughs A, Feagan B (eds) (1999) Evidence Based Gastroenterology and Hepatology. London: BMJ Books.

Rockall T, Logan R, Devlin H, Northfield T (1995) Incidence of and mortality from acute upper gastrointestinal haemorrhage in the United Kingdom. British Medical Journal 311: 222–6.

Rockall T, Logan R, Devlin H, Northfield T (1996) Risk assessment after acute upper gastrointestinal haemorrhage. Gut 38(3): 316–21.

Travis S, Taylor R, Misiewicz J (1998) Gastroenterology, 2nd edn. Oxford: Blackwell Science.

Further reading

Cotton P, Williams C (1996) Practical Gastrointestinal Endoscopy, 4th edn. Oxford: Blackwell Science.

Kumar P, Clark M (1998) Clinical Medicine, 4th edn. London: WB Saunders.

Munro J, Campbell I (eds) (2000) MacLeod's Clinical Examination, 10th edn. London: Churchill Livingstone.

Weatherall D, Ledingham J, Warrell D (eds) (1996) Oxford Textbook of Medicine, 3rd edn. Oxford: Oxford University Press.

CHAPTER 11

Extremity pain and swelling

IAN WOOD

Aims

This chapter will:

- describe the questions to ask when taking a history from a patient with extremity pain and swelling
- discuss the causes, pathophysiology, investigation and treatment of patients with the following conditions: deep vein thrombosis, thrombophlebitis and cellulitis

Immediate management – initial stabilising measures

An assumption has been made in this chapter that the patient has had an overall initial assessment and that any immediately life-threatening problems have been identified and treated.

Patients presenting with painful or swollen extremities can be nursed on a trolley-stretcher, in a bed or in a chair. The principle of nursing care is that the patient will be in a position comfortable for them with their leg elevated and supported on a pillow. Elevation encourages venous drainage.

The clinical features associated with disorders of the extremities are outlined in Box 11.1.

Initial assessment of painful and/or swollen limbs

Clinical assessment starts when the nurse first sees the patient and begins with a visual inspection and physical examination (Box 11.2).

Box 11.1. Common presenting features associated with extremity pain and swelling

Oedema
Calf pain
Tenderness
Swelling
Increased skin temperature
Engorgement of superficial leg veins
Slight fever
Positive Homan's sign (discomfort in calf muscles on forced dorsiflexion)

Box 11.2. Initial assessment by observation and examination

Observation
- Observe and record skin colour. Compare with unaffected side.
- Is the area swollen? Compare with unaffected side.
- Is oedema present?
- Is the area painful? Check for pain at rest or on movement.
- Is the area reddened? Compare with unaffected side.
- Are any wounds present? If so, how long have they been present? Have they been treated? By whom?

Physical examination
- Check and record presence of distal pulses on the affected limb and compare with the unaffected side.
- Check and record heart rate, respiratory rate and depth, blood pressure and temperature.
- Is the area hot? Compare with unaffected side.
- Palpate the area for pain or tenderness. Compare with the unaffected side.
- Check for range of movement of proximal and distal joints. Does this increase pain?
- Can the patient walk normally on the affected limb(s)?

Verbal questioning to collect a history of the current problem supports this assessment (Box 11.3).

Conditions most commonly causing lower limb pain and swelling are:

- deep vein thrombosis
- thrombophlebitis
- cellulitis
- heart failure (see Chapter 8 – Shortness of breath)

Box 11.3. Information to be collected during history taking

Information to be collected verbally
- History of present problem:
  How long has it been present?
  When did it start?
  Is it constant or intermittent?
  Is it worse today than usual?
- Is there any previous history of same or similar problem?
- Is there any recent history of injury to the affected area?
- Has there been any recent long distance travel (>4 hours) in last 4 weeks?
- Has there been any previous surgery especially orthopaedic, pelvic or abdominal?
- Is the area painful? If so, does anything relieve the pain or make it worse?
- Has any medication been taken to relieve the problem?

Deep vein thrombosis

Deep vein thrombosis (DVT) and its sequela pulmonary embolism (PE) (see Chapter 9 – Chest pain) are important and potentially preventable causes of mortality and morbidity in hospitalised patients. It is estimated that 1 in 10 000 men and 1.5 in 10 000 women die each year from DVT and PE (Hopkins and Wolfe 1991). Medical patients who have suffered myocardial infarction (MI) or cerebrovascular accident (CVA) have a 25–30% incidence of developing a DVT if prophylactic preventative measures are not taken (Karwinski and Svendsen 1989).

Causes

The causes of DVT centre on pathophysiological changes that occur most commonly in the veins of the lower leg. An individual patient's likelihood of developing a DVT increases when they possess one or more predisposing risk factors (Box 11.4).

Although figures for patients in MAUs are not readily available, for those attending A&E departments, the prevalence of DVT correlates with the number of risk factors identified. Patients who have no identified risk factors have an incidence of confirmed DVT of only 11% (Schreiber 2001).

Pathophysiology

A combination of factors is thought to lead to the development of DVT. Known as Virchow's triad, these factors comprise venous stasis, vessel wall injury and hypercoagulability of the blood. The relative importance of

---

Box 11.4. Risk factors associated with the development of DVT (Perkins and Galland 1999, Schreiber 2001)

Age >40 years
Obesity
Immobilisation longer than 3 days
Pregnancy and post-partum period
Plane or car journey >4 hours in previous 4 weeks
Major surgery (especially hip, pelvis or leg)
Previous DVT or PE
Varicose veins
High dose oestrogen therapy/oral contraceptives
Malignancy
Recent myocardial infarction
Cerebrovascular accident
Heart failure
Paralysis of leg(s)
IV drug abuse
Infection

---

each of these factors is still not fully understood but the mechanism for the formation of DVTs is best summarised as the activation of coagulation factors in areas of reduced blood flow (Schreiber 2001).

DVT usually starts in the veins of the calf with coagulation originating around valve cusps. Calf DVTs are probably not dangerous if they remain isolated distally. However, between 5% and 20% of calf DVTs will progress proximally. In these cases, the primary thrombus extends within and between the deep and superficial veins of the leg and, as a result, can cause venous obstruction, valvular damage and, possibly, thrombo-embolism (Gorman et al 2000). Half of all proximal vein thromboses embolise to the lungs if left untreated (Moulton and Yates 1999). More rarely, cases of primary DVT can arise in the ileo-femoral veins, primarily after vessel wall damage from orthopaedic surgery or venous catheterisation.

Presenting features

The classic presenting features of DVT include boring, unilateral calf pain with swelling, tenderness to touch/palpation, localised warmth and skin erythema. This 'textbook' presentation is, however, rare. In reality, the presenting features of DVT relate to the degree of venous obstruction and inflammation of the vessel wall. Many thrombi do not cause enough obstruction to reduce blood flow significantly and collateral circulation can develop to ensure adequate venous return. Inflammation of vessel walls may not cause significant pain or swelling and, consequently, patients suffering from DVT can often be asymptomatic and the findings of a physical examination alone are often inconclusive. According to Jenkins and Braen (2000), clinical features of DVT are misleading, unreliable or absent in approximately 50% of patients.

The clinical features that may be present are outlined in Box 11.5 and these, linked with the predisposing factors above, give a clearer indication of the likelihood of DVT being present.

Box 11.5. Possible presenting features of DVT

Oedema, often unilaterally
Calf pain (occurs in 50% of cases but is non-specific to DVT)
Tenderness (occurs in 75% of cases of DVT but is also found in 50% of patients without confirmed DVT)
Swelling below knee in distal DVTs and up to groin in proximal DVTs
Increased skin temperature
Engorgement of superficial leg veins (only in minority of cases)
Slight fever
Positive Homan's sign* (in less than 20% of cases)

*Homan's sign: Discomfort in calf muscles on forced dorsiflexion of the foot with the knee
            straight.

Immediate management and investigations

Patients with suspected DVT are nursed on a stretcher-trolley, in a bed or in a chair. Elevate the affected leg with some flexion of the knee (to encourage venous drainage) and support it on a pillow in the position most comfortable for the patient. Take a history (Boxes 11.2 and 11.3), measure vital signs, gain intravenous (IV) access and take bloods for full blood count (FBC), urea, electrolytes and clotting screen. In addition, oxygen saturation may be measured and oxygen given if required. Measurement of calf circumferences to provide a baseline for further evaluation may be carried out 10 cm below the tibial tuberosity. A swelling of 3 cm greater than the asymptomatic side is a relative indicator of DVT but is not definitive. Application of graded compression stockings can reduce post-thrombotic syndrome by up to 60% (Gorman et al 2000). Explain procedures to the patient and assess their potential for early discharge.

The principle of managing patients with a DVT is early initiation cf effective anticoagulant therapy with the aim of preventing further progression of the thrombosis to the proximal veins and, thereby, pulmonary embolism. Given that diagnosis on the basis of clinical features is often inconclusive, management of suspected DVT is based on the results obtained from one or more objective diagnostic investigations. To support this, clinical risk factors (Box 11.1) are also assessed and taken into account, as confirmation rates of DVT rise with the number of factors present. Identification of an underlying cause, if present, will also guide the treatment and prevention of further episodes (Gorman et al 2000).

The standard radiographic investigation for DVT is contrast venography (Gorman et al 2000) but the painful, invasive nature of this procedure, its technical difficulty and the time taken for completion make it inappropriate for use in acute settings. Technological advances in recent years have led to the introduction of non-invasive ultrasonography as a first-line investigation for DVTs. Known as pulsed Doppler ultrasound, this technique measures the velocity of moving objects (such as red blood cells) in comparison to other objects. Scanning time can be further reduced by the use of colour Duplex ultrasonography. In the case of venous thrombosis, colour Duplex scanning has a 90–100% accuracy for detecting proximal DVTs (from the common femoral vein to the popliteal vein) but is less reliable for diagnosing calf vein thrombosis (Donnelly et al 2000). Impedance plethysmography (IPG) is a non-invasive investigation used in some centres. This procedure is based on recording changes in blood volume in a limb, which are directly related to venous outflow. IPG has been shown to be sensitive and specific for proximal vein thrombosis but it is insensitive for calf vein thrombosis, non-occluding proximal vein thrombus and ileo-femoral vein thrombosis above the inguinal ligament. False positive results can occur in the presence of significant congestive heart failure and raised central venous pressure (CVP) (Schreiber 2001).

In most centres, ultrasonography is combined with measurement of circulating D-dimer concentrations (a normal by-product of fibrin degradation). When combined with ultrasound investigations, D-dimers are up to 98% sensitive for proximal DVTs with a high negative predictive value (Gorman et al 2000, Ofri 2000, Bernardi et al 1998). However, D-dimer tests are less accurate when detecting calf vein thrombosis and have poor specificity as other conditions (such as malignant neoplasms, liver failure and disseminated intravascular coagulation) can cause raised levels.

In addition to ultrasonography and D-dimer measurement, prediction of probability for DVT can be undertaken. Box 11.6 (from Anand et al 1998, Gorman et al 2000, Ofri 2000) gives a clinical model for this prediction:

Box 11.6. The Wells clinical prediction guide for DVT (Anand et al 1998)

Clinical feature	Score
Active cancer (treatment ongoing or within 6 months or palliative)	1
Paralysis, paresis or plaster of Paris on lower leg	1
Recently bedridden >3 days or major surgery within 4 weeks	1
Localised tenderness along distribution of deep vein system	1
Calf diameter >3 cm larger than the asymptomatic leg*	1
Pitting oedema	1
Entire swollen leg	1
Collateral superficial veins (non-varicose)	1
Alternative diagnosis (as likely or greater than that of DVT)	-2

Adding the scores with a total as follows indicates probability of DVT:

0	= low probability	= 3% frequency of DVT
1–2	= medium probability	= 17% frequency of DVT
3+	= high probability	= 75% frequency of DVT

*Measured 10 cm below tibial tuberosity

In summary, a combination of diagnostic investigations (such as ultrasonography alongside D-dimer measurement or pre-test probability testing, or both) gives better accuracy than any single approach in detecting distal as well as proximal DVTs.

Rapid, effective anticoagulant therapy is important in the initial management of DVT. Treatment usually starts with an intravenous dose of heparin (5000 units) followed by subcutaneous low molecular weight heparin (LMWH) for 5 days. LMWH has been shown to be at least as effective as the traditionally used unfractionated heparin in preventing recurrent venous thromboembolism. In addition, it significantly reduces the occurrence of major haemorrhage during initial treatment and reduces overall mortality at the end of the patient's follow-up period (van den Belt et al 2000). Oral warfarin is usually started on day 1 with the dose determined by algorithm.

Ongoing assessment and treatment

Gorman et al (2000) suggest that the patient's activated partial thromboplastin time (aPTT) is checked every 6 hours until the target of 1.5–2.5 is reached or according to a heparin algorithm. Once reached, this should be checked daily to maintain this range. Platelet count should also be measured at the start of treatment and on day 5 to rule out thrombocytopenia. Duration of treatment for DVT varies from 3 to 12 months depending upon the risk of recurrence of thrombosis.

Many patients who are referred with DVT can be discharged once initial investigations and treatment have been completed. Pout et al (1999) give an example of how a nurse-led outpatient clinic has successfully been introduced to treat patients with daily doses of LMWH. This approach has been adopted in other centres with the aim of improving the service to patients and relieving pressure on individual MAUs.

Thrombophlebitis

Thrombophlebitis is an inflammatory response that may affect superficial or deep veins of either the upper or lower limbs. It is characterised by pathophysiology that is similar to DVT involving venous stasis, hyper-coagulability and vessel wall injuries.

Causes

Thrombophlebitis can occur spontaneously or as a result of invasive interventions such as venepuncture or intravenous administration of medication (either therapeutically or illegally). The most important identifiable clinical risk factors associated with thrombophlebitis are a previous history of superficial phlebitis, DVT or pulmonary embolism (Feied 2000). In the lower limbs, it is associated with superficial varicosities, pregnant or post-partum women as well as recent surgery, prolonged immobilisation or underlying malignancy.

Presenting features

Features of superficial thrombophlebitis include a gradual onset of tenderness, inflammation and swelling of the superficial veins. The area may be hot and erythema may be present along the path of the affected vein. A history of local trauma may be evident.

Thrombophlebitis should be assumed to be DVT until proven otherwise as clinical examination cannot satisfactorily exclude deep vein involvement. As with DVT, visual examination is unreliable as the features present could be attributed to a number of conditions such as venous complications of liver disease, heart failure, renal disease, infection or trauma. Palpation usually indicates a painful or tender area and may reveal a firm, thickened and thrombosed vein (Feied 2000).

Immediate management and investigations

Management of lower limb inflammation centres on the exclusion of underlying DVT (see section on deep vein thrombosis, above). Nurse the patient in the most comfortable position for them, ideally with their leg raised, slightly flexed at the knee and elevated on a pillow. Record vital signs and take bloods for FBC, urea, electrolytes and clotting screen. Calf measurements may be recorded for comparison with the unaffected side. If the upper limb is affected, it too can be elevated and supported in a position most comfortable for the patient.

Once DVT has been excluded, superficial thrombophlebitis can be treated with a short course of an appropriate non-steroidal anti-inflammatory agent (Wyatt et al 1999).

Infective thrombophlebitis must be considered in patients who have a fever, raised white cell count, cellulitis or who have had recent venepuncture (including illicit drug use) or cannulation.

Ongoing assessment and treatment

If it is not possible to exclude infection, re-examination within 24–48 hours is recommended. If confirmed, patients with infective thrombophlebitis require admission for IV antibiotics.

Cellulitis

Causes

Cellulitis literally means inflammation of cellular tissue. This common condition is caused when microorganisms enter a break in the skin and lead to the spread of an acute infection usually caused by group A *Streptococcus* or *Staphylococcus aureus* (Jenkins and Braen 2000). It can occur anywhere on the body and may be associated with minor or unrecalled trauma or IV drug use. Patients with diabetes mellitus, immune deficiency disorders or systemic illness are prone to cellulitis (Curtis 2000).

Presenting features

Classic signs of cellulitis include a warm, reddened, swollen area that is tender to touch. Red 'track' marks may be visible on the skin proximal to the area of cellulitis. These are characteristic of lymphangitis, an indication that infection is being carried through the lymph system.

Immediate management and investigations

Mild cellulitis can be treated with oral antibiotics on an outpatient basis. Systemic infection can be a sequela to undiagnosed or untreated cellulitis. Patients who have systemic signs including fever, dehydration, altered mental status, tachypnoea, tachycardia and hypotension require management associated with a shocked patient (see Chapter 6 – Shock) (Curtis 2000).

Ongoing assessment and treatment

Arrange follow-up either with the patient's GP or in the outpatients department 24–48 hours later to monitor the effectiveness of this treatment. It is useful to mark the margins of the infection with a pen so that any changes are more obvious when the patient is reviewed. Give details of where to seek advice if the condition deteriorates. Patients who do not respond to oral antibiotics may require admission for IV antibiotics.

Less common conditions causing extremity pain and swelling are:

- arterial embolism
- ruptured Baker's cyst
- intra-arterial injection
- acute compartment syndrome

Summary

This chapter has focused on the assessment and management of patients referred to the MAU with painful and/or swollen lower limbs. As a group of patients, these individuals can place considerable demands on the resources available within the acute admissions system. As new roles in nursing develop, the care of these patients has been identified as an area in which MAU nurses can have a positive impact on improving the service delivered.

References

Anand S, Wells P, Hunt D, Brill-Edwards P, Cook D, Ginsberg J (1998) Does this patient have deep vein thrombosis? Journal of the American Medical Association 279: 1094–9.

Bernardi E, Prandoni P, Lensing A, Agnelli G, Guazzaloca G, Scannapieco G, Piovella F, Verlato F, Tomasi C, Moia M, Scarano L, Girolami A (1998) D-dimer testing as an adjunct to ultrasonography in patients with clinically suspected deep vein thrombosis: prospective cohort study. British Medical Journal 317: 1037–40.

Curtis D (2000) Cellulitis. Emedicine. www.emedicine.com/EMERG/topic88.htm. Published: 9 December 2000.

Donnelly R, Hinwood D, London N (2000) Non-invasive arterial and venous assessment. British Medical Journal 320: 698–701.

Feied C (2000) Superficial thrombophlebitis. Emedicine. www.emedicine.com/EMERG/topic582.htm. Published: 20 March 2000.

Gorman W, Davis K, Donnelly R (2000) ABC of arterial and venous disease: swollen lower limb 1: general assessment and deep vein thrombosis. British Medical Journal 320: 1453–6.

Hopkins N, Wolfe J (1991) Thrombosis and pulmonary embolism. British Medical Journal 303: 1260–1.

Jenkins J, Braen G (eds) (2000) Manual of Emergency Medicine. Philadelphia: Lippincott/Williams & Wilkins.

Karwinski B, Svendsen E (1989) Comparison of clinical and post-mortem diagnosis of pulmonary embolism. Journal of Clinical Pathology 42: 135–9.

Moulton C, Yates D (1999) Lecture Notes on Emergency Medicine, 2nd edn. Oxford: Blackwell Science.

Ofri D (2000) Diagnosis and treatment of deep vein thrombosis. Western Journal of Medicine 173: 194–7.

Perkins J, Galland B (1999) Venous thrombosis and pulmonary embolism: Part 1. Prevention. Care of the Critically Ill 15(4): 140–3.

Pout G, Wimperis J, Dilks G (1999) Nurse-led outpatient treatment of deep vein thrombosis. Nursing Standard 13(19): 39–41.

Schreiber D (2001) Deep vein thrombosis and thrombophlebitis. Emedicine. www.emedicine.com/EMERG/topic122.htm. Published: 1 March 2001.

van den Belt A, Prins M, Lensing A, Castro A, Clark O, Atallah A, Buriham E (2000) Fixed dose subcutaneous low molecular weight heparins versus adjusted dose unfractionated heparin for venous thromboembolism (Cochrane Review). In The Cochrane Library, vol 4. Oxford: Update Software.

Wyatt J, Illingworth R, Clancy M, Munro P, Robertson C (1999) Oxford Handbook of Accident & Emergency Medicine. Oxford: Oxford University Press.

Further reading

Advanced Life Support Group (ALSG) (2001) Acute Medical Emergencies: The Practical Approach. London: BMJ Books.

http://www.emedicine.com/emerg/contents.htm

Index